From Spectacle-Making Trade to Scholarly Profession

From Spectacle-Making Trade to Scholarly Profession

A History of Optometry in the United States

David A. Goss, OD, PhD

Emeritus Professor of Optometry
Indiana University
Bloomington, Indiana

Formerly Professor of Optometry
Northeastern State University
Tahlequah, Oklahoma

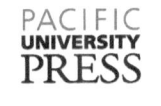

FOREST GROVE, OREGON

PACIFIC UNIVERSITY PRESS
2043 College Way
Forest Grove, Oregon 97116

© 2022 by David A. Goss

This book is distributed under the terms of a Creative Commons Attribution-NonCommercial-No Derivatives License, which permits non-commercial use, distribution, and reproduction in any medium in unadapted form only, provided the original author and publisher are credited.

Images provided courtesy of other rightsholders, as noted in the book, may require additional permissions or fair use determinations prior to re-use.

Cover design by Alex Bell

ISBN (pbk) 978-1-945398-06-3
ISBN (PDF) 978-1-945398-11-7

Published in the United States of America

To
Diane

Contents

Preface	ix
Acknowledgments	xi
PART I: A Brief Survey of Optometry History	**1**
Chapter 1: *The First Six Centuries of Optometry*	3
Chapter 2: *Development of Professionalism in Optometry and Related Early Twentieth-Century Developments*	35
Chapter 3: *Continuing Twentieth-Century Challenges and Changes*	65
Chapter 4: *The Profession Advances and Gains in Recognition*	113
PART II: Some Elements of the Development of Optometry as a Scholarly Profession	**145**
Chapter 5: *Maturation of the Optometric Examination*	147
Chapter 6: *Optometric Education*	187
Chapter 7: *Optometry Publications*	249
Appendices	
Appendix 1: *A Historical List of Optometry Schools in the United States*	265
Appendix 2: *The Changing Optometry Student Body: Data on Optometry Students and Graduates*	279
Appendix 3: *A History of Selected Optometric Periodicals*	295
Appendix 4: *Notes on the History of Optometry Books*	319
About the Author	341
Index	343

Preface

This book is intended to give the reader an awareness and appreciation of some of the processes and persons responsible for optometry's advancement from a trade to a scholarly profession. Part I provides a brief general survey of optometry history from its conceptual beginning with the invention of spectacles and extending to more recent developments. Part II documents some of the factors that have led to optometry's rise from a spectacle-making craft to the scholarly profession it had become by the late twentieth century. Factors such as the maturation of the optometric examination, the development of optometric education, and optometric publications are discussed. The European origins of optometry are considered in the first chapter, but subsequent coverage is almost exclusively on optometry in the United States.

Many other historical accounts could be written on this subject, hence the subtitle of *A* History Of Optometry rather than *The* History of Optometry. Most of the books relating to optometry history published in the last 50 years have been histories of organizations or companies, institutional histories, or histories of relevant objects such as spectacles. Such books have been important, and this discussion offers an appreciation for some aspects of optometry's development that haven't been emphasized previously.

A knowledge of the history of optometry is important for the continuing advancement of the profession and the well-being of its practitioners and patients. The most obvious reason is that everyone learns from the past. Probably the most famous statement of that concept is from George Santayana: "Those who cannot remember the past are condemned to repeat it." Second, by learning about the history of a profession, one can learn about its perennial problems, its ethics, the cultural atmosphere that influenced its development, and the nature of professional life. Third, understanding the contributions and the unique heritage of optometry can enhance a feeling of pride in the profession and improve the image and the self-image of its practitioners. In addition, communication of the contributions of optometry to public welfare can enhance the status and respect enjoyed by the profession. Finally, a study of history can be a means of honoring those who have made contributions, and it helps in advancing the correct attribution for such contributions. I hope that this book will help to advance those ends in some small way.

Acknowledgments

Numerous individuals at libraries, archives, optometry schools, and optometric organizations have patiently answered inquiries and provided information and photographs. In particular, I thank Doug Freeman and Laura Robinson of the Indiana University Optometry Library, and Linda Draper and Kirsten Hébert of the Archives and Museum of Optometry and the American Optometric Association Foundation. My graduate school advisor, Henry Hofstetter, has served as an excellent example and inspiration for my history research. Colleagues in the Optometric Historical Society provided occasional information and encouragement for my research, especially Jerry Abrams, John Amos, R. Norman Bailey, Irving Bennett, Jack Bennett, Gary Campbell, Linda Casser, Jay Enoch, Ronald Ferrucci, Ted Grosvenor, and Doug Penisten. I thank my wife Diane for her enduring support and assistance with photographs. Lastly, I enjoyed working with Isaac Gilman of Pacific University Press, and I appreciate his dedication to the publication process. Initial research and drafts of Chapters 1, 2, and 3 were completed while on a sabbatical granted by Indiana University. Much of the content of Chapters 5 and 6, and Appendices 1, 2, and 3, was adapted from articles I published between 2008 and 2019 in *Hindsight: Journal of Optometry History*, the quarterly publication of the Optometric Historical Society.

PART I
A Brief Survey of Optometry History

We have to know who we were if we're to know who we are and where we're headed. —David McCullough[1]

Full knowledge of the past helps us in dealing with the future. —Theodore Roosevelt[2]

A confidence in the future depends on a reverence for the past. —Arthur Herman[3]

Monroe Hirsch and Ralph Wick[4] suggested that the history of optometry can be divided into an early optometry period covering the fourteenth through the nineteenth centuries and a modern optometry period beginning in about 1890. This review of optometric history reveals not only advances in science and practice but also optometry's transformation from a trade into a profession. A trade is often seen as "the business of buying and selling or bartering commodities" and "an occupation requiring manual or mechanical skill."[5] In contrast, a profession has been defined as "a calling requiring specialized knowledge and often long and intensive academic preparation."[6] Among the other attributes of a profession are establishment of professional organizations, creation of regulatory agencies that evaluate qualifications for certification of licensure, a literature supporting its practice, and formulation of ethical standards.[7] As seen in its history, while optometry's origins lie in the spectacle making trade, it has continually evolved and its transition to scholarly profession was complete by the later decades of the twentieth century.

Part I: Notes

1. McCullough D. *The American Spirit: Who We Are and What We Stand For.* New York, NY: Simon & Schuster, 2017:111.
2. Roosevelt T. The Progressives, past and present. *Outlook* Sept. 3, 1901;96(1):19-30.
3. Herman A. *How the Scots Invented the Modern World: The True Story of How Western Europe's Poorest Nation Created Our World and Everything in It.* New York, NY: Crown Publishers, 2001:429.
4. Hirsch MJ, Wick RE. *The Optometric Profession.* Philadelphia, PA: Chilton, 1968:2-3.
5. www.merriam-webster.com/dictionary/trade
6. www.merriam-webster.com/dictionary/profession
7. Wilensky HL. The professionalization of everyone? *Am J Sociol.* 1964;70:137-158.

Chapter 1

The First Six Centuries of Optometry

Optometry is a centuries-old occupation that has ministered to the vision care needs of millions of people. It has developed independently of other health care professions though at times it was influenced by them, and it experienced parallel developments to other health care professions. Optometry's early development was driven by practical and empirical forces rather than scientific advances although later it would embrace science. The craft, albeit a distinguished one, of spectacle making gradually developed into the learned profession of optometry that we know today.

Many people think that optometry is a relatively new profession, beginning in the early twentieth century. It is true that American optometry licensure laws began to be passed at that time. It is also true that in the early twentieth century, those who prescribed and fit spectacles started calling themselves *optometrists*. However, it was the optometrists themselves who pushed for licensure laws and who started calling themselves by that name. It wasn't the other way around. Optometry did not appear because licensure laws were passed or because the term *optometry* began to be used. Perhaps the best way to explain this is to say that optometry became a more clearly defined practice because of events that occurred around the beginning of the twentieth century.

The invention of spectacles is the logical conceptual beginning of optometry. As word of the existence of spectacles spread and the demand for them increased, testing methods and conventional wisdoms for determining their optimum power for an individual developed. Methods of lens manufacture and the quality of lenses improved. Visual function and its relation to wearing lenses became better understood. Spectacle prescribers formed organizations and raised their levels of education. The practitioners who had started calling themselves optometrists expanded their expertise into binocular vision, contact lenses, low vision, and other areas of vision practice. These and other developments have continued in interrelated cycles.

The invention of spectacles made it possible for their wearers to better perform visual tasks. Optometrists of all eras have helped those who sought their care to have improved clarity, comfort, and efficiency of vision. This was true even of the first spectacle-making craftsmen although their ability to improve vision was surely relative rather than optimal. It is easy to assume that optometrists today have more treatment and management tools at their disposal, and more and better testing procedures and diagnostic capabilities than the earliest practitioners could ever have imagined. Today's optometrists also have the benefit of a rigorous and challenging education.

THE INVENTION OF SPECTACLES

Scholars[1,2,3,4] agree that the most exhaustive and definitive work on the invention of spectacles was done by Edward Rosen, who concluded that an unknown artisan in northern Italy, in or near Pisa, invented spectacles in about 1286.[5] It seems likely that the inventor remains unknown because he most likely kept his methods secret to protect his profits from potential competitors.

Rosen sorted through various myths and false claims about the origins of spectacles. He derived the date of 1286 from a sermon delivered in Florence, Italy, on February 23, 1306 by Friar Giordano da Pisa (also called Giordano da Rivalto). An excerpt from the sermon reads: "It is not yet twenty years since there was found the art of making eyeglasses which make for good vision, one of the best arts and most necessary that the world has. So short a time is it since there was invented a new art that never existed....I have seen the man who first invented and created it and I have talked to him."[5]

The means of making such a useful invention could not remain secret for long. The initial spreading appears to have been hastened along by Friar Alessandro della Spina of Pisa, who died in 1313. The *Ancient Chronicle of the Dominican Monastery of St. Catherine in Pisa*[6] stated that: "Friar Alessandro della Spina was a modest and good man....Whatever had been made, when he saw it with his own eyes, he too knew how to make it. Eyeglasses were first made by someone else, who was unwilling to share them. Spina made them, and shared them with a cheerful and willing heart"[5]

One person sometimes incorrectly credited with the invention of spectacles was Roger Bacon. Bacon was born in England sometime between 1210 and 1220, lived to 1292 or 1294, and undertook university studies in Oxford and Paris.[7] He composed significant works on optics, including *Perspectiva* and *De multiplicatone specierum*.[8] His *Perspectiva* was part of his *Opus maius*, completed in 1267 or 1268. In *Perspectiva*, Bacon wrote about magnifying print with a plano-convex lens placed on it.[9] He stated that lenses "will prove to be a most useful instrument for old persons and all those having weak eyes, as they can see in this manner the small letters." Bacon was obviously correct in his statement about the usefulness of lenses, but there is no indication that he was writing about spectacles, that is, an appliance with a frame to hold corrective lenses conveniently on the face in front of the eyes.

Another incorrect attribution for the invention of spectacles is Salvino degli Armati, who may have lived in Florence. A memorial, which was placed in Florence probably in the mid-nineteenth century, reads: "Here lies Salvino degli Armati, son of Armato, of Florence, inventor of eyeglasses. May God forgive his sins. A.D. 1317." In his detailed study of the origins of spectacles, Rosen devotes some fifteen pages to showing that this memorial was based on a hoax that attempted to credit the invention to a Florentine.[5]

After spectacles were first made in Italy, the craft of spectacle making spread very rapidly. By the early fourteenth century, there were spectacle making businesses not only in Italy but also in Nuremberg in Germany and Haarlem in the Netherlands. There is evidence that spectacle makers guilds existed in France in 1465, in Nuremberg in 1483, and in England in 1563.[10]

There have been some suggestions that spectacles may have been invented in China earlier than in Italy; however, scholars who have attempted to find reliable evidence for the Chinese attribution have been unsuccessful.[11,12,13] One paper stated that "glass spectacles were rare and precious in the Ming Dynasty [which started in 1368] and most likely were brought into China from abroad."[14] Rosenthal,[15] in his book on the history of spectacles, suggested that all that can be said with certainty is that by the fifteenth century, developments in the manufacture of spectacles in China paralleled those in Europe.

EARLY SPECTACLES

The first spectacles were plus (convex) lenses made for presbyopia. These lenses in the first few centuries of their manufacture usually were made from quartz or glass. Frames were made from many different materials, including leather, bone, horn, and wood. At first, spectacles did not have temples extending to the ears. They were held by hand or perched precariously on the nose. One common early frame design had round frames around each lens with handles from those frames joined by a rivet. If print was particularly small, the lenses could be taken from the nose and rotated around the rivet so that they were superimposed, allowing viewing through both lenses at the same time. With the frame folded up like that, they could also be placed in a pouch suspended from the belt.

Within the first 200 years of spectacle production, the use of minus

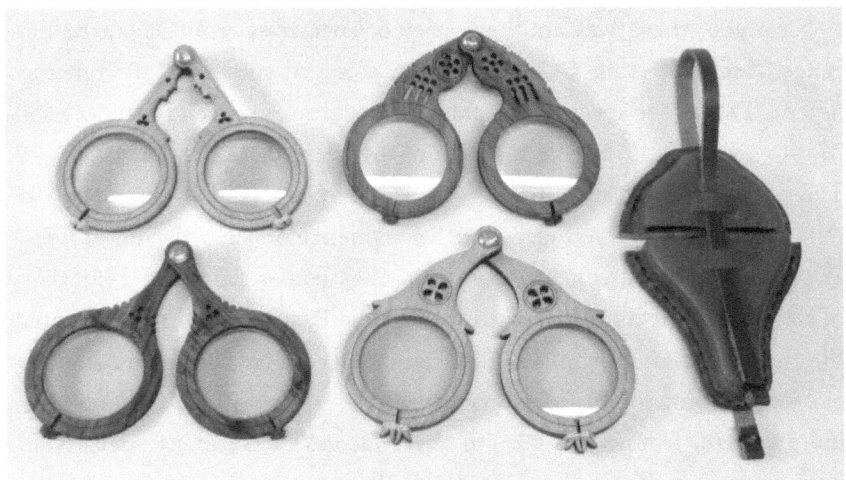

Figure 1.1. Reproductions of original rivet spectacles dated from the fourteenth to the sixteenth century and a reproduction of a leather case for rivet spectacles. Photo from www.ocularheritagesociety.com/galleryadverti. (Image courtesy Ocular Heritage Society)

(concave) lenses for myopia and the recognition of the need of different powers of plus lenses for presbyopia arose. This is documented through an order of spectacles in 1462 to be made in Florence, discovered by Ilardi.[16] That order, placed by Duke Francesco Sforza of Milan, stated:

> …we wish and charge you to send us three dozens of the aforesaid eyeglasses placed in cases so that they will not break; namely one dozen of those apt and suitable for distant vision, that is for the young; another [dozen] that are suitable for near vision, that is for the elderly; and the third [dozen] for [more] common vision. We inform you that we do not want them for our use because, thank God, we do not need them, but we want them in order to please this one and that one who asks us for them…[16]

The eyeglasses for "distant vision" are clearly minus (concave) lenses; those for "common vision" would appear to be for early presbyopia, while those "for the elderly" are obviously for advanced presbyopia.

In 1466, there was another order of spectacles from Milan to Florence, this time from Galeazzo Maria, son and successor of Francesco Sforza. This order specified 15 pairs of spectacles for each of the ages 30, 35, 40, 45, 50 and; 15 pairs for each of the ages 40, 45, 50, 55, 60, 65, 70. Ten pairs were for "medium vision for the young" and 10 pairs for "distant [vision] for the young."[17] Further evidence of the ordering of lenses at powers for presbyopia by age groupings comes from the 1488 diary of the Florentine ambassador to the Middle East in an entry that stated: "Remember what I promised the friars at Jerusalem, especially the eyeglasses. First for the Commissary [of the friars], from [age] 40 to 50. For the guardian, from 35 to 40. For Friar Iacopo of Germany [della Magnia], from 60 to 70. For Friar Egidio da Piacenza, from 50 to 60. For Friar Gabriel, from 35 to 45. And [for] the others, up to twelve pairs."[18]

Thus, by the mid-fifteenth century it was recognized that increasing lens power was needed for presbyopia as it advanced with age. The documents further show that there was a capability of making lenses of different powers and the ability to measure lens power to some approximation. It seems unclear how much of an active diagnostic role was played by the spectacle makers at that time beyond providing lenses based on patient age and through trial and error.

THE FIRST OPTOMETRY BOOK

The first book that can be identified as being on the subject of optometry was published in 1623 by a Spaniard, Benito Daza de Valdes. Although a later chapter will discuss optometry publications, it is worthwhile to discuss the Daza de Valdes book in some detail here because it offers a fascinating glimpse into what seventeenth-century optometry may have been like.

Daza de Valdes identified five categories of vision defects that could be treated with spectacles. His names for these categories (with our terms for them today in parentheses) are: (1) "blurred or weak vision in old people" (presbyopia); (2) "natural nearsightedness of the young" (myopia); (3) "unaccustomed vision" (refractive amblyopia); (4) "uneven vision" (anisometropia, unequal refractive errors in the two eyes); and (5) "opposite vision" (mixed anisometropia or antimetropia, hyperopia in one eye and myopia in the other eye).[19] When speaking about presbyopia, he said, "Of all types of imperfect vision–and these are innumerable–the most common and most prevalent is blurred vision, which is created by aging. Therefore, this affliction is found in almost all people of advanced years. Blurred vision is first noticed when one is forty years old–fifty at the latest."[20] Daza de Valdes was aware of a phenomenon that optometrists today know well: that nearsighted children most often don't know that they have a vision problem until they find out that their friends can see better than they do. A common scenario today is that children notice classmates can read what the teacher is writing on the board at the front of the room and they can't. He explained this as follows:

> Every day we encounter children who learn to read and write well, but whose vision deficiency frequently goes unnoticed. Upon reaching the age of reason, however, these young people with deficient vision discover their lack themselves. They do so by measuring and comparing their vision with that of others who have perfect vision. It is then that they realize that their vision is short because they cannot see far away as well as others.[21]

According to Daza de Valdes, the types of eyeglass lenses were *convex*, *concave*, and *conservative*. Today we call convex and concave lenses *plus* and *minus* lenses, respectively. Convex or plus lenses converge light rays, while concave or minus lenses diverge light rays. Daza de Valdes described conservative lenses as "plain-glass lenses, which are neither convex nor concave," being "of the same thickness throughout. Thus they allow vision to pass without adding or subtracting anything."[22] Today we call such lenses *plano lenses*. Plano lenses have no optical power.

Daza de Valdes used a unit of lens power based on a Spanish measure of linear distance, the *vara*. One vara is equal to about 0.835 meters. Daza's lens power unit, the *grado*, often translated as degree, is a reciprocal vara. Today's diopter (D) is a reciprocal meter, so Daza's grado or degree was equal to about 1.20 D.

Daza de Valdes also described methods for determining lens power. For plus lenses, there are two circles, a larger one labeled X and a smaller one labeled Q. Circle Q is viewed through the plus lens and the lens is moved toward and away from circle Q until the two circles are the same size. The distance of the lens from the chart containing the circles is noted on a scale, which gives the power of the lens in grados or degrees. There are two similar charts for determining minus lens power (one for minus up to 10 degrees and one for minus more than 10 degrees), with the minus lens held over the larger of the two circles on each of the charts. There is an additional chart to mark the punctum remotum (far point of clear vision) of a person with myopia. The location of the punctum remotum could then be converted into the number of degrees of needed lens power. The chart covered 5 to 30 degrees.

There are also recommendations for how to order lens power, in absentia, according to age and gender. It may be noted that the powers recommended by Daza de Valdes are much greater than we would think appropriate for nearpoint plus adds for presbyopes today. For men, the recommended lens recommendations were ages 30 to 40 years, 2 degrees (about 2.4 D); 40 to 50 years, 2.5 degrees (about 3.0 D); 50 to 60 years, 3 degrees (3.6 D); 60 to 70 years, 3.5 degrees (4.2 D); 70 to 80 years, 4 degrees (4.8 D); and over 80 years, 5 degrees to 6 degrees maximum (6.0 to 7.2 D). For women, ages 30 to 35 years, 4 degrees (about 4.8 D); ages 35 to 40 years, 5 degrees (6.0 D); 40 to

45, 6 degrees (7.2 D); 50 to 60 years, 8 degrees (9.6 D); and over 60 years, 9 degrees to 10 degrees maximum (10.8 to 12.0 D).[23] Perhaps the different lens powers for men and women that Daza de Valdes recommended reflected his views concerning gender differences in visual needs, as later he talked about the vision of women becoming weak due to needlework.[24]

Next Daza de Valdes presented a series of dialogs in which an optometrist (maestro) holds illustrative consultations with patients with various vision problems. The consultations are also attended by a "doctor." Some of the information contained in these dialogs illustrates that one of the ways of determining the power of presbyopic lenses for a given patient was the use of ranges of clear vision with lenses. The optometrist had the patient use lenses of 2.5 degrees and stated to the patient: "Move the book farther and closer away and tell me at what distance you see best with those eyeglasses. Then I will know which glasses to give you." Based on those measurements, the optometrist increases the power to 3 degrees, and being satisfied with the result at that power, reports to the patient: "Those are the glasses you need because you see the print as it is and you read it well and with ease at the distance where one usually puts a book."[25] The optometrist goes on to say that one should not wear lenses with any greater power than necessary. Even though higher powers would make print appear larger, "too many degrees weaken the vision."[26]

Also in the dialogs are recommendations about wearing only well-made spectacles. For example, Daza de Valdes warned against lenses with unwanted cylinder power (at that time only spherical lenses were used): "...raise the glasses over the print. Twist them around and if the print is sometimes long and narrow and at other times short and wide, the lenses are badly ground."[27]

BEGINNINGS OF THE SPECTACLE INDUSTRY AND OPTOMETRY IN THE UNITED STATES

In colonial America, the need for spectacles was met by imports from Europe. Details on the development of spectacle making in America are unclear. Warner[28] identified the widow of Balthasar Sommer as the first person known to have done optical work in America, based on her 1753 advertisement in the *New York Gazette* that she was a "grinder of all sorts of optical glass." The first American of some renown to work in optics was David Rittenhouse (1732-1796). Rittenhouse was an instrument maker, astronomer, mathematician, and surveyor. He taught astronomy at the University of Pennsylvania from 1779 to 1782, and he succeeded Benjamin Franklin as president of the American Philosophical Society in 1791. He also held other public offices, being state treasurer of Pennsylvania from 1777 to 1789 and first director of the U.S. Mint from 1792 to 1795. He invented a collimating telescope and is credited with introducing the use of cross hairs in telescopes.[29] Rittenhouse imported optical glass from Europe to grind lenses for telescopes and surveying equipment. In 1783, Rittenhouse made a pair of spectacles for George Washington.[30]

In the late eighteenth century, American optical workers began referring to themselves as *opticians*. William Richardson was listed in Philadelphia city directories 1789 to 1799 as an "optical instrument maker" or "optician." Richardson sold several pairs of spectacles to Thomas Jefferson before selling his stock of spectacles to John McAllister, Sr., in about 1799.

The McAllister family of opticians is important in optical history. John McAllister, Sr., (1753-1830), was born in Scotland and immigrated to the United States in 1775. He was trained in Scotland as a woodworker, and in 1781, he established a business in Philadelphia making hickory walking sticks. He soon also started making riding whips and selling them and various sundry items. In the 1790s, McAllister added spectacles to the goods that he sold. John McAllister, Jr., (1786-1877) graduated from the

University of Pennsylvania in 1803 at 17. He received a Master of Arts from the University of Pennsylvania in 1816, but that may have been an honorary degree.[31] John McAllister, Jr., started working for his father in 1807 and became his partner in 1811. He was also a collector of books and historical documents. He assembled a significant library and was a member of the Library Committee of the Historical Society of Philadelphia. He is also known for the system of house numbering using 100s, 200s, 300s, etc., to indicate separate blocks.[32]

In 1815, the McAllisters started making spectacle frames, fitting imported lenses into them. Some time after that, they started grinding lenses themselves. Later, they also started doing vision testing to determine spectacle prescriptions. John McAllister, Jr., was followed in business in Philadelphia by two of his sons, William Young McAllister (1812-1896), and for a shorter time, Thomas H. McAllister (1824-1898). Two of William Young McAllister's sons, James Cook McAllister (1853-1928) and William M. McAllister (1843-1912), continued the business in Philadelphia, with William leaving the firm in 1883. Although the McAllister optical business ended in Philadelphia when James Cook McAllister died in 1928, another of William Young McAllister's sons, Francis W. McAllister, started an optical business in Baltimore, which, in turn, was carried on by two of his sons.[33,34] John McAllister, Jr., and his sons referred to themselves as *opticians*[30] although with the addition of vision testing to their services, they were among the optometrists of their day.

Among the important legacies of the McAllisters was that they trained many persons in spectacle making and vision testing. James Queen was one of their apprentices. Queen entered into partnership with William Young McAllister in 1836 and then opened his own business in 1853.[30] Queen was highly successful on his own and, in turn, taught many persons in the optical field. Some of those trained by Queen included John W. Jarvis, who became a president of the New York Optometric Association, and Harry E. Pine, Sr., whose son, Harry E. Pine, Jr., was president of the American Optometric Association from 1936 to 1938.[33]

In the nineteenth century, the optical industry and optometry in the United States were highly influenced by immigrants from Europe, who had been trained in optics before leaving their native countries. Among the many German opticians who came to the United States in the mid-nineteenth century were John Jacob Bausch, Henry Lomb, Joseph Zentmayer, John L. Borsch, Sr., William Bohne, and William Gerhardt.[30,33,35] Included among foreign-trained opticians from England were Benjamin Pike, Sr., and James Prentice. Pike trained several opticians, and Pike's sons, Benjamin Pike, Jr., and Daniel Pike, followed him into optical work.[31] Benjamin Pike, Jr., opened his own business in 1839, in which he manufactured spectacle frames, ground spectacle lens, and fitted the finished spectacles as well as selling a variety of scientific instruments.[36]

James Prentice arrived in the United States in 1842 and started doing optical work and making precision instruments in New York. He sold optical, metereological, mathematical, engineering, and drawing instruments.[37] During the Civil War, he started emphasizing his optical shop and he identified himself as an optician. He won several medals for his drafting and engineering instruments at American Institute exhibitions in New York City from 1848 to 1861 and at the 1876 World's Fair in Philadelphia.[38] In 1867, he patented a self-adjustable pince-nez spectacle frame and a spectacle frame called an "anatomical eye glass," which was marketed by Bausch & Lomb for several years.

James Prentice's son, Charles F. Prentice (1854-1946), went on to have immense importance for optometry. Being of the opinion that opticians of the future would need a strong education and knowing that there were no schools for opticians in the United States, James sent Charles to Germany to study mechanical engineering. From 1871 to 1874 Charles attended the Royal Polytechnicum in Karlsruhe.[39] Upon his return to New York in 1874, Charles worked for some months as a mechanical engineer and draftsman, but in 1875, he started working for his father.[40] At that time, James was "preoccupied with fitting and prescribing spectacles," and one of Charles' duties was preparing the 192-page "elaborately illustrated" catalog of the instruments they made and imported.[41]

As Charles Prentice started doing more work in optometry and reading the available literature, he decided there was a need for work on spectacle lens optics. The result was his 48-page book, *A Treatise on Simple and Compound Ophthalmic Lenses*, published by James Prentice & Son in 1886. Charles was the first to use the term *ophthalmic* to describe lenses used in spectacles. In 1888, he published another small book, *Dioptric Formulae for Combined Cylindrical Lenses*. He also published several papers in optical and ophthalmological journals. Among these was "A Metric System of Numbering and Measuring Prisms" published in the *Archives of Ophthalmology* in 1890. It was in that paper that he proposed the unit *prism dioptry* that we now know as the *prism diopter*. Soon after he suggested the prism diopter, the American Optical Company started using that unit, and shortly thereafter other companies did as well.[42] Charles Prentice is also known for Prentice's Rule, the formula with which the prismatic effect of the decentration of lenses can be calculated.

In 1888, James Prentice died and Charles took over the business, which he transformed into what we might think of today as a more professional practice. Charles gained recognition for his optical writings, and increasingly, as time would pass, for his crusading efforts for professionalism and licensure in optometry. It is for these latter efforts that he is particularly known today.

INVENTION OF BIFOCALS

Prior to the invention of bifocals, those needing optical correction for both distance and near had to have two pairs of glasses. Benjamin Franklin is usually given credit for the invention of bifocal spectacles, and based on their close examination of the documentary evidence, Levene[43] found no one with a better claim to the invention and Letocha[44] argued strongly for Franklin as the inventor. In a 1784 letter to George Whatley of London, Franklin wrote,

> Your Eyes must continue very good, since you can write so small a Hand without Spectacles. I cannot distinguish a Letter even of Large Print; but am happy in the invention of Double Spectacles, which serving for distant objects as well as near ones, make my Eyes as useful to me as ever they were....I imagine it will be found generally true, that the same Convexity of Glass, through which a Man sees clearest and best at the Distance proper for Reading, is not the best for greater Distances. I therefore had formerly two Pair of Spectacles, which I shifted occasionally, as in travelling I sometimes read, and often wanted to regard the Prospects. Finding this Change troublesome, and not always sufficiently ready, I had the Glasses cut, and half of each kind associated in the same Circle...By this means, as I wear my Spectacles constantly, I have only to move my Eyes up or down, as I want to see distinctly far or near, the proper Glasses being always ready...[45]

It is of interest that Thomas Jefferson wrote a letter to noted Philadelphia optician John McAllister, Sr., in which he said,

> You have heretofore furnished me with spectacles, so reduced in size as to give facility to looking over their top without moving them....This is a great convenience, but the reduction has not been sufficient to do it completely....Those who are obliged to use spectacles know what a convenience it would be to have different magnifiers in the same frame. Dr. Franklin tried this by semicircular glasses joined horizontally, the upper and lower semicircles of different powers, which he told me answered perfectly. I wish to try it, and therefore send you a drawing.[43]

Later, in 1807, he wrote to the painter Charles Willson Peale, "I have adopted Dr. Franklin's plan of half-glasses of different focal distances, with great advantage."[46]

The Franklin bifocal with two lenses joined at a horizontal line continued to be made until the late nineteenth century.[47] In 1888, the so-called perfection bifocal was introduced by August Morck. The perfection bifocal, like the Franklin bifocal, was made with two pieces of glass, but in the perfection bifocal the juncture was rounded. At about this time, the first cemented bifocal, in which a thin piece of glass was cemented to the back of a lens with the distance correction, was introduced. Subsequent variations of cemented bifocals were the Optifex bifocal and the cemented Kryptok bifocal.[47] The cemented Kryptok bifocal was patented by John Borsch, Sr., in 1899.[48] The next development was the fused bifocal in which a piece of flint glass was fused by heating into a ground-out area on the front of a crown glass lens. The first fused bifocal was the Kryptok fused bifocal patented by John Borsch, Jr. in 1909.[48] Additional types of fused bifocals, including the panoptic patented by J. H. Hammon in 1939 and the flat-top bifocal, were subsequently developed.[47] The Ultex one-piece bifocal was made of one piece of crown glass with the back surface of the lens ground to yield reading power in the bottom of the lens. Another one-piece bifocal was the Executive bifocal with two different powers ground on the front surface with a horizontal line demarcating distance and near powers, somewhat reminiscent of the Franklin bifocal. The newest multifocal lens design is the progressive addition lens.[47] Further refinements of progressive addition lens design continue today.

The invention of trifocals was announced in an 1827 paper by John Isaac Hawkins. Hawkins was born in England but lived for a while in the United States as a young man and then again in old age.[49] He might be best described as an engineer and inventor as he published descriptions of new devices or improvements in numerous areas, such as lathes, paper-cutting machines, musical instruments, saws, stoves, etc.[50] The power of the lenses in Hawkins' own spectacles worn in 1826 at age 54 were +1.50 D for distance, +3.25 D in the intermediate portion of the lenses, and +5.62 D in the reading portion. It is worth noting that Hawkins also described a gauge for the measurement of interpupillary distances. He observed that interpupillary distance was seldom taken into account, at that time, when people purchased spectacles.[49] If the separation of the optical centers of the lenses did not match the interpupillary distance of the patient, unwanted prism couldresult.

DISCOVERY AND CORRECTION OF ASTIGMATISM

Until the early nineteenth century, spectacle lens corrections were spherical lenses. The first published report of astigmatism was by Thomas Young in 1801. Young, who had trained as a physician, had an amazing intellect and made contributions to numerous fields, including physics, medicine, linguistics, optics, vision science, and engineering.[51,52,53,54,55] He also improved upon an optometer made by William Porterfield and used it to measure his own astigmatism. Young wrote this about his astigmatism:

> My eye, in a state of relaxation, collects to a focus on the retina, those rays which diverge vertically from an object at the distance of ten inches from the cornea, and the rays which diverge horizontally from an object at seven inches distance. For, if I hold the plane of the optometer vertically, the images of the line appear to cross at ten inches; if horizontally, at seven....I have never experienced any inconvenience from this imperfection, nor did I ever discover it till I made these experiments; and I believe I can examine minute objects with as much accuracy as most of those whose eyes are differently formed.[56]

Young had compound myopic astigmatism. At the suggestion of scientific instrument maker William Cary, he tilted the minus lens for his myopia (thus inducing a cylinder effect), and he found that he could improve the clarity of his vision. However, apparently because the astigmatism didn't seem to bother him, he did not pursue a more permanent correction for it.

It might be mentioned that John Isaac Hawkins, previously discussed as the inventor of trifocals, also made a measurement of his own astigmatism.[57] Using an optometer based on Young's design, he found 1.37 D of astigmatism in his right eye and 0.12 D of astigmatism in his left eye. He suggested that Young's optometer would be helpful in the prescription of spectacles. Hawkins used spherical lenses in trifocals, basing the distance correction on the spherical equivalent.[57] Hawkins and John F. W. Herschel appear to have been the first to put forward the cornea as the source of astigmatism.

Credit for the development of the first spherocylinder lens to correct astigmatism goes to British astronomer George Biddell Airy. During his long life, Airy held distinguished positions such as Lucasian Professor of Mathematics and Plumian Professor of Astronomy at Cambridge and Astronomer Royal.[58] Airy had long-standing poor vision in his left eye and noticed that a distant bright point of light, such as a star, appeared elliptical rather than circular. Like Young, Airy had compound myopic astigmatism. Airy found the distances of his far points of clear vision in the meridians in which the far points were maximum and minimum; he then computed the needed surface curvatures of a glass spherocylindrical lens to correct his astigmatism.

Airy recorded his far points in inches, and based on those measurements, Levene[59] calculated that Airy had 4.69 D of astigmatism when he made his first measurements. With that amount of astigmatism, it is easy to understand why Airy, an astronomer, might have been motivated to design a lens for his own eye! A lens was made for Airy in 1824 by someone named Fuller, about whom little is known. Airy published his measurements and the design of the lens in 1827 in a paper titled "On A Peculiar Defect in the Eye and a Mode of Correcting It." In a follow-up report in 1849, Airy used the term *astigmatism*, which had been suggested to him by a Cambridge colleague, William Whewell.[58]

In 1828, the first description of the correction of astigmatism in the United States was made by Chauncey Enoch Goodrich.[60-61] It appears that Goodrich was not aware of Airy's paper, so his work was an independent announcement of the wearing of a corrective lens for astigmatism. Goodrich graduated from Union College in 1825, and from 1825 to 1828 he attended Princeton Theological Seminary. He served in a number of different ministerial positions in his life, but he was also noted for his scientific research, particularly for his development of some disease-resistant varieties of potatoes. In 1825, Goodrich obtained concave spherical lenses, and he observed that without the lenses he could see vertical lines better than horizontal lines, but with the lenses he could see horizontal lines better. He realized that he needed a lens with different curvatures in different meridians. In 1827, Goodrich obtained cylindrical lenses from John McAllister, Jr., and he may well have been the first to wear them in America. It is often been suggested that these cylinder lenses were ground by McAllister,[62-63] but Levene[60] makes a case for McAllister having had them ground in France. Goodrich's 1828 paper on his astigmatism and its correction was entitled "Notice of a Peculiarity in Vision." It would actually be a few decades before it was realized how common astigmatism actually is.

If the McAllisters didn't make the first cylinder lens in the United States, we could ask who did. Levene[64] suggested that it was Joseph Zentmayer, who completed an apprenticeship as an optician in Germany and came to the United States at age 22. Zentmayer established a business in Philadelphia making scientific and optical instruments, for which he won numerous awards from scientific organizations.[65] He was particularly known for making high-quality lenses for microscopy and photography.[66] Zentmayer made spherocylindrical lenses for the James Queen Optical Company until 1874, when, seeing an increased demand for cylinder lenses, the Queen Company began making them themselves.

According to Charles Prentice,[67] by the 1860s and later, the opticians who were testing and prescribing for astigmatism included John McAllister and J.W. Queen of Philadelphia, Widdefield of Boston, Charles Lembke and James Prentice of New York, and others. Test targets and procedures developed, as practitioners realized that astigmatism was more common than originally thought. Cylinder lenses began to be included in trial lens sets in the mid-nineteenth century.[68]

A test lens for astigmatism that was introduced in 1849 was the Stokes lens.[69,70,71] George Gabriel Stokes was a mathematician and physicist at Cambridge. He held the Lucasian Chair in Mathematics at Cambridge, the position once held by Isaac Newton, from 1849 until his death in 1903. Stokes studied a wide range of topics in mathematical physics, including various studies on the nature of light.[72] The Stokes lens consisted of a planoconvex cylinder and a planoconcave cylinder mounted with the flat surfaces almost touching each other. The two cylinders, which were about four diopters each, rotated in a linked fashion in opposite directions. The maximum resultant cylinder power (+4 D sphere with -8 D cylinder) was achieved when the power meridians of the two cylinders were perpendicular, and the minimum power (plano) was attained when the power meridians were superimposed. The Stokes lens did not see wide usage, perhaps because it didn't offer a great advantage over trial lens set cylinders or because the sphere changed as the cylinder changed, requiring neutralization of the induced sphere power.[73] It has been suggested that the main importance of the Stokes lens was as the precursor for the Jackson cross cylinder test for astigmatism; in the twentieth century, the Jackson cross cylinder test became the standard subjective test for astigmatism.[69,70,71] In a paper presented in 1887, ophthalmologist Edward Jackson stated that he used a cross cylinder to determine whether a patient had astigmatism. In 1907, he published a paper showing how a cross cylinder could be used to find the astigmatic axis.[74]

AN 1837 DESCRIPTION OF THE OPTICIAN

In 1837, an American, Edward Hazen, published a book titled *The Panorama of Professions and Trades; Or Every Man's Book*. Written to aid the reader in the choice of an occupation, it described seventy professions and trades, including printer, baker, carpenter, cooper, architect, physician, dentist, teacher, bookseller, silversmith, and others. There was also a chapter on "The Optician." On the first page of the chapter, there is an engraving illustrating an optician's shop. In the center, there is a counter on which there are several pairs of spectacles. On one side of the counter is presumably the optician, holding up one pair of spectacles for inspection. On the other side of the counter are a seated woman, probably a customer, and a child. To one side, another seated optician, perhaps an apprentice, appears to be grinding lenses. To the other side another assistant is working on a telescope. On the wall behind the optician, there are some tools and on the shelves behind the counter there are various instruments.

The chapter on the optician in Hazen's book contains thirty-nine numbered paragraphs. These paragraphs discuss optics, optical instruments, definitions of presbyopia and myopia and their "palliation" by convex and concave glasses, microscopes, telescopes, and some history of optics discoveries. The chapter gives the following description of an optician: "The word *optician* is applicable to persons who are particularly skilled in the science of vision; but especially to those who devote their attention to the manufacture of optical instruments; such as – the spectacles, the camera obscura, the magic lantern, the telescope, the microscope, and the quadrant."[75] It was also noted that "opticians have their spectacles numbered to suit different periods of life; but as the short-sighted and long-sighted conditions exist in a thousand different degrees, each person should select for himself such as will enable him to read without effort at the usual distance."[75]

The First Six Centuries of Optometry

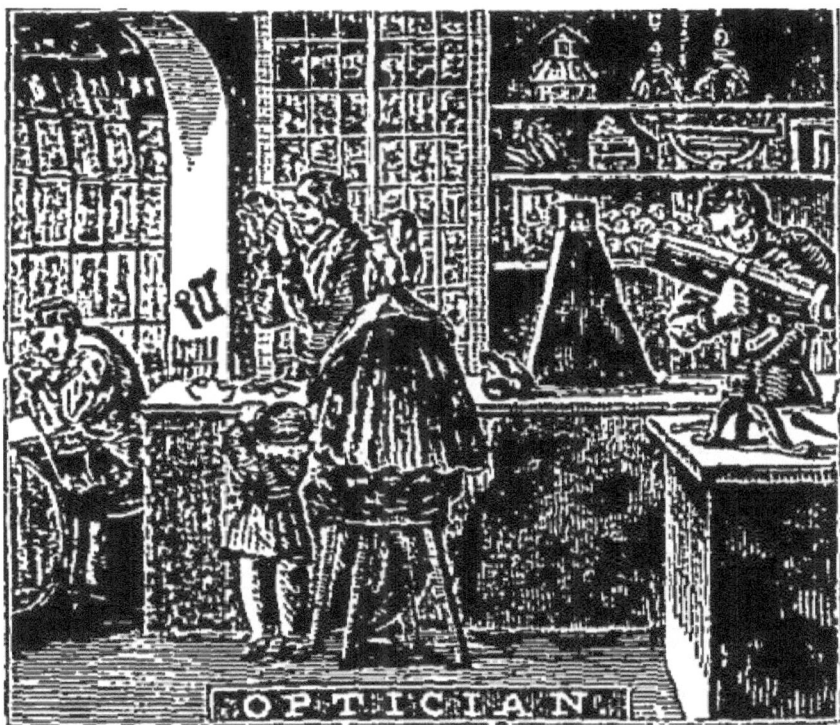

Figure 1.2. Engraving of an optician's premises from the 1837 book *The Panorama of Professions and Trades; Cr Every Man's Book*, by Edward Hazen.

MEDICAL PRACTITIONERS ENTER THE FIELD OF OPTOMETRY

The field of medicine didn't start to have a significant interest in spectacle prescribing until about the mid-nineteenth century. For more than five centuries, the general attitude of medicine toward spectacles was one of opposition. Physicians recommended remedies to avoid their use. For example, Piero Ubertini da Brescia wrote a treatise translated as *Prescriptions for the Eyes* (1361) as part of a medical and surgical manual. He recommended the treatment compiled by a colleague from Florence, who prescribed pills composed of chamomile, colocynth, quince, leeks, and other herbs for persons who needed eyeglasses.[76] In 1363, surgeon and professor of medicine at the University of Montpellier in France, Guy de Chauliac, published *Chirurgia magna*, which served as a standard medical textbook for the next two hundred years. He suggested that eyeglasses should be used only as a last resort if remedies or potions such as fennel seeds did not clear vision.[77]

Sixteenth-century Spanish physician Cristóbal Méndez opposed spectacles because with them the eyes did not expend the effort they should for proper health. In 1553, he wrote, "Besides the eyes not dissipating something produced by lack of exercise (because the spectacles prevent it), many superfluities and vapors of the body cannot come out through the eyes which have those doors in front of them....if it were possible that no spectacles existed it would be a good thing, because their constant use...produces great harm to the eyes."[78]

One of the most famous early books on the medical and surgical care of the eyes was *Ophthalmoduleia* by the German surgeon George Bartisch. Bartisch was not formally educated and he learned surgical care by apprenticeship to a barber surgeon, starting at age 13.[79] Instead of wearing glasses, he recommended remedies such as potions, pills, eye powders, ear washes, charms, and purges. One of his treatments was wearing the tongue of a fox around the neck.[79] In his 1583 book, Bartisch wrote, "It is better and more useful that one leaves spectacles alone. For naturally a person sees and recognizes something better when he has nothing in front of his eyes than when he has something there. It is much better that one should preserve his two eyes than he should have four."[80]

Thus, while the manufacture of spectacles and the refractive testing for their prescription was being developed by opticians (optometrists), medicine avoided that field for centuries. However, some physicians did refer patients to opticians for the prescription of glasses. For example, the physicians at the Wills Eye Hospital in Philadelphia referred patients to John McAllister, Jr., for vision testing and prescription of spectacles as well as for the grinding of the lenses.[81] Significantly, there was no direct financial competition in the prescription of spectacles between optometry and medicine, but that began to change in the nineteenth century.

According to Levene[82], the first physician to suggest that refractive testing should be occur in the domain of medicine may have been the British ophthalmic surgeon James Ware. Ware presented a paper on refractive errors to the Royal Society in 1813. In 1846, Ferdinand Ritter von Arlt, who was then at the University of Prague, suggested that medicine should fit spectacles because such an important function should not be left to opticians.[83,84]

According to Albert,[85] the development of eye care as an independent medical specialty had its origins in the early nineteenth century. Physicians who drifted into eye care without substantial training in eye conditions were generally known as *oculists*, but it also appears that some persons proclaimed themselves oculists without the benefit of medical training. In the United States, some oculists started learning refraction testing procedures from refracting opticians in the second half of the nineteenth century, including those in Philadelphia who were taught by William Young McAllister and James Queen in the early 1870s.[86] Charles Prentice observed that "prior to the year 1865 the optician had...exclusively exercised his traditional right to adapt glasses to the sight. But oculists were quick to perceive the opportunity for extending their line of practice to include that of the optician, and soon took advantage of it by providing themselves with the necessary test-types and lenses."[67]

According to the Oxford English Dictionary, the first uses of the terms *ophthalmology* and *ophthalmologist* appeared in the British journal *The Lancet* in 1825 and 1826, respectively. The term *ophthalmologist* came to be associated with someone who had completed medical school and had some training in eye care beyond medical school. In the nineteenth century, that advanced training for American ophthalmologists likely consisted of studying for a while at a prominent eye clinic in the Eastern

United States or perhaps traveling overseas to study with a European ophthalmologist. In the twentieth century, qualification in ophthalmology came to mean completion of a formal residency program in ophthalmology. According to Truhlsen,[87] the first American physician to practice only ophthalmology was Henry Willard Williams (1821-1895).

In the mid- and late-nineteenth century, many states were passing medical licensure laws that granted medical practitioners all-inclusive rights to practice in all areas of health care.[88] As a consequence, spectacle prescribing legally became a part of medicine. However, ophthalmologists, being trained in medicine and not in optics, did not all flock to the practice of spectacle prescribing. This led ophthalmologist Casey Wood to write in 1918:

> There can be no doubt but that if the medical profession as a whole does not in some effective manner provide for the needs (or demands) of that rather large percentage of the laity who continue to frequent the shops of the optician the so-called "optometrist" will, sooner or later, under pressure of public opinion, receive legal recognition, either through legislative action or, as in the case of Columbia University, by the establishment of optical (or optician's) courses. For good or evil, that portion of the public that goes (or is sent by physicians) to the optician believes that much of the oculist's work is as well done by the "optometrist" as by the ophthalmologist....doctors...are opposed to "simple refracting" by a "qualified" optometrist and still refuse to do the work themselves.[89]

In the late nineteenth century, there was also often medical opposition to the prescription of plus lenses for conditions other than presbyopia, even though many did recognize that correction of hyperopia could alleviate eyestrain. American ophthalmologist Thomas Hall Shastid, a prolific writer on ophthalmology history and other topics,[90,91] wrote about the medical thinking of the time: "The M.D.s generally would not recognize even the existence of such a thing as eyestrain....they called 'quacks' all of us who fitted glasses to the eyes of the young....Hardly anything that now I can recall served so much to weaken the standing and influence of physicians in any community than this absurd, ridiculous, hard-headed, stubborn...opposition to the fitting of glasses."[92]

The entry of the medical profession into the practice of optometry precipitated recurrent "turf battles" and episodes of ill will between optometry and ophthalmology that continued for decades. The fact that medicine by itself did not manage the refractive problems of the public, though legally allowed to do so, meant that the development of optometry would continue unabated, and, in fact, interference from ophthalmology would spur optometrists to improve education and press for licensure laws. One positive aspect of the entry of medicine into the field of refraction, however, was that the vast resources of the medical profession were used to address refractive problems, resulting in a number of important developments and publications. The most important of these was *On the Anomalies of Accommodation and Refraction of the Eye* by Frans Cornelis Donders in 1864.

DONDERS' BOOK

The famed Dutch physician Frans Cornelis Donders completed medical school at 22. In his early 30s, after publishing widely in medicine and physiology, he started practicing mostly ophthalmology.[93,94,95] In 1858 and 1860, he published papers on spectacles and refraction that received considerable notice, and in 1862, he published a book on astigmatism and cylindrical glasses in Dutch and then in a German translation.[96] Because of the acclaim received by those publications, the New Sydenham Society of London asked Donders to write a book on refraction.[97] The result, his 635-page *On the Anomalies of Accommodation and Refraction of the Eye*, was published in 1864 in English, based on a translation of his Dutch manuscript. It essentially summarized and codified the field of clinical optometry at that time. His clear writing, depth of coverage, command of the field, clinical insight, and application of scientific principles and experimental findings to clinical care made it an instant classic and the standard reference work in clinical refraction for years to come.

The book included geometrical and physiological optics background for the understanding of refraction, instructions on clinical procedures and analysis, characteristics of clinical conditions, and case reports. In the discussion of accommodation, he presented a graphical procedure for showing ranges of accommodation and convergence, and relationships between accommodation and convergence. Levene credited Donders with the first scientifically and clinically sound description of hypermetropia and for coining that term (the synonym *hyperopia* was suggested by Helmholtz).[98] His coverage of astigmatism, which largely reproduced his earlier monograph on astigmatism,[96] stimulated practitioners to look for astigmatism in addition to spherical refractive errors. Donders' book also served as an inspiration to others, including Edward Jackson in his work on retinoscopy and cross cylinder astigmatism testing procedures.[95]

Joseph Bruneni's book on the history of the American ophthalmic industry includes a five-page memoir of nineteenth-century optometrist Thomas M. Heard, which illustrates the impact of Donders' book.[98] After Heard was discharged from the United States Army at the close of the Civil War in 1865, he decided to study medicine and started working for a physician in central Ohio. The physician developed difficulty reading and was not able to find glasses that helped him adequately. At age 57, this physician was starting to accept that his eyes were "simply wearing out," so Heard read to him by candlelight. This led Heard to study spectacle prescribing and try to find out why the physician could not find adequate spectacles. Heard traveled to Cleveland and Boston to learn what he could. It was in Boston that he heard about Donders' book. Heard wrote to Donders to request a copy, to which Donders responded that he was sending a copy and that Heard could contact him if he had questions after reading it. Heard wrote in his memoir about his excitement in getting the book and that he "kept studying my book night and day for at last I had found what I wanted." After reading the book, Heard returned to see and examine his physician friend. Heard fit the physician with spectacles containing a high astigmatic correction, which were ordered from Europe. When the glasses arrived, Heard found that they were the first glasses the physician "had ever been able to read with for any length of time." Heard set up an office in Warren, Ohio, and later practiced in Cleveland. Heard had a son and grandson who graduated from optometry school in the early twentieth century.

DIFFERENTIATION OF TYPES OF OPTICIANS

The first use of the term *optician* cited by the Oxford English Dictionary was in 1672 and was attributed to Sir Isaac Newton. By the nineteenth century, it had become the common term applied to someone knowledgeable in optics and its applications, such as making spectacles and optical instruments, or, as we noted earlier in the 1837 definition from Hazen, to "persons who are particularly skilled in the science of vision." By the late nineteenth century, there began to be a differentiation of opticians into *manufacturing opticians, dispensing opticians*, and *refracting opticians*. Examples of manufacturing opticians were John Jacob Bausch and Henry Lomb, who founded the company of Bausch & Lomb, and George Washington Wells, who took over as president of American Optical Company in 1891.[99]

Dispensing opticians, or *prescription opticians* as they were also known, did not do vision testing. They ground the lenses and filled the lens prescriptions written by others. According to Bruneni,[100] Joseph Zentmayer was the first to limit his business in that way. Refracting opticians did the vision testing to derive a lens prescription as well as grinding the lenses and fitting the spectacles to the patient. Examples of prominent refracting opticians include James and Charles Prentice, some of the members of the McAllister family, and Andrew Jay Cross.

Beginning in the 1890s and continuing into the twentieth century, the refracting opticians struggled with improving their professional and educational standing and with deciding what to call themselves (they soon began calling themselves *optometrists*). By the end of the nineteenth century, they had established a niche earned through the preceding centuries caring for the visual needs of the population through refraction and provision of spectacles. The twentieth century would also mark the broadening of the concept of vision care into other areas such as binocular vision, contact lenses, low vision, vision therapy, and management of ocular disease. Yet they also were faced with external challenges, notably a threat to Charles Prentice for charging an examination fee. These struggles and the continuing development of the identity of the optometrist are examined next.

Chapter 1: Notes

1. Levene JR. *Clinical Refraction and Visual Science*. London, UK: Butterworths, 1977:56, 85.
2. Letocha CE. The origin of spectacles. *Surv Ophthalmol*. 1986;31:185-188.
3. Rosenthal JW. *Spectacles and Other Vision Aids: A History and Guide to Collecting*. San Francisco, CA: Norman, 1996:395.
4. Ilardi V. *Renaissance Vision from Spectacles to Telescopes*. Philadelphia, PA: American Philosophical Society, 2007:4.
5. Rosen E. The invention of eyeglasses. *J Hist Med Allied Sci*. 1956;11:13-46, 183-218.
6. Ilardi, 6.
7. Goss DA. Thirteenth-century European authors and manuscripts on the eye and vision. *Hindsight*. 2007;38:85-94.
8. Lindberg DC. Lines of influence in thirteenth-century optics: Bacon, Witelo, and Pecham. *Speculum* 1971;46:66-83. In: Lindberg DC. *Studies in the History of Medieval Optics*. London, UK: Variorum Reprints, 1983.
9. Weimer MF, Bernard Becker. Collection in Ophthalmology: Catalog of the

Bernard Becker, M.D., Collection in Ophthalmology at the Washington University School of Medicine Library, 1979.
10 Hofstetter HW. *Optometry: Professional, Economic, and Legal Aspects.* St. Louis, MO: Mosby, 1948:22-24.
11 Chiu K. The introduction of spectacles into China. *Harvard J Asiatic Studies* 1936;1:186-193.
12 Gasson W. The evolution of spectacles. Part 1. The Chinese contribution. *Ophthalmic Optician* 1980;20:490-492.
13 Shirayama S. Spectacles in Chinese history. *Ophthalmic Antiques* 1991;36:2-3.
14 Chan E, Mao W. The history of spectacles in China. Proceedings of the XXVth International Congress of Ophthalmology 1986:731-734.
15 Rosenthal, 62-65.
16 Ilardi, 82.
17 Ilardi 90-91.
18 Ilardi, 92-93.
19 Daza de Valdes B. *The Use of Eyeglasses.* English translation edited by Paul E. Runge. Oostende, Belgium: J. P. Wayenborgh, 2004:79.
20 Daza de Valdes, 81.
21 Daza de Valdes, 83.
22 Daza de Valdes, 101.
23 Daza de Valdes, 117-118.
24 Daza de Valdes, 164.
25 Daza de Valdes, 128.
26 Daza de Valdes, 128.
27 Daza de Valdes, 167.
28 Warner DJ. Presentation on the history of lens grinding in America given at the 1984 Ocular Heritage Society meeting. In: Rosenthal, 50-54.
29 Von Doren C, ed. David Rittenhouse. *Webster's American Biographies.* Springfield, MA: Merriam-Webster, 1984:877-878.
30 Warner DJ. Optics in Philadelphia during the nineteenth century. *Proc Am Phil Soc.*1985;129:291-299.
31 Levene, 260-265
32 Bruneni JL. *Looking Back: An Illustrated History of the American Ophthalmic Industry.* Torrance, CA: Optical Laboratories Association, 1994:29-31.
33 Cox ME. *Optometry, the Profession: Its Antecedents, Birth, and Development*, rev. ed. Philadelphia, PA: Chilton, 1957:15-16.
34 The Library Company of Philadelphia. The John A. McAllister Collection. http://www.librarycompany.org/mcallister
35 Sullivan L. *Bausch & Lomb: Perfecting Vision, Enhancing Life for 150 Years—A Brief History of Bausch & Lomb's First 150 Years.* Rochester, NY: Bausch & Lomb, 2004:4-5.
36 Bettman OL. Benjamin Pike, Jr., pioneer in American optics. *Optical J Rev Optom.* 1941;78(17):23-24.

37 Kidwell PA. James Prentice's rectangular protractor. *Am Scientific Instrument Enterprise* 1987;1(3):61-63.
38 Prentice CF. *Legalized Optometry and the Memoirs of its Founder*. Seattle, WA: Casperin Fletcher Press, 1926:236.
39 Hofstetter HW. Prentice at Lahr and Karlsruhe. *J Am Optom Assoc.* 1978;49:921-924.
40 Christensen J. Chronology of Charles Prentice's life. *Hindsight* 2000;31:2-5.
41 Prentice, 241.
42 Bruneni J. Charles F. Prentice, Opticist. *Hindsight* 1999;30:1-7.
43 Levene, 141-165.
44 Letocha CE. The invention and early manufacture of bifocals. *Surv Ophthalmol.* 1990;35:226-235.
45 Finger S. *Doctor Franklin's Medicine*. Philadelphia, PA: University of Pennsylvania Press, 2006:261-262.
46 Finger, 264.
47 Rosenthal, 258-265.
48 Bruneni, 85-88.
49 Levene, 166-189.
50 Levene, 317-321.
51 Wood A, Oldham F. *Thomas Young, Natural Philosopher 1773-1829*. Cambridge, UK: Cambridge University Press, 1954.
52 Levene JR. Thomas Young, 1773-1829. In: Olby RC, ed. *Early Nineteenth Century European Scientists*. Oxford, UK: Pergamon Press, 1967:67-93.
53 Morse EW. Thomas Young. In: Gillispie CC, ed. *Dictionary of Scientific Biography*. New York, NY: Charles Scribner's Sons, 1976:562-572.
54 Gauger GE. The great mind of Thomas Young (1773-1829). *Documenta Ophthalmologica* 1997;94:113-121.
55 Goss DA. Five eighteenth and nineteenth century books significant in vision science selected from the collection of the Lilly Library at Indiana University. *Hindsight* 2007;38:68-75.
56 Robinson A. *The Last Man who Knew Everything: Thomas Young, The Anonymous Polymath Who Proved Newton Wrong, Explained How We See, Cured the Sick, and Deciphered the Rosetta Stone, Among Other Feats of Genius*. New York, NY: Pi Press, 2006:74.
57 Levene, 214-219.
58 Levene, 223-251.
59 Levene, 224-228.
60 Levene, 258-280.
61 Hofstetter HW. The Rev. Chauncey Enoch Goodrich, 1801-1864. *Newsletter Optom Hist Soc.* 1977;8:60-61.
62 Hirsch MJ, Wick RE. *The Optometric Profession*. Philadelphia, PA: Chilton, 1968:115.
63 Bruneni, 31.
64 Levene, 272.

65 Hofstetter HW. Joseph Zentmayer (1826-1888). *Newsletter Optom Hist Soc.* 1976;7:11.
66 Oliver CA. Obituary notice of Joseph Zentmayer. *Proc Am Phil Soc.* 1893;31:358-364.
67 Prentice, 44.
68 Levene, 230.
69 Levene, 242-246.
70 MacKay K. The astigmatic lens of George Gabriel Stokes. *Newsletter Optom Hist Soc.* 1980;11:20-23.
71 Wunsh SE. The cross cylinder. In: Safir A, ed. *Refraction and Clinical Optics.* Hagerstown, MD: Harper & Row, 1980:177-186.
72 Wood A. George Gabriel Stokes 1819-1903. In: McCartney M, Whitaker A, eds. *Physicists of Ireland: Passion and Precision.* Bristol, UK: Institute of Physics Publishing, 2003:85-94.
73 Bannon RE, Walsh R. On astigmatism: Part I – Historical Survey. *Am J Optom Arch Am Acad Optom.* 1945;22:101-110.
74 Newell FW. Edward Jackson, MD: A historical perspective of his contributions to refraction and to ophthalmology. *Ophthalmol.* 1988;95:555-558.
75 Hazen E. *The Panorama of Professions and Trades, or Every Man's Book.* Philadelphia, PA: Uriah Hunt, 1837:245-251.
76 Ilardi, 54-55.
77 Ilardi, 64.
78 Ilardi, 247-248.
79 Ilardi, 249-250.
80 Levene, 70.
81 Kelly C. McAllister: 5 generation optometrics. *Optical J Rev Optom.* 1975;112(13):10-17.
82 Levene, 42.
83 Hofstetter, 31.
84 Hirsch & Wick, 120-121.
85 Albert DM. The development of ophthalmic pathology. In Albert DM, Edwards DD, eds. *The History of Ophthalmology.* Cambridge, MA: Blackwell Science, 1996:65-106.
86 Hirsch & Wick, 136-137.
87 Truhlsen SM. The American Academy of Ophthalmology. In: Albert DM, Edwards DD, eds. *The History of Ophthalmology.* Cambridge, MA: Blackwell Science, 1996:323-358.
88 Classé JG. *Legal Aspects of Optometry.* Boston, MA: Butterworths, 1989:3,4,26.
89 Hirsch & Wick, 121.
90 Hofstetter HW. Tramping to failure. *Newsletter Optom Hist Soc.* 1975;6:14-15.
91 Newell FW. Thomas Hall Shastid (1866-1947): America's forgotten historian of ophthalmology. *Doc Ophthalmol.* 1992;81:53-58.

92 Shastid TH. *Tramping to Failure*. Ann Arbor, MI: George Wahr, 1937:166-167.
93 Pfeiffer RL. Frans Cornelis Donders, Dutch physiologist and ophthalmologist. *Bull New York Acad Med.* 1936;556-581.
94 ter Laage RJCV. Franciscus Cornelis Donders. In: Gillispie CC, ed., *Dictionary of Scientific Biography*. New York, NY: Charles Scribner's Sons, 1971;4:162-164.
95 Albert DM. *Men of Vision: Lives of Notable Figures in Ophthalmology*. Philadelphia, PA: Saunders, 1993:142-160.
96 Hofstetter HW. Astigmatism and cylindrical glasses. *Newsletter Optom Hist Soc.* 1988;19:22-24.
97 Duke-Elder S, Abrams D. Ophthalmic optics and refraction. In: Duke-Elder S, ed. *System of Ophthalmology*. St. Louis, MO: Mosby, 1970;5:255.
98 Bruneni, 125-129.
99 Bruneni, 25-29.
100 Bruneni, 21.

Chapter 2

Development of Professionalism in Optometry and Related Early Twentieth-Century Developments

In the later decades of the nineteenth century, those doing optical work tended to become more specialized, some doing either manufacturing or dispensing alone, and some doing vision testing. Toward the end of the nineteenth and the beginning of the twentieth century, those doing vision testing, practicing what we would recognize as optometry, were usually referring to their field of practice as optics. Yet they didn't know what to call themselves, sometimes using terms like *refracting optician* or *sight-tester*. Besides establishing a more consistent identity, they were struggling with a number of issues that are often part of the development of a professional status.

CHARACTERISTICS OF A PROFESSION

The elements of transition from trade to profession have been identified[1,2,3] as including the following: (1) a body of systematic knowledge learned through specialized standardized education in training schools or universities; (2) the ability to deliver a unique service that is in the general public interest and for which a fee may be charged; (3) formal qualifications and licensure based on education and examination, overseen by a regulatory body; (4) formation of professional associations and organizations that may perform a variety of cultural, social, ethical, educational, political, or promotional functions; and (5) control of the body of knowledge, ethical standards, and qualifications for practicing the profession by the members of the profession. Many of these characteristics began to surface during the events leading up to Charles Prentice's crusading efforts to establish licensure.

CHARLES PRENTICE AND AN EXAMINATION FEE

For the first few centuries after the invention of spectacles, those who made and fit spectacles earned their living by marking up the cost of the spectacles themselves. Today, practitioners expect to charge a fee for their services rather than making a profit on goods. The gradual adoption of this mode of thinking was part of the professionalization of optometry.

As noted earlier Charles Prentice worked for his optician father in the 1870s and 1880s and then took over the business in 1888.[4] In the 1880s, he consulted opticians and ophthalmologists to advance his practical learning, and he was influenced by John Ailman of Boston, whom he described as "a very competent and successful optician." Prentice was particularly impressed by Ailman's "dignified attitude toward his clients, with the confidence they seemed to place in him, and with the practical arrangement of his premises."[5] So that he could refer patients with eye disease to physicians, Prentice learned about ocular disease from William F. Mittendorf, who identified himself as an ophthalmic surgeon (see the title page of his book, *A Manual on Diseases of the Eye and Ear*). Prentice has been described as an "idealist" who "deplored anyone who compromised" and who had an "intense desire to excel."[6] By the early 1890s, Prentice was noted by both opticians and ophthalmologists for his books and articles on the optics of lenses, and for his invention of the prism diopter unit. Prentice may have been the first refracting optician to charge a fee for his examination services.

In 1892, Prentice got a letter, dated December 16, from New York ophthalmologist Henry D. Noyes, who had learned that Prentice charged

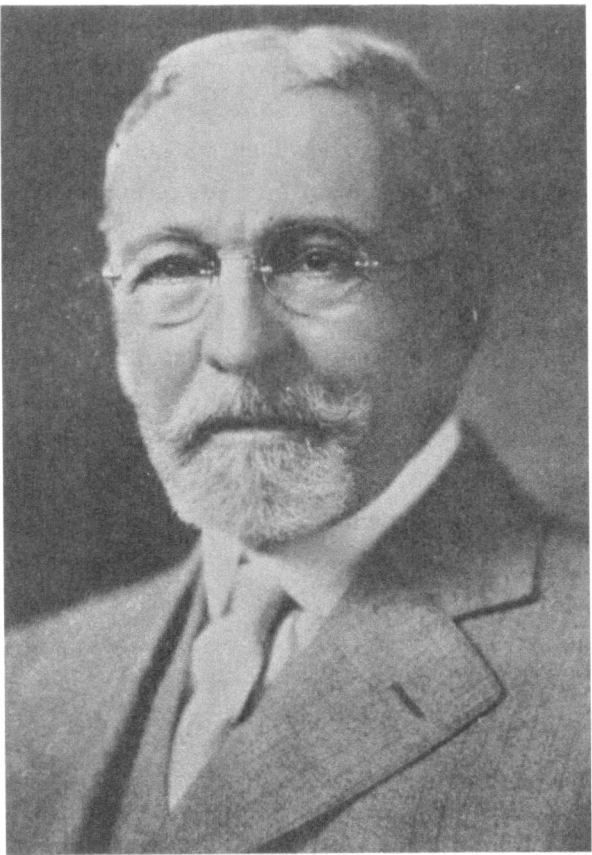

Figure 2.1. Charles Prentice (1854-1946). (Image courtesy of the Archives & Museum of Optometry and The AOA Foundation)

an examination fee. Noyes told Prentice that by charging an examination fee, Prentice was placing himself "in direct competition with [oculists], not only, but you assume their functions without having their training and general education. I think you must see the impropriety of such practice....an injustice is done the public by the fact that in charging a fee you assume that you have the qualifications which entitle you to a fee for advice."[7]

The next day Prentice wrote back to Noyes that for the past five years he had been charging:

a fee of $3.00 for my services, comprising the time and skill necessary in ascertaining the proper optical correction for persons not afflicted with disease of the eyes...All my patrons are distinctly given to understand that I am not a physician, that I do not prescribe medicine, or give advice in a medical sense; but that the fee is intended to cover my scientifically conducted mechanical services...if I did not charge a fee for services rendered, I should be obliged to exact an extortionate price for the glasses, which is the method of the charlatan. As far as my patrons are concerned, you must, therefore, admit that my dealings with them in this respect are irreproachable and just. I have but one price for glasses whether they are executed according to an oculist's formula or my own.[8]

In the meantime, Noyes sought the opinion of fellow ophthalmologist D. B. St. John Roosa. When Roosa wrote back to Noyes, he said this about Prentice: "I am inclined to think that he is violating the law in measuring a cornea, and in adjusting a glass, and giving a positive opinion to the patient in regard to the glasses that they ought to wear..."[9] Angry over the Noyes correspondence and over Noyes having brought Roosa into their correspondence, Prentice sought medical and legal support for his position. Georgetown University ophthalmologist Swan M. Burnett wrote to Prentice that "the interference of Roosa is an impertinence of which, he alone, I believe, is capable" and that "I know how scrupulous you have been in regard to assumption of responsibilities." Burnett further warned Prentice that he shouldn't expect anything different from the New York oculists because "they consider you their rival."[10] Support for Prentice by many physicians can also be seen in the fact that sixty general medical practitioners sent him patients for optical care.[10]

In February 1895, a physician friend of Prentice informed him that Roosa had pushed a resolution through the New York County Medical Society that any member who referred a patient to an optician for exami-

Development of Professionalism in Optometry 39

nation for glasses be ejected from the society. Roosa had also declared that "he would have the medical practice act so amended as to deprive men of Prentice's cult from meddling in ophthalmology." Roosa seemed to have ignored the facts that Prentice had far more training in optics than the vast majority of oculists and that opticians had been providing optical care for centuries. Prentice became determined to solidify his position and those of his colleagues. One of these was Andrew J. Cross.

Although born in New York State, Andrew J. Cross practiced in the field of refraction in Visalia, California, from 1876 to 1881; in Walla Walla, Washington, from 1881 to 1884; and then from 1884 to 1889, he covered sixteen cities in New York, Pennsylvania, and Connecticut for Hartzog and Company of Philadelphia.[11] In 1889, Cross opened an office in New York City. He was the first treasurer of the Optical Society of the State of New York and became its president in 1898. In 1900-1901, he was president of the American Association of Opticians, the organization that became the American Optometric Association. Cross was an instructor in the optometry school at Columbia University from 1911 to 1924. He became known as one of the developers of dynamic retinoscopy, publishing books on retinoscopy and dynamic retinoscopy procedure in 1903 and 1911. Cross is said to have been "an enthusiastic research worker, a teacher, and a lecturer, full of earnest zeal in the cause of his profession, and strong in the power of imparting both his enthusiasm and his knowledge to others."[11]

THE FIRST EFFORT TO ACHIEVE LICENSURE

In 1895, Prentice became convinced that for refracting opticians to protect themselves from attacks by people like Roosa, they needed to form a national organization. Prentice told Frederick Boger, the editor of *The Optical Journal*, a national periodical for opticians, of the threat from Roosa, and Boger's call for the formation of a national organization in the March issue of his journal was

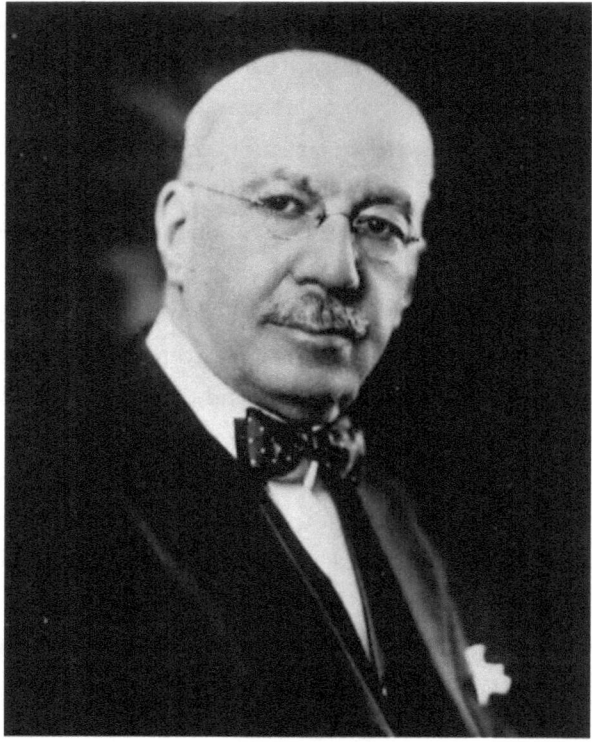

Figure 2.2. Andrew Jay Cross (1855-1925). (Image courtesy of the Archives & Museum of Optometry and The AOA Foundation)

greeted with a good response from opticians around the country. Boger and Prentice formed a steering committee with additional prominent members: Andrew J. Cross and J. J. Mackeown.[12] All four were from New York City.

Mackeown's attorney, T. Channon Press, expressed the opinion that it could be possible to incorporate an organization that would serve to regulate opticians' practice, similar to a society for dentistry. Rather than working immediately on a national organization, it was decided to first to form a state group to push for licensure. While other states had already formed state optometric associations, this was the first to be formed for the purpose of seeking licensure.

Both refracting opticians and dispensing opticians became involved in planning the New York state organization. When the dispensing opticians heard that Prentice's plan was to seek licensure, they asked the New York Ophthalmological Society for their opinion of the legislation that was going to be proposed. The first meeting of the Optical Society of the State of New York was held in February 1896 at Cross's office. Roosa's response was reported thus: "I know who is at the bottom of this – that man Prentice, he is foxy, and I'm only waiting for the opportunity to put him behind prison bars; and if any optician undertakes to join this movement, I shall see that he is punished. Besides, I shall fight you in Albany to the last ditch."[13] Learning this, the dispensing opticians left the meeting because they were dependent for their work on the prescriptions ophthalmologists wrote. Thus, the goals and interests of the refracting opticians and the dispensing opticians were diverging.

The eleven refracting opticians who remained at the meeting plus Boger elected officers among themselves: Charles Prentice, president; George R. Bausch of Rochester, vice-president; Andrew J. Cross, treasurer; Frederick Boger, secretary. The Executive Committee consisted of Bausch, Cross, W. W. Bissell also of Rochester, J. J. Mackeown, M. E. Kenney of Utica, and E. R. Mason of Binghamton.[14] Within a week, the bill that would allow the Optical Society of the State of New York to regulate practice by refracting opticians was introduced into the state legislature in Albany. Drafted by T. Channon Press and containing the provisions set forth by Prentice, it was entitled "An Act to Regulate the Practice of Optometry in the State of New York." It defined the practice of optometry as "the employment of subjective and objective means to determine the accommodative and refractive states of the eye and the scope of its functions in general, or the act of adapting glasses to the eye by using such skilled means as will determine their choice."[15]

In a hearing before the state legislature's Committee on Public Health, the refracting opticians presented a petition with 600 signatures in favor of the bill and letters from prominent physicians who praised the work of the opticians.[16] Press, the lawyer for the refracting opticians, made a presentation and introduced Prentice. Then Prentice gave his paper, "Defense of the Optician."[17] Prentice's presentation has been described as "a masterpiece of logic,"[18] a document that embodied "much of the reasoning on which optometry bases its claim to professional status,"[19] written in a style that was "vigorous and the language forthright with no sparing of medical feelings."[19] Some of the points of emphasis made by Prentice (partially in his own words) were as follows[17]:

1. Spectacles were invented about 1300, but medical practitioners didn't start giving spectacles their attention until about 1865, after the publication of Donders' book. Opticians developed the testing procedures for the correction of astigmatism before the entry of medicine into refraction. "He [the refracting optician] was then the only eye refractionist known to the world, and always has been since the invention of spectacles, a period of more than 500 years."
2. After Donders' book, "...oculists were quick to perceive the opportunity for extending their line of practice to include that of the optician, and soon took advantage of it by providing themselves with the necessary test-types and lenses." The oculists then sought to control opticianry by limiting the opticians to filling the prescriptions written by oculists. "The favored, though intimidated, dispensing opticians,...are declared to be the only type of opticians that the oculist is prepared to recognize."
3. Oculists often learned refraction and treatment of eye diseases in a short course after they completed medical school. These courses did not include geometrical optics, and oculists were not trained adequately in optics. "Long before medical eye-specialists became their own curse, as well as that of the optician, by dabbling in the latter's education, many opticians were credited with being men of learning and skill. It is only since oculists have invaded the province of the optician that even the skilled optician, who exercises his traditional right

to make optical investigations and adapt glasses, has been placed under the ban of charlatanism by oculists."
4. Many optical instruments were designed based on the work of physicists and opticians. These included optical instruments adapted for use in eye examinations. "If a medical education should now be insisted upon, it would prevent non-medical experts in optical science from contributing anything to ophthalmology, through being disbarred from gaining a practical knowledge of the eye, its defects and requirements...A medical education has not been essential to the acquirement of a thorough knowledge of optics."
5. Oculists who did happen to study physics generally did not object to the formal recognition of refracting opticians. Two oculists, Herman Knapp and George Stevens of New York, informed Prentice that they would prefer that opticians did the refractions so that physicians could devote their time to surgery and the treatment of disease.
6. "...The most essential requirement to the art of adapting glasses is a knowledge of optics...So long as it can be shown that opticians can adapt glasses to the sight as skillfully, or more so, than oculists, the vested right of the optician should not be interfered with....Oculists, in denouncing the optician, do not, as a rule, accuse him of incompetency in optics, for they know this to be their own vital point of weakness."
7. In response to the assertion of some oculists that atropine, which could not be used by the refracting opticians, was necessary in refraction, Prentice countered that: "the glasses that are adapted to an eye in this condition can never be worn by the patient when the effects of the drug have become dissipated. The oculist who uses atropine is, therefore, compelled to make an [e]mpirical allowance for a toning of the ciliary muscle, medical opinions differing as to the amount, and to compel the patient to wear the glasses *guessed* at."
8. Opticians should refer patients with disease to physicians. An optician should be instructed in the use of the ophthalmoscope "to the extent

that would qualify him to detect, not to differentiate between, diseased conditions of the interior of the eye....Opticians using the ophthalmoscope would act as vigilant detectives among the public at large, thereby protecting it against possible neglect of disease, in every instance where spectacles are demanded of skilled opticians....The oculist who would deny the optician the right to make use of the ophthalmoscope clearly has not the public welfare at heart."

9. Oculists were divided in their opinions about the existence of "muscular asthenopia" and its causes. "My own experience has been that, while the medical profession has been floundering about in its efforts to settle the disputed question, I have successfully fitted a number of persons with prisms who had previously been in the care of oculists without securing relief."

10. "During the past ten years, I have personally adapted glasses for over 12,000 persons...In all that time, I have not been obliged to refer more than 200 of them to oculists, while fully half of my patrons had been in the care of oculists before applying to me. In fact, it is this class that recommends my services most highly to others."

11. "Of course, there are good as well as unqualified opticians, and some of the latter may be charlatans, yet none so despicable as the optical incompetent who seeks to traffic under protection of his medical degree." The refracting opticians should be protected "against the threat of a small minority of the medical profession to relegate opticians to a position of serfdom in the interests of oculists."

12. The optician who achieved certification would "occupy an analogous position to that of the Dentist in his relations to medical science."

A few days after the presentations by the refracting opticians, the New York Assembly's Committee on Public Health gave a hearing to oculists and dispensing opticians who opposed the bill. The refracting opticians were so eager to have the bill passed that they agreed to several concessions. Originally, the bill was to regulate all persons practicing optometry, whether they were oculists or opticians. One concession was that physicians be exempted from the law. Another concession was that one of the four persons on the licensing board was to be a physician, and later, that all four members would be physicians.[20] The bill did not pass. It was probably fortunate for optometry that it was not passed in the negotiated form. Having optometry regulated by four physicians would have established a precedent of medicine controlling optometry.

In 1897, Prentice's thinking seemed to diverge from that of most other refracting opticians. While continuing to distribute copies of his "Defense of the Optician" talk, he also explored the idea of a specialist who would combine the abilities of both the refracting optician and the eye physician.[21] That same year, he noted that opticians and medical practitioners "now practice optometry upon divergent lines" but that they should be led "upon convergent lines of practice to a point where in time their interests, both educational and otherwise, will have become so amalgamated as to have created the legalized ideal eye-specialist."[22] Such an idea appears to be different from his declaration the year before that "the optician treats light—the oculist treats disease."[23] After 1897, Prentice became less involved in the effort to pass an optometry licensure law.

It has been suggested that while Prentice was dynamic, brilliant, and forceful, it was fortunate that someone more tactful, but just as enthusiastic, took the leadership role in the fight for recognition of optometrists: Andrew J. Cross.[24] Cross had excellent leadership skills and was adept at getting people to work together.[25] With the efforts of Cross and others, such as E. E. Arrington of Rochester, the New York optometrists finally obtained a licensure law in 1908. The optometrists in New York had been the first to attempt to have a licensure law passed, but due to staunch opposition, they were the thirteenth state to achieve it.

THE FIRST LICENSURE LAW

The first licensure law for American optometrists was enacted in 1901 in Minnesota and was described as "an act to regulate the practice of optometry."[26] The Minnesota refracting opticians faced the same problems that beset those in New York, opposition from physicians and dispensing opticians. One of the leaders of the Minnesota optometrists, Hiram M. Hitchcock, noted that "the chief purpose of all of our organized effort is to encourage and promote among opticians a higher degree of professional attainment" and not protection of their business interests from competition.[27] Just as in the bill originally proposed in New York, optometry was defined as "the employment of subjective and objective means to determine the accommodative and refractive states of the eye and the scope of its functions in general."[26]

The Minnesota law established a licensing board of five opticians. It had been necessary to make two political compromises to achieve passage of the law: physician exemption and a grandfather clause.[27] Physician exemption meant that licensed physicians could practice optometry without any formal testing of their skills in the field. The part of the law that came to be called the *grandfather clause* was a provision that persons who were already practicing optometry did not have to pass the licensure examination. The law stated, "Every person who is engaged in the practice of optometry in the State of Minnesota at the time of the passage of this act shall within six months thereafter file an affidavit in proof thereof with said board, who shall make and keep record of such person, and shall in consideration of the sum of three dollars, issue to him a certificate of registration."[26] Persons who were not practicing at the time the law passed had to pay ten dollars to take the licensure examination and then pay an additional five dollars for a certificate if they passed. Grandfather clauses were viewed as defensible in that experience, prior achievements, and recognition of skill by the public were reasonable criteria in lieu of an examination, and that a law should not force anyone out of an established livelihood in which he had been effective.[28] An unfortunate consequence of the grandfather clause was that it allowed licensure of persons who viewed refraction as a lucrative sideline to their jewelry, watchmaking, or other business and thus may not have been imbued with the ideal of professionalism as some of those who practiced optometry on a full-time basis.[27] Physician exemption and grandfather clauses became parts of the licensure laws subsequently passed in other states.

The five persons on that first optometry licensing board in Minnesota—and in the United States—were Joseph W. Grainger, of Rochester; Hiram M. Hitchcock, of Redwood Falls; Clifton A. Snell, of Minneapolis; Alexander Sweningson, of Moorhead; and Frank A. Upham, of St. Paul.[27,29] At the second meeting of the board, on June 11, 1901, sixty-five persons received the first optometry licenses. The first licensed optometrist in the United States was Grainger, a member of the board. Grainger, whose father was in the spectacle business, was born in Yorkshire, England. Grainger came to the United States in 1868. He completed a course at the Northern Illinois College of Ophthalmology and Otology, receiving a Doctor of Optics credential.[30]

OTHER LICENSURE LAWS FOLLOWED

Two more states passed licensure laws in 1903 (California and North Dakota), and by 1924, all 48 states and the District of Columbia had optometry licensure laws. Thus, it took 24 years for optometry laws to be in place in all states, a little less than the 32 years (1868 to 1900) it took dentistry to do so.[31] The years in which the optometry laws were passed are shown in Table 2.1.[32]

The struggles were similar from state to state in that there was opposition from oculists. Arrington[33] observed that the arguments the oculists used could be placed into six categories: (1) The eye is a part of the human body, thus making any form of care of the eye the province of physicians.

(2) Legal recognition of optometry could open the door for persons so licensed to practice medicine without medical training, or it could create the impression that optometrists could treat eye disease. (3) Optometrists completed fewer years of education than physicians. (4) Eye drops are needed for proper refraction. (5) Optometrists are not competent in the recognition of eye disease and they may overlook pathological conditions. (6) The legal recognition of optometrists could produce public confusion and thus lead to quackery and health abuses.

Arrington[33] also classified the arguments that were used to counter those objections. (1) Refraction of the eye has never been a medical procedure; it was developed as an applied optical science through the efforts of physicists and opticians. Spectacles do not treat the eye, but rather they affect the light to allow the eye to focus it with minimal exertion. (2) Optometry does not seek to practice medicine but rather the legal acceptance of the profession. (3) Although it is true that the medical school curriculum is longer than that of optometry training, the minimal instruction in optics and refraction in medical training is inadequate for the practice of refraction. Optometric training is designed to provide intensive training in optics and ocular refraction. (4) It is not only possible, but preferable, to do refractions without eye drops, as opposed to with them, as shown by both optometric and medical authorities. (5) The legal recognition of the already existing profession of optometry would clear, rather than create, confusion in the minds of the public.

Table 2.1. Years in which optometry licensure laws were passed[32]

Year	States Passing a Licensure Law
1901	Minnesota
1903	California, North Dakota
1905	New Mexico, Oregon
1907	Arizona, Idaho, Indiana, Montana, Nebraska, Tennessee, Utah

Development of Professionalism in Optometry

1908	New York
1909	Delaware, Florida, Iowa, Kansas, Maine, Michigan, North Carolina, Rhode Island, Vermont, Washington, West Virginia
1911	New Hampshire, Oklahoma
1912	Massachusetts
1913	Colorado, Connecticut, Nevada, South Dakota
1914	Maryland, New Jersey
1915	Arkansas, Wisconsin
1916	Georgia, Virginia
1917	Alaska, Hawaii, Pennsylvania, South Carolina, Wyoming
1918	Louisiana
1919	Alabama, Illinois, Ohio
1920	Kentucky, Mississippi
1921	Missouri, Texas
1924	District of Columbia

The content of the original state licensure laws varied from state to state. They served mainly to define optometry, establish how the licensing boards would be constituted, and set forth procedures for examination and registration of applicants. Most states introduced amendments to their optometry laws from the 1920s through the 1940s, which were designed to advance professionalism by measures such as regulating corporate practice, limiting advertisement, establishing educational requirements, and restricting the sale of ready-made spectacles.[34]

LEGAL CHALLENGES

The opening decades of the twentieth century were marked by some legal challenges from authorities in medicine.[35] Two of those are briefly discussed here because they established legally what the refracting opticians already knew: that optometry was separate from the practice of medicine.

In about 1900, a traveling refracting optician named Lincoln Smith was charged in Illinois with practicing medicine without a license. Smith had advertised that he treated people with symptoms such as blurring, dizziness, neuralgia, or headaches, but his advertisement also stated that he did not use medical or surgical treatments. In 1904 the Illinois State Supreme Court ruled that the prescription of spectacles, which can relieve ailments such as headaches or dizziness caused by vision problems, does not constitute the practice of medicine.

Another case occurred in 1914, when the Pennsylvania Bureau of Medical Education and Licensure established a regulation that optometry was a "minor branch" of medicine, and therefore that the licensure and regulation of optometrists would fall within its function.[5] The optometrists in Pennsylvania had been trying to have an optometry licensure law passed for sixteen years, so to many this case appeared to be a way to establish licensure. A dissenting opinion was presented at a meeting of optometrists in Philadelphia by Albert Fitch, who would become founder and long-time president of the Pennsylvania State College of Optometry. Fitch recalled later:

> I pointed out that we could not trust the Medical Profession. For, I said in effect, if the Medical Profession had been sincere in its friendship to Optometry, their leaders could have shown their friendship before this and at least conferred with us before having the Medical Act amended so as to include Optometry as a minor branch of medicine. To me, I said, this procedure looked as

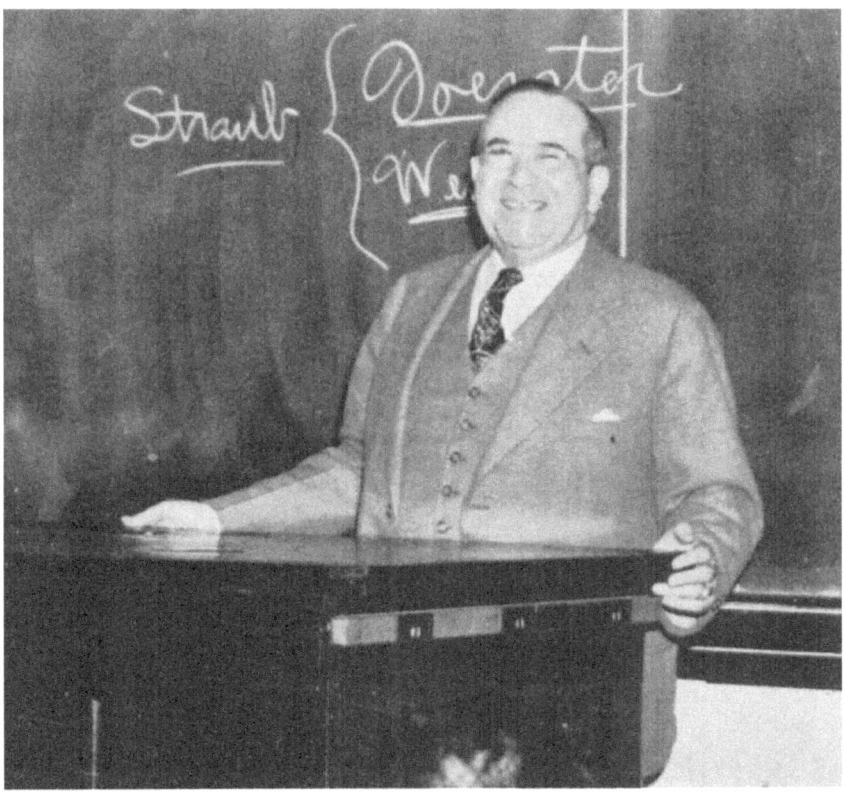

Figure 2.3. Albert Fitch (1879-1960), long time president of the Pennsylvania State College of Optometry and important optometric leader. (Image courtesy Salus University)

if they now worked out a legal means of eliminating Optometry. I also pointed out that it didn't make any difference how the optometrists voted at this meeting, for all the Medical Board needed to do was to license a few optometrists and to put the law into operation and then under one pretext or another to prosecute the rest of us for practicing unlawfully. I maintained urgently that what was needed now was for us to attack the Amendment in the Courts, because I believed the amendment to be unconstitutional insofar as it applied to Optometry.[36]

After much disagreement, the optometrists who made up the Pennsylvania Optical Society decided to fight the medical bureau. They were heartened when they received a resolution from the American Optical Association (which would become the American Optometric Association) that the association approved "the stand taken by the Pennsylvania Optical Society, against the contention of the Bureau of Medical Education and Licensure of that State—that Optometry 'is a minor branch of medicine.'"[37] In the summer of 1914, the Pennsylvania Optical Society went to court, requesting an injunction against the medical board. It was at these proceedings that James Cook McAllister testified that his grandfather, John McAllister, Jr., had done the first refractions in Pennsylvania and that the oculists in Philadelphia first learned refraction from his father, William Young McAllister, and James W. Queen. In October, 1914, the Pennsylvania Court of Common Pleas ruled that "the Practice of Optometry is separate and distinct from the practice of Medicine."[38] That decision was later affirmed by the Pennsylvania Supreme Court.

FORMATION OF STATE OPTOMETRIC ASSOCIATIONS

The first state to form an optometric association was Colorado in 1892, led by Jacob C. Bloom.[39] A regional organization, the New England Association of Opticians, was formed in 1894. By 1905, most states had formed associations. The July 6, 1905, issue of *The Optical Journal* listed optometric organizations for 29 states. By the publication of the August 1, 1907, issue, the list had increased to 39 state associations. There were also 20 local organizations, such as the Buffalo Optical Society and the Chicago Optical Society. In 1907, most of the state groups used the word "Optical" in the name of the association rather than optometric or optometrist. The exceptions were the California State Association of Optometrists, the Michigan Society of Optometrists, the Minnesota State Association of Optometrists, the New Mexico Association of Optometrists, the Rhode

Island Society of Optometry, the Utah Association of Optometrists, and the Wisconsin Association of Optometrists. According to *The Optical Journal* in 1907, the state associations formed before 1900 were the Pennsylvania Optical Society (1895), Indiana Optical Society (1896), New York State Optical Society (1896), Iowa Optical Society (1897), Illinois Optical Society (1898), and California State Association of Optometrists (1899).

FORMATION OF A NATIONAL OPTOMETRIC ASSOCIATION

The 1895 suggestion of Frederick Boger, editor of *The Optical Journal*, to form a national society was met with interest by optometrists around the country. An organizational meeting was held in St. Louis in 1897.[40] Charter membership in the American Association of Opticians, which would become the American Optometric Association, was 183 persons from 31 states and Canada. The first official meeting was held October 10, 1898, in New York City. Both refracting opticians and dispensing opticians were in the organization initially. There were no educational presentations at the first meeting, but many exhibits, among them ophthalmometers, test cards, a new optometer, books, and a DeZeng refractor. There were also exhibits by camera distributors, by *Jeweler's Review*, and by *Jeweler's Circular*.[40,41]

Officers elected at the first meeting were Charles Lembke, President; Henry Borsch, Vice President; William Bohne, second Vice President; Charles A. Longstreth, Treasurer; and Frederick Boger, Secretary. Most discussions of this era of American Optometric Association history state simply that Lembke was a dispensing optician.[42,43] However, Prentice mentions Charles Lembke (spelled Lempke in Prentice's book[44]) as one of the few opticians testing for astigmatism in the 1860s. Perhaps Lembke had limited himself to dispensing by 1898. However, he was a person of some prominence as election to national office would suggest. He was born in Karlsruhe, Germany, and came to the United States at 18. He learned optical work from Charles Alt of New York City and opened his own business in New York in 1857. When the building his business occupied was destroyed by fire nine or ten years later, he established a partnership with Julius Gall, also of New York. Patrons of Gall and Lembke included Mrs. Ulysses S. Grant, President James Garfield, and President Grover Cleveland.[45] When Gall died, Lembke was joined in business by his sons, Charles Jr. and Emil. Lembke was a member of the New York Academy of Sciences and the Brooklyn Astronomical Society, which elected him to go to North Carolina to collect data on a total eclipse of the sun. He also developed a new way of regulating and manufacturing sun dials.[45] Lembke was re-elected president of the American Association of Opticians in 1899.

Starting in 1900, the American Association of Opticians was evolving into an organization of mostly refracting opticians. Andrew J. Cross was elected president and served in that capacity for two years. In his communications with the membership, Cross emphasized the importance of improved education, better cooperation among members, and the passage of licensure laws.[46]

In 1904, the national association worked out a system of affiliation of state associations.[47] In 1907, 22 state societies were members of the national association, and in 1910, 42 state associations were members. This provided a valuable method of exchanging ideas, and it was helpful in the development of optometric legislation.[42] The 1910 national meeting was notable for the badge members wore. It contained the slogan "A lens is not a pill" coined by Charles Prentice, to emphasize that optometry was not the practice of medicine. In 1909, the name of the organization was changed from the American Association of Opticians to the American Optical Association, and in 1919, it became the American Optometric Association.

ETHICAL STANDARDS

As noted earlier, one of the criteria separating a profession from an occupation or a trade is the establishment of ethical standards. In 1908, the American Association of Opticians formed a committee to compose a code of ethics. The three committee members were Andrew J. Cross as chairman, John Eberhardt, and William Huston. All of them were active in the organization – Cross as president in 1900-1901, Eberhardt as president in 1903-1904, and Huston as secretary in 1905-1910. The code of ethics that they drew up and which was subsequently adopted is as follows:

Each member should fully appreciate the responsibilities assumed by him and endeavor by unceasing study to qualify in the important work of ministering to the visual needs of his fellow men.

He should at all times emphasize the fact that optometry is a purely technical profession based upon a comprehensive knowledge of the mechanism of the human eye, the skillful manipulation of instruments for its adequate examination, and a knowledge of the properties of light and the relative effects thereon of lenses.

He should cultivate those sensibilities which permit the formation of standards for the generous appreciation of the work of others and the criticism of his own.

He should discourage the use of titles calculated to mislead or cause confusion in the public mind.

His methods of publicity should rigidly adhere to a dignified and modest statement of fact.

He should value his services commensurate with his ability, special preparation and skill, always welcoming the opportunity to be generous with his knowledge where it is needed, thereby realizing in fullest measure the true success which lies in the consciousness that the world has profited by his work.[48]

Subsequent adoptions or modifications of codes of ethics by the American Optometric Association were effected in 1935, 1944, 2005, and 2007.[49,50,51,52]

Beginning in the early twentieth century and continuing throughout it, there were discussions of the outward appearances of professionalism that might be considered of an ethical nature, such as the nature of advertising or the restriction of its use, restriction of types of signage, charging a fee for service instead of making a profit on goods, and location of office. The concern about location of office was that the professional office was more likely to be on the second floor of a city office building than on the first floor. An upstairs office put one in a professional atmosphere as compared to the more commercial atmosphere one might expect in an office on street level, where daily commerce was conducted. However, the location of an office upstairs did not always guarantee that the practitioner had a more professional practice.[53]

ADOPTION OF THE TERMS *OPTOMETRY* AND *OPTOMETRIST*

Not specifically stated as a criterion for a profession is a specific identity, but the importance of having a uniform identity can be implied from several of those criteria. As has been discussed, optometric forebears can be traced from early spectacle makers and those who tested vision for the power needed in spectacles to refracting opticians. By the late nineteenth century and early twentieth century, refracting opticians could be distinguished from dispensing opticians, but there didn't seem to be much agreement over what refracting opticians should call themselves. In addition to *refracting optician,* some of the terms that had been suggested or used were *sight-testing optician, eyeglass specialist, physical eye specialist, opticist,* and *optometrist.*[54,55,56] Although what a group of professionals calls themselves is only a term, the lack of a uniform term can correlate with a lack of a uniform identity.

Charles Prentice liked the name *opticist* and went so far as to have the title registered as a trade mark by the United States Patent Office.[4] Prentice said that he "practiced under this appellation from 1886 until the enactment of the optometry law in 1908."[56] He cited a definition of *opticist* as "a person skilled or engaged in the study of optics."[57]

The terms *optometry* and *optometrist* derive from the term *optometer*, which was coined by William Porterfield in a 1737 paper. Porterfield's optometer was a simple device he used to measure refractive error and amplitude of accommodation. Discussion of his optometer also appeared in his famous 1759 book, *A Treatise on the Eye, the Manner and Phaenomena of Vision*.[58]

Optometers en Optometrie was the title of an 1865 dissertation on refraction published in the Netherlands by J. W. Verschoor.[59] The first appearance of the word *optometry* in English appears to have been the English translation of Landolt's 1886 book, *The Refraction and Accommodation of the Eye*. In the introduction, Landolt states, "All the principles of Optometry are explained, but he [the author] has abstained from entering into a description of all the different kinds of Optometers."[60]

It is unclear when the first use of the word *optometrist* occurred. John H. Ellis of South Bend, Indiana, president of the American Association of Opticians in 1902, suggested that it was important to establish a name for refracting opticians. Some sources suggest that Emmanuel Klein of Cincinnati, a charter member of the American Association of Opticians, suggested the term *optometrist* to John C. Eberhardt.[61,62] It was Eberhardt who would then became the champion for its adoption.

Eberhardt was born in Muhlhausen, Germany, and came to the United States when he was 9.[63] His family settled in Dayton, Ohio, where as a teenager, he apprenticed in an optical shop while studying civil engineering. For several years, he served as a civil engineer and then as a surveyor in the Western United States. Returning to Dayton in 1882, he took a position with a jewelry firm fitting glasses. Not satisfied with the crude procedures being used, he took short courses in optics in Kansas City and Cleveland, and a correspondence course from the Northern Illinois College of Ophthalmology and Otology. Eberhardt joined the American Association of Opticians in 1899 and soon became involved with many of its activities. He was elected the first president of the Physiological Section of the association, a group set up to advance educational standing. In that capacity, he helped start the association's library, which would eventually become the International Library, Archives, and Museum of Optometry. Eberhardt was elected president of the American Association of Opticians in 1903. Hofstetter[63] described Eberhardt as "in so many ways...the role model of the pioneer professional optometrist. Scholarly, forthright, scientific, and personable, he was widely accorded numerous optometric honors here and abroad. He contributed frequently and constructively to the technical and professional optometric literature of his era."

Eberhardt was aware that a word for the refracting opticians seeking licensure regulations should be established in order to obtain the needed legislation.[64] In 1903, Eberhardt suggested that the American Association of Opticians discuss, and consider for future adoption, the words *optometry*, which he defined as "the science which treats of the philosophy of light and sight and the art of determining the visual status of the human eye and the neutralization of abnormal conditions by lenses," and *optometrist*, defined as "one skilled in the practice of optometry."[65] In 1940, an optometrist from Virginia, John Buchanan, recalled attending the 1903 meeting where Eberhardt asked the association to consider the term *optometrist*. Buchanan said that he returned home and put the word *Optometrist* on his office door. He claimed to be the first to do so in Virginia and thought he might be the first in the country. Buchanan also recalled that at the time, the term was pronounced *op-to-meet-rist*, with the accent on *meet*.[66] Eberhardt convinced the editors

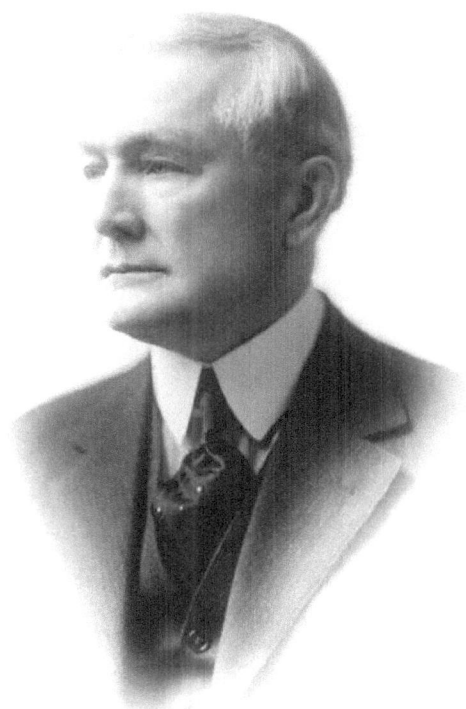

Figure 2.4. John C. Eberhardt (1857-1927), president of the American Association of Opticians in 1903-1904, and leading advocate for use of the term optometrist. (Image courtesy of the Archives & Museum of Optometry and The AOA Foundation)

of *Webster's Dictionary* to include the two words in its Spring 1904 edition.[64] At the 1904 convention, the American Association of Opticians officially adopted the term *optometrist*.

The actual usage of these two terms spread very gradually. The name of the national association of optometrists was not changed to the American Optometric Association until 1919. The optometry school at The Ohio State University was started in 1914 as a program in Applied Optics, and the 1915 bulletin for the school did not mention the word *optometrist* anywhere in its 12 pages.[67] Even as late as the 1940s, some practitioners identified themselves as "optometrist and optician."[68] In 1942, the American Optometric Association passed a resolution that members use only the word *optometrist*, and not *optician* or any other designation, in order to avoid the implication that optometry was a business instead of a profession.[69]

DISAPPEARANCE OF THE SPECTACLE PEDDLER AND THE JEWELER OPTICIAN

On the nineteenth-century American frontier, there were not enough optometrists to care for the visual needs of the people. To fill the void, some entrepreneurial individuals started traveling from town to town selling ready-made spectacles. These individuals came to be known as *spectacle peddlers*. The phenomenon of spectacle peddlers did not originate in the United States as it already existed in parts of Europe. Spectacle peddlers are typically portrayed as charlatans who sold their wares for prices much greater than the wares were worth.[70] However, some were honest because they counted on repeat business the next time they came to a town.

Among the latter was an individual named Ephraim Weiss. Hirsch and Wick[71] told of having conversations with Weiss in the late 1930s when Weiss was in his 90s. Among Weiss's repeat clients was the noted California scientist Luther Burbank. Hirsch and Wick noted:

> Weiss had learned many useful rules for prescribing lenses. Each quarter diopter of minus lens added to the prescription, he told us, should increase the acuity one line of Snellen type or else it was an overcorrection. Although we never understood how he determined muscle balance, he knew that one should "add a little plus if the eyes tend to turn in and a little minus if they tend to turn out." Self-taught, he practiced a most acceptable brand of sight-testing

for the time, seemingly with great patient satisfaction.[71]

As optometry licensure laws were passed and the distribution of optometrists across the country expanded, the spectacle peddler gradually disappeared. Some spectacle peddlers settled down in one location and became optometrists or dispensing opticians. By about 1930, the spectacle peddler had passed from the scene.[70] It seems likely that the questionable practices of some spectacle peddlers led to some lack of trust among the public concerning the prescription of spectacles.

Another commercial taint to the efforts to professionalize optometry was the involvement of jewelers in the sale of spectacles. In the nineteenth century, there were several jewelry firms in the business of importing spectacles or manufacturing spectacle frames.[72] Many jewelers and watchmakers got involved in vision testing and the dispensing of spectacles as a sideline to their primary business, perhaps because many of the tools used in jewelry or watchmaking could also be used in working with spectacles. Some turn-of-the-century schools in horology (clock and watch-making), also offered courses in vision testing. Many of the optometrists grandfathered with the early licensure laws were jewelers who also practiced optometry. An optometrist who attended the Massachusetts College of Optometry in the late 1920s recalled that several of his classmates were "students whose parents or friends owned jewelry stores. They were convinced there was a future for them. I think fully a quarter of my class [of about 27] fell into this category."[73] However, the jeweler who also practiced some optometry too gradually faded from the scene, and by the mid-twentieth century, had disappeared. The disappearance of the spectacle peddler and the jeweler optometrist was another factor, along with passage of licensure laws, formation of professional organizations, establishment of ethical standards, and adoption of the term optometrist, helping to clarify the identity and advance the professional status of the optometrist.

Chapter 2: Notes

1. Wilensky HL. The professionalization of everyone? *Am J Sociol.* 1964;70:137-158.
2. Denzin NK, Mettlin CJ. Incomplete professionalization: The case of pharmacy. *Social Forces* 1968;46:375-381.
3. Cruess SR, Cruess RL. Professionalism must be taught. *Br Med J.* 1997;315:1674-1677.
4. Christensen J. Chronology of Charles Prentice's life. *Hindsight* 2000;31:2-5.
5. Prentice CF. *Legalized Optometry and the Memoirs of its Founder.* Seattle, WA: Casperin Fletcher, 1926:242.
6. Hirsch MJ, Wick RE. *The Optometric Profession.* Philadelphia, PA: Chilton, 1968:131.
7. Prentice, 20.
8. Prentice, 22-23.
9. Prentice, 27-28.
10. Prentice, 31.
11. Arrington EE. *History of Optometry.* Chicago, IL: White Printing House, 1929:113-116.
12. Prentice, 33.
13. Prentice, 38.
14. Prentice, 40.
15. Prentice, 131.
16. Prentice, 41.
17. Prentice, 43-62.
18. Hirsch & Wick, 136.
19. Cox ME. *Optometry, the Profession: Its Antecedents, Birth, and Development,* 1st ed., rev. Philadelphia, PA: Chilton, 1957:36.
20. Classé JG. *Legal Aspects of Optometry.* Boston, MA: Butterworths, 1989:5-6,28.
21. Hirsch & Wick, 138.
22. Prentice, 143.
23. Prentice, 94.
24. Gregg JR. *The Story of Optometry.* New York, NY: Ronald Press, 1965:188-192.
25. Hirsch & Wick, 139.
26. Hirsch & Wick, 315-317.
27. Classé, 6-7.
28. Hofstetter HW. Licensed by exemption. *Newsletter Optom Hist Soc.* 1989;20:45-47.
29. Fisher EJ. Some historical tidbits. *Newsletter Optom Hist Soc.* 1973;4:22-23.
30. Hofstetter HW. First registered optometrist. *Newsletter Optom Hist Soc.* 1972;3:38-39.
31. Hirsch & Wick, 180.
32. Arrington, 26-27.
33. Arrington, 23-25.

34 Classé, 12-15,31.
35 Classé, 7-12.
36 Fitch A. *My Fifty Years in Optometry*. Philadelphia, PA: Pennsylvania State College of Optometry, 1955;1:7-8.
37 Fitch, 11.
38 Fitch, 29.
39 Fair RD. Letter to the editor. *Rev Optom.* 1991;128(5):23.
40 Koetting RA. *The American Optometric Association's First Century.* St. Louis, MO: American Optometric Association, 1997:9.
41 Gregg JR. *American Optometric Association: A History.* St. Louis. MO: American Optometric Association, 1972:11.
42 Hirsch & Wick, 149.
43 Gregg, 10.
44 Prentice, 44.
45 Hofstetter HW. Concerning the first AOA president. *Newsletter Optom Hist Soc.* 1977;8:30-31.
46 Gregg, 12-15.
47 Gregg, 26.
48 Koetting, 11-12.
49 Hofstetter HW. *Optometry: Professional, Economic, and Legal Aspects.* St. Louis, MO: Mosby, 1948:133.
50 Gregg, 143-144.
51 *American Optometric Association Code of Ethics.* www.aoa.org/x4878.xml
52 Bailey RN. The history of ethics and professionalism within optometry in the United States of America 1898-2015. *Hindsight* 2016;47:14-31, 52-71, 78-95, 112-133.
53 Hofstetter, 129-131.
54 Gregg, 13.
55 Bruneni JL. *Looking Back: An Illustrated History of the American Ophthalmic Industry.* Torrance, CA: Optical Laboratories Association, 1994:14.
56 Prentice, 18.
57 Prentice, 119.
58 Levene JR. *Clinical Refraction and Visual Science.* London, UK: Butterworths, 1977: 1,15.
59 Hofstetter, 90.
60 Landolt E. *The Refraction and Accommodation of the Eye and Their Anomalies.* Culver CM, translator. Edinburgh, Scotland: Pentland, 1886:vii.
61 Cox, 30.
62 Gregg, 206.
63 Hofstetter HW. John C. Eberhardt (1857-1927). *Newsletter Optom Hist Soc.* 1987;18:43-44.
64 Eberhardt JC. Letter to the editor. *Optical J Rev Optom.* 1920;45:844.

65　Gregg, 22-27.
66　Hofstetter HW. Op-to-meet'-rist and 1842 asthenopia. *Newsletter Optom Hist Soc.* 1979;10:68-69.
67　Hofstetter HW, Penisten DK. The curriculum in 1915. *Newsletter Optom Hist Soc.* 1990;21:2-3.
68　Hofstetter HW. Interpreting history. *Hindsight* 1997;28:22.
69　Gregg JR. *American Optometric Association: A History.* St. Louis, MO: American Optometric Association, 1972:180.
70　Cox, 25-28.
71　Hirsch & Wick, 126-127.
72　Cox, 23-26.
73　Moline SW. *Century of Vision: The New England College of Optometry, An Anecdotal History of the First Hundred Years.* Boston, MA: The New England College of Optometry, 1994:17.

Chapter 3
Continuing Twentieth-Century Challenges and Changes

With the passage of licensure laws, the formation of a national association, the codification of ethical standards, and the development of a more uniform identity, optometry was poised for further advances. Throughout the twentieth century, as optometry continued to develop as a profession, changes were necessitated by different challenges, but leaders within the profession also introduced changes. Many factors influenced the continuing evolution of the identity and status of the optometrist, including the question of the doctor title, the broadening of treatment options for vision problems, increasing educational standards, an increase in scholarly work in optometry, and the expansion of scope of practice into areas traditionally solely the province of medicine.

THE DOCTOR TITLE AND THE DOCTOR DEGREE

Before about 1915, officials of the American Optical Association were opposed to the use of the title *doctor* by optometrists.[1] Of course, persons legally had the right to use the term if they had received a doctor's degree from an entity officially authorized to grant such degrees. Some of the schools offering instruction in optometry around the beginning of the twentieth century offered doctor's degrees. For example, starting in 1889, the Philadelphia Optical College offered a Doctor of Optics degree to those who successfully completed a short course in refraction.[1] But it wasn't until 1923 that a non-proprietary optometry school offered a Doctor of Optometry (OD) degree approved by a state legislature, and not until 1970 that all accredited optometry schools granted the OD for a minimum of six years of college work.

The term *doctor* is derived from the Latin *docere*, to teach or to inform. The term was originally applied to teachers. The Oxford English Dictionary gives many definitions for *doctor*, including a teacher or instructor, one eminently skilled in a field of knowledge or a craft, one who has achieved the highest degree conferred by a university, one who is proficient in knowledge of theology or the law, or a doctor of medicine. Because in the early twentieth century the term *doctor* was often used to address those who worked in many fields related to health care and because it was used by physicians who practiced refraction, some optometrists felt it appropriate that they be referred to as *doctor*.[1] Furthermore, there were many practitioners in other health care fields, including medicine, without doctorate degrees but who identified themselves as doctor. In 1912, Andrew J. Cross wrote to Charles Prentice that he favored the use of the term because it "means a man of learning and is purely a courteous word."[2] But the prevailing opinion among optometrists for the first two or three decades of the twentieth century was against the use of the title.

One of those who ardently resisted the use of the doctor title was Charles Prentice. In writing back to Cross, he said that "the only apparent foundation for the use of the doctor title is an inordinate and unpardonable conceit."[3] Prentice apparently had a habit of correcting people who addressed him as doctor, as he recalled in his memoirs:

> Many years ago, at the time the Hon. Frederick R. Coudert was Minister to France, Mr. Coudert called upon me for a re-examination of his visual powers, addressing me as "Doctor." Endeavoring to tactfully remind him that I was not a doctor, he said: "Well,

you have done more for me than some oculists; your ability and the recognition you have received from medical authorities, in my opinion, justifies my having thus addressed you, *sir*." His emphasized, *sir*, caused me to apologize for having corrected him, when he laughingly reassured me by saying: "Doctor, let us proceed, I am in somewhat of a hurry this morning."[4]

The title *doctor* for optometrists became more common in the 1920s, but debate over its use continued through the first half of the twentieth century. Arguments for and against its use can be classified into the following categories:

(1) Dentists, osteopaths, chiropractors, and veterinarians refer to their fellow practitioners as doctor, so it would be appropriate for optometrists to do so as well.[5]

(2) Optometrists should not use the title until they hold a doctor of optometry degree based on at least four years of university work.[6]

(3) The term *doctor* increasingly came to be synonymous with someone who practiced medicine. As a result, there was concern that by using the title *doctor*, optometrists could be confused with medical practitioners. There were two reasons for this concern. First, it might mean that the public wouldn't recognize the unique training and background of optometrists in optics and vision care; this seems largely to have been Prentice's stance. Second, it might mean that optometrists could be construed as, or could represent themselves as, fraudulent pretenders to the practice of medicine. To avoid this situation, it became common practice, as recommended by the American Optometric Association and as required by some state laws, to append the term *Optometrist* after one's name, if the abbreviation for doctor was used before the name, as in Dr. John Smith, Optometrist.[7,8]

(4) Medical doctors should not feel that they have exclusive right to the use of the term *doctor*. This was expressed by an anonymous university professor:

> "There is no group of doctors who are so jealous of their titles as the medicos. There is no profession that attempts to arrogate to itself, as its own exclusive property, any and everything with which it has been associated...from the Middle Ages the word 'doctor' has meant, first of all, a master teacher, one competent to teach, and...it is a title subsequently taken and claimed by the medicos..."[9]

(5) There are other health care workers, including some medical practitioners, who had no more educational experience than optometrists, but they referred to themselves as *doctor*. This opinion was held by Albert Fitch, who, in 1919, founded the Pennsylvania State College of Optometry, later known as Pennsylvania College of Optometry. In 1913, when Fitch was practicing in Philadelphia, he resigned for a while from the Philadelphia Optical Association, in part because the leaders of that optometric organization objected to him using the title *doctor*. Fitch later noted that

> in regards to my assumption of the title of "Doctor," it must be remembered that many medical doctors of that day also assumed the doctorate title. These doctors had never attended a medical school, but instead they had read medicine under the tutelage of another doctor. In fact, it would have been almost as easy for me to have undertaken to become a physician as to become an optometrist, as there were many courses available at that time of short duration for either day or evening attendance whose entrance requirements were easy to meet. I would like to mention here that the first high school graduation requirement for entrance into medical school was not made compulsory by law in Pennsylvania until 1906.[10]

(6) The use of the title *doctor* helps to establish the confidence of the public and rapport with patients.[11]

(7) Because the title *doctor* implies a high level of training to the public, it becomes an economic disadvantage to those who do not use the title.[12]

(8) The title *doctor* should not be used by persons who do not have a Doctor of Optometry degree. Even into the late 1940s, in some locations where the majority of optometrists did not have the OD degree, there were objections to optometrists with the OD using the *doctor* title.[13]

The Pennsylvania State College of Optometry started granting the OD degree to its graduates in 1923, as authorized by the state of Pennsylvania.[14] In 1948, four of the nine accredited American optometry schools awarded the OD degree: Northern Illinois College of Optometry, Pacific University, Pennsylvania State College of Optometry, and Southern College of Optometry, while the Los Angeles School of Optometry awarded a doctor degree for a year of graduate work beyond the bachelor degree in optometry.[11] The Los Angeles School of Optometry changed its name to the Los Angeles College of Optometry in 1949, and in 1951, it started awarding the OD degree to students who successfully completed the optometry curriculum.[15] In 1953, the Massachusetts College of Optometry, now known as the New England College of Optometry, conferred its first OD degree.[16]

In 1955, the first optometry graduates of the University of Houston received an OD degree after five years of college study. Starting with the 1956 entering class, the University of Houston required six years of college study for the degree, although initially a certificate adequate for optometry licensure could be obtained after five years, with the sixth year of study to earn the OD being optional.[17] Clanton W. Williams, the president of the University of Houston in 1956, insisted on the increase to six years because he saw it as important for the recognition of the OD as "a fully respectable professional doctorate."[18] He noted that every doctorate that came historically after the PhD, even the MD, "went through a period of relatively low academic prestige."[18] He felt that a minimum of six years of college study should be required for persons to be able to call themselves *doctor*.

Entering the 1960s, there were three optometry schools that did not offer the OD degree: Indiana University, The Ohio State University, and the University of California at Berkeley. During the 1960s, their change from five years of college study (pre-optometry studies plus optometry school) to six years made it possible for these schools to gain approval from their respective university administrative boards to grant the Doctor of Optometry degree. Indiana University and The Ohio State University awarded their first OD degrees in 1968 and University of California at Berkeley in 1970.[19] All American optometry schools founded after 1970 have granted the OD degree starting with their first graduating classes. Today American optometry schools require four years of undergraduate pre-optometry study and four years of optometry school for the OD degree.

In the late 1950s and early 1960s, some state optometry licensing boards started requiring the OD degree for licensure, effectively eliminating the graduates of some schools from taking their board examinations.[20] Also at that time, the Pennsylvania State College of Optometry and the Massachusetts College of Optometry started offering courses to non-OD optometry school graduates to provide an opportunity to earn an OD and thus allow them to refer to themselves as *doctor*.

FORMATION OF ORGANIZATIONS PROMOTING EDUCATION AND RESEARCH

While the American Optometric Association in its early years did have educational sessions, much of its time was spent on organizational matters. This led some optometrists to suggest the formation of associations that would have the purpose of promoting education and research.

In 1905, E. LeRoy Ryer, who was then president of the Optical Society of New York, proposed an American Academy of Optometry. Ryer's concept of the nature of such an organization is much the same as the American Academy of Optometry as it exists today. However, it appears to have been an idea before its time and there was some opposition to forming another organization.[21] It wasn't until 1922 that the Academy was formed.

Morris Steinfeld of Paducah, Kentucky, called a meeting in January of 1922, with 10 of his colleagues from Illinois, Indiana, Kentucky, and Missouri to organize a national academy. By June 1922, the organization had been formed, with Steinfeld as chairman.[22] The first meeting with presentation of papers was held in December 1922 in St. Louis, with 10 people in attendance.

The founders of the American Academy of Optometry sought to promote professional practice as well as to advance education and research. At first, the basic requirements for membership in the Academy were that the candidate had a practice location that was in an office rather than a retail establishment, charged an examination fee of at least three dollars, and did not engage in any form of advertising. The organizers also invited a few educators to join. In 1923, there were 40 charter members, which included educators G. W. McFatrich, W. B. Needles, Charles Sheard, A. P. DeKeyser, and A. J. Cross. Steinfeld was chairman of the Academy in 1922 and 1923. The first officers along with Steinfeld were C. S. Brown, Vice-Chairman; Carel C. Koch, Secretary; E. E. Fielding, Treasurer; and Ernest Petry, Charles Sheard, and E. LeRoy Ryer, Council Members. Eugene Wiseman was chairman of the Academy from 1924 to 1928 and a very important figure in its early years.[23] Wiseman was also active in the American Optometric Association, and he wrote and lectured frequently on professionalism in optometry. He was awarded honorary life fellowship in the American Academy of Optometry in 1962.

In addition to an annual meeting, which over the years became a high-quality, well-attended meeting, the Academy produced publications. From 1925 to 1939, it published 13 volumes of the papers presented at the annual meetings in the *Transactions of the American Academy of*

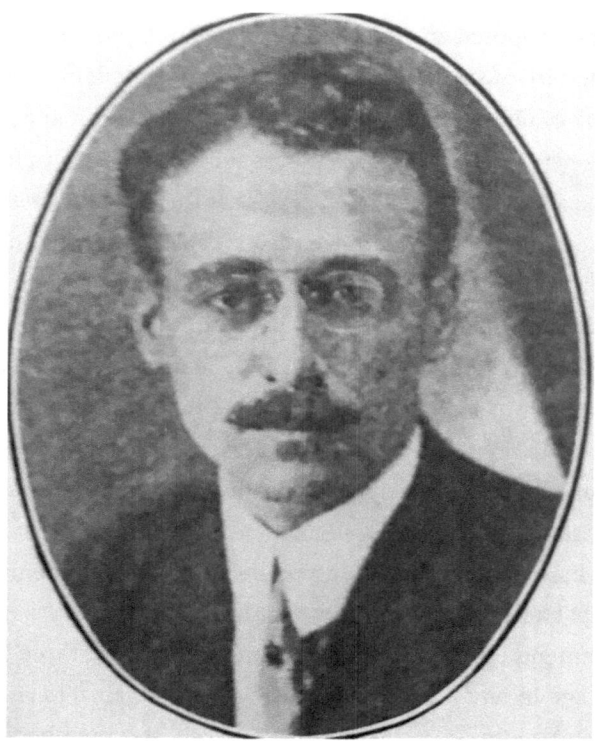

Figure 3.1 Eugene G. Wiseman (1885-1967). (Image from *Optical Journal and Review of Optometry* 1912;29:180)

Optometry. In 1942, it sponsored publication of Ewald Hering's *Spatial Sense and Movements of the Eye*, translated by Carl A. Radde, an optometrist from Cleveland, Ohio. From 1959 to 1979, the Academy published a series of "post-graduate courses" in soft cover book form: *Synopsis of Glaucoma for Optometrists* by Arthur Shlaifer (1959, 88 pages); *Synopsis of Corneal Contact Lens Fitting* by Bernard Mazow (1962, 87 pages); *Synopsis of Jurisprudence for Optometrists* by George P. Elmstrom and Harold Kohn (1964, 103 pages); *Synopsis of the Refractive State of the Eye* edited by Monroe J. Hirsch (1967, 104 pages); *Synopsis of Glaucoma*, 2nd edition, by Arthur Shlaifer and John H. Carter (1970, 162 pages); and *Synopsis of Health Science Terminology for Optometrists* by Margaret S. Gilbert (1970, 57 pages).

The Academy started its association with the *American Journal of Optometry* in 1928. The Academy's journal underwent name changes in 1941 and 1974, becoming *Optometry and Vision Science* in 1989. The Academy journal is viewed as the most eminent journal in optometric science by many readers. The Academy also gives out many prestigious awards. Throughout its existence, the Academy has emphasized professionalism, education, and research. The history of the American Academy of Optometry has been detailed in two books.[24,25]

Another organization, important at one time but now largely forgotten, was the Distinguished Service Foundation of Optometry. It sought to encourage education and research through publications, and the awarding of fellowships and medals, in order to facilitate the conservation of vision.[26,27,28] It existed from 1927 to 1979 but was most active in the 1930s and 1940s. It was founded in 1927 by George Stevens Houghton.[26,29,30]

Houghton practiced optometry in Boston and was heavily involved in optometric organizations. He was president of the Massachusetts State Optometric Association, was a member of the Massachusetts Board of Registration in Optometry, and organized the New England Council of Optometrists.[31] He served as president of the American Optometric Association from 1928 to 1930. He was Director of the Distinguished Service Foundation of Optometry (DSFO) from its beginning until his death in 1933. The DSFO Consulting Board in 1933 consisted of many well-known persons in optometry and optics: Charles Sheard, Edwin H. Silver, Howard C. Doane, James P.C. Southall, Frederic A. Woll, Arthur E. Hoare, Ernest H. Kiekenapp, Clinton R. Padelford, Matthew Luckiesh, Thomas McBurnie, and Chester Johnson.[29]

The director of the DSFO in the late 1930s and in the 1940s was Clinton R. Padelford, who practiced optometry in Fall River, Massachusetts. He was a president of the Massachusetts and New England optometric societies.[32] Serving as secretary-treasurer of the DSFO in the 1940s was Laurence P. Folsom of South Royalton, Vermont. Folsom had also served as a president of the New England Optometric Association and of the International Association of Boards of Examiners in Optometry.[33]

In 1958, Theodore A. Brombach was installed as director of the DSFO.[30] Brombach practiced optometry in San Francisco for many years, and was a lecturer at the University of California Berkeley School of Optometry. He served on the California State Board of Examiners for 10 years.[34,35] Brombach received an honorary DOS degree from Pacific University in 1956. During the time that Brombach was director of the DSFO, John R. Uglum was the secretary-treasurer. Uglum had served several years as secretary of the National Board of Examiners in Optometry.[36]

Following the death of Brombach, James F. Wahl (1901-1982) took over as director of the DSFO.[36] Wahl received a BS degree from the United States Military Academy at West Point in 1920, and in 1923 he graduated from optometry school at the Needles Institute.[37] Wahl was president of the American Optometric Association from 1952 to 1954. He practiced optometry from 1923 to 1955 and was Dean of the Pacific University College of Optometry from 1955 to 1963. He received honorary DOS degrees from Northern Illinois College of Optometry in 1952 and from Los Angeles College of Optometry in 1953.

The DSFO granted fellowships to invitees who submitted an acceptable thesis or to individuals who were voted to Fellowship unanimously by the DSFO Council by virtue of their outstanding contributions. Fellowship was limited to 100 active members.[30] The Foundation did not collect dues and was "self-supporting."[30] The DSFO also awarded medals for meritorious contributions to vision science. A list of DSFO Gold Medal winners was published in *Hindsight: Journal of Optometry History*.[38]

From 1932 to 1949, the DSFO published several monographs: *Annals of the Distinguished Service Foundation of Optometry* (1932, 62 pages; 1935, 78 pages; 1937, 158 pages); *Visual Fields* by Theodore A. Brombach (1936, 228 pages); *An Introduction to the Mathematics of*

Ophthalmic Optics by Paul Boeder (1937, 244 pages); *Seeing Dramatized: The Human Eye Demonstrator. How We See, Why We See, What We See* by Frederick Hamilton (1937, 54 pages); *The Diagnosis and Elimination of Visual Handicaps Preventing Efficient Reading* by George A. Parkins (1941, 142 pages); and *The Philosophy and Science of Health* by E. E. Rogers (1949, 153 pages).

After a period of inactivity in the 1970s, the decision was made to dissolve the Foundation in 1979. Its documents and papers were turned over to the International Library, Archives and Museum of Optometry (ILAMO) in St. Louis, Missouri (now the American Optometric Association Archives and Museum of Optometry). Maria Dablemont, librarian for ILAMO, wrote the following about the DSFO: "The Foundation was a good, sound optometric organization concerned with optometric research...Its awards were prestigious...There have been attempts to revive the Foundation and I believe economic reasons, along with satisfaction with the role of the Academy, have prevented it."[39]

Recognizing the need for faculty with advanced degrees and research skills at optometry schools, the American Optometric Foundation (AOF) was formed in 1947. The leader in the years of planning efforts for establishing the AOF, and its president for its first 14 years, was William C. Ezell. Ezell received his optometry degree from the Northern Illinois College of Ophthalmology and Otology. He was president of the American Optometric Association from 1944 to 1946 and was president of the South Carolina Board of Examiners in Optometry from 1922 to 1971.[40]

Over the years, the main contributors to the AOF have been optometrists, but donations have also come from corporations, other foundations, state optometric associations, and individuals interested in vision care.The primary focus of the AOF has been the provision of fellowships to graduate students pursuing MS and PhD degrees in physiological optics and vision science. These fellowships came to be known

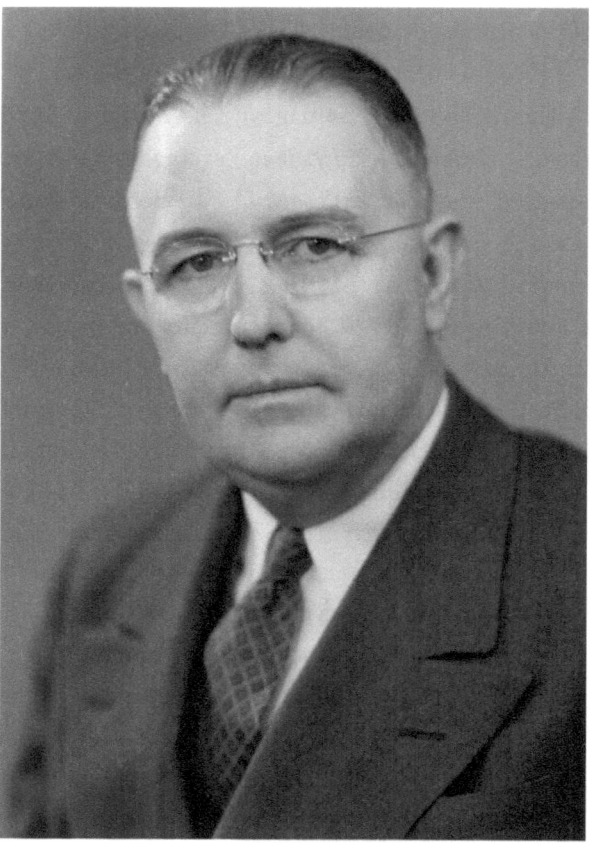

Figure 3.2. William C. Ezell (1893-1977), leader in the formation and activities of the American Optometric Foundation. (Image courtesy of the Archives & Museum of Optometry and The AOA Foundation)

as Ezell Fellowships. The first fellowship from the AOF was awarded in 1949 to Charles R. Stewart, who received his PhD in physiological optics from The Ohio State University in 1951 and who became the founding Dean of the College of Optometry at the University of Houston in 1952.

An online historical listing of Ezell Fellows, as of 2018, contains the names of more than 300 individuals, many of whom can be recognized as optometry school deans, presidents, and faculty members as well as leading optometric researchers.[41] In addition to the Ezell Fellowships, the AOF has funded small research grants, scholarships, travel stipends, named awards, and the publication of textbooks.[42]

In 1992, the management and governance of the AOF was transferred to the American Academy of Optometry. In 2017, the name of the Foundation was changed to the American Academy of Optometry Foundation.

Another organization that promoted education was the Optometric Extension Program (OEP), which was founded in 1928. One of its contributions was work towards standardizing the optometric examination with its 21-point sequence. For many years, OEP encouraged local study groups. It has published literature on functional vision care for decades and has organized numerous regional and national seminars.

CONTINUING DEVELOPMENT OF PROFESSIONALISM

One aspect with which optometry continued to struggle through much of the twentieth century was the commercial atmosphere of many optometric establishments. An unfortunate consequence of the grandfather clauses in the initial licensure laws was that they resulted in the optometric licensure of many who had taken short courses in refraction and established businesses that made profits from the sale of spectacles rather than earning a living from fees for services.

At the 1918 meeting of the American Optical Association, an advertising specialist, Charles H. Mackintosh of Washington, DC, expressed his ideas on the promotion of professionalism and the reduction of commercialism. He noted:

> An optometrist should be known as an expert upon errors in vision, not as a vendor of glasses. Offering free examinations as a sales help to the eyeglass business...is proof positive to the public that the advertiser is a seller of spectacles and not a professional

man....this association should set up certain standards of practice which would eliminate entirely both the use of [advertising] and occupation of stores.[43]

Mackintosh also suggested that a fee-for-service system was essential for optometry rather than a fee system that was based on the sales of glasses.

Also in 1918, W. H. Kindy of St. Paul, Minnesota, then chairman of the American Optical Association Bureau of Optometric Information, observed that "optometry can never become a profession if we continue advertising ourselves as we have been doing. Newspaper copy signed by an individual is unethical and the buying public knows it."[43]

Despite efforts to promote professional practice, many optometrists continued to use advertising and emphasize sales of glasses. These commercial aspects were publicized in a damaging 1937 article in *Readers Digest.*[44] The article, based on visits to "shops,...department stores,...and chain stores," claimed that optometrists appeal to the public "with all the wiles of sales psychology" to sell unneeded glasses. The article said that the paths to optometrists' doors "are well marked with newspaper advertisements, neon signs, shop window displays, huge spectacles hung over the sidewalks." Worse yet, the article accused optometrists of being incompetent to conduct vision examinations. Although the article did begrudgingly state that "there are many conscientious and skilled optometrists" and despite the fact that the article was obviously biased to any intelligent reader, the damage was done.

In 1948, Hofstetter wrote of the *Readers Digest* article:

Late in 1937 the profession received an awakening blow from which it has not yet ceased to stagger....allegedly supported by documented statements and statistics, the author of the article led the reader through a step-by-step, but purportedly fruitless, search for the slightest trace of honesty and capability in any optometrist anywhere. Even today no optometrist who was in practice at the time has forgotten the ordeal he sustained in the glare of the public eye. The subsequent half-hearted attempts on the part of the author of the article to present the actual facts in an unbiased manner afforded small comfort. The long-lasting lowered morale among optometrists is well remembered. The organized optometrists found themselves without an effective program to deal with the situation, and, while such a program was being formulated, were only able to fight the interests that had dealt the blow by simple counter propaganda.[45]

An editorial in the *Journal of the American Optometric Association* responded to the *Readers Digest* article, stating:

While some of the things cited in the article purporting to be actual experiences of the investigators may have been true, official and unadulterated optometry refuses to accept the verdict of any biased investigation based upon alleged misconduct of certain individuals arbitrarily named by the investigators as the standard bearers for optometry. Obviously medicine refuses to be judged by the physician narcotic-peddler...The legal professional refuses to accept, endorse or even condone the acts of its ambulance chasers. Official dentistry...vociferously disowns its unethical and unscrupulous practitioners.[46]

Officials of the American Optometric Association, including then President Harry Pine, met with representatives of *Readers Digest* to present information refuting allegations in the articles and requesting that optometry be allowed to address that attack upon it. There appeared to have been some understanding on the part of the optometric officials that *Readers Digest* would publish a reply article with information from the

American Optometric Association, but that article was never published.[47] Eventually the *Readers Digest* article was forgotten, and as organized optometry's continuing efforts toward professional practice took root and many of the more commercially oriented optometrists who had originally been licensed by the grandfather clause retired, optometry became more professionally oriented.

A 1963 article in another national popular magazine, *Coronet*, was more favorable to optometry than the *Readers Digest* article had been 25 years before. The main emphases of the article were to decry the "senseless conflict" between ophthalmologists and optometrists, and to educate readers concerning the difference between optometrists and ophthalmologists.[48] The article concluded that optometrists have better results in strabismus with visual training than ophthalmologists do with surgery and that it was optometrists who had pioneered optical treatments in low vision. The article also noted that "the accusation that optometrists are ignorant of pathology doesn't seem to hold up," and "in contrast, medical students specializing in ophthalmology concentrate on eye surgery and medicine, spending little time on the vision sciences."[48] The author suggested that a good model for cooperation between optometry and ophthalmology was found in the U.S. Army "where there's no conflict between ophthalmologists and optometrists, each group expert in its field...so there's mutual recognition and respect—presumably because there's no dollar factor involved."[48] The *Coronet* article concluded: "Until peace is declared in the sight-saving professions, you and I will have to be on guard. The best objective advice is this: If you think you may have an eye disease or may need surgery, consult an eye physician—an ophthalmologist recommended by the family doctor you trust....But if you are certain that all you need is glasses, go to a reliable optometrist."[48]

Challenges to optometry laws against commercial practice and advertising went to the United States Supreme Court in 1955 and 1963. In both cases the Supreme Court ruled that the laws were constitutional.[49] The challenged 1955 law was an Oklahoma law that prohibited, among other things, the advertisement of spectacles, frames, and optical appliances, and the provision of space in retail stores to persons doing eye examinations or rendering eye care. Supreme Court Justice William O. Douglas expressed the following opinion about the restriction on leasing of space in retail stores: "This regulation is on the same constitutional footing as the denial to corporations of the right to practice dentistry. It is an attempt to free the profession, to as great an extent as possible, from all taints of commercialism. It certainly might be easy for an optometrist with space in a retail store to be merely a front for the retail establishment."[49] By the 1970s, 45 states had restrictions on advertising and/or other aspects of commercial practice.[49]

Starting in the late 1970s, there was a relaxation of the attitude of the public toward advertising by professionals, perhaps related to the changes in consumer attitudes, sometimes referred to as *the consumerism movement*. In addition, the United States Federal Trade Commission (FTC) struck down optometry laws that had been established with great effort in order to protect the public from commercialism.[50] For example, the FTC established a regulation in 1978 allowing advertising by optometrists and ophthalmologists. The American Optometric Association initiated efforts to prevent the FTC from pre-empting state laws that regulated advertising by optometrists, but ultimately the association was unsuccessful.

The FTC also overturned the decades-long prohibition of advertising by the American Academy of Optometry among its membership. This struck at the core of what many Academy leaders saw as an essential component of a professional practice. Furthermore, a study conducted by the FTC on the quality of care by optometrists, as a function of advertising and organization membership, seemed to support the traditional stance of the Academy. The FTC found the quality of care to be highest among Academy members, next best with American Optometric Association members, next with non-American Optometric Association members who did not advertise, next among those who advertised locally, and lowest among those who advertised nationally.[51] Bradford W. Wild, president of the Academy in 1979, said, "We are confident that all Academy Fellows will continue to adhere to our traditional tenets of practice despite the necessity of dropping, hopefully temporarily, the enforcement of the prohibition of advertising from our code of conduct."[51] The Academy fought the rule of the FTC, but the dropping of the prohibition of advertising was not temporary. Gradually, in the later years of the twentieth century, tasteful advertising became a more accepted practice in all health care professions.

OPTOMETRIST CYRUS BASS'S SUIT AGAINST THE AMERICAN MEDICAL ASSOCIATION

In 1954, the American Optometric Association (AOA) passed a resolution at its annual meeting stating in part that "the field of visual care is the field of Optometry and should be exclusively the field of Optometry..."[52] A second resolution urged that "encroachments by untrained, unqualified and unlicensed persons into the exclusive field of Optometry be prevented..." The resolutions were intended to prevent lay persons from doing refractions. Optometrists were seen as experts in refraction and functional aspects of vision, an expertise lacking in lay persons.

Unfortunately, many ophthalmologists interpreted the resolution to mean that the AOA was suggesting that ophthalmologists should not be doing refractions. The American Medical Association (AMA) convention of 1955 was the site of a great deal of anti-optometry fervor. At that convention, the AMA passed a resolution that it was unethical for an ophthalmologist or any other physician to teach in an optometry school, to lecture to any optometry group, or to impart knowledge in any way to optometrists. Other resolutions criticized lay organizations for having relations with optometry, demanded that commissions to optometrists in the Armed Forces be revoked, and denounced referrals by optometrists to any health care provider other than an ophthalmologist.[52]

In response, the AOA issued a clarifying resolution in 1955 that stated that the AOA had no intention of eliminating refraction by ophthalmologists or of expanding optometric practice into medical eye care. However, the 1955 AOA resolution did not reverse the medical profession's reaction to the 1954 resolution.[52] Relations between optometry and ophthalmology remained highly contentious for several years.

In 1964, optometrist Cyrus Bass filed a lawsuit against the AMA and nine ophthalmologists.[49,53,54,55] Bass alleged "that the defendants had conspired to monopolize the examination of the eyes and the production, marketing, and sale of ophthalmic eyewear..."[49] Bass had been trained in clinical psychology before attending the Northern Illinois College of Optometry, from which he graduated in 1939. He practiced optometry in Chicago, and in 1959 he completed a law degree.[54] In 1965, Bass amended the complaint to make it a class action suit on behalf of practicing optometrists in the United States. Five optometrists joined Bass in the amended complaint. Bass had hoped for more optometrists to enter into the suit, and he had to bear most of the financial burden himself.

Bass did not consult the AOA concerning the lawsuit, and the AOA took no position on it. In February 1966, the AOA filed a separate 63-page memorandum with the Antitrust Division of the United States Department of Justice, which contained the complaint that organized medicine had hindered and restrained the profession of optometry.[56]

In June 1966, the AMA changed its resolution to allow medical doctors to teach in optometry schools. In May 1967, the Bass lawsuit was dismissed on the basis that actions of the AMA had effectively resolved the issues in the original complaint. It seems likely that both the Bass lawsuit and the AOA action were important in the reversal of the AMA stance.[56]

ASPECTS OF PRACTICE

Along with changes in the educational, research, and legal landscape for optometry, the twentieth century also saw the broadening of treatment options for vision problems, including vision therapy, contact lenses, low vision care, an increased interest in environmental vision concerns in optometric care, and the expansion of the optometric scope of practice to include the use of diagnostic and therapeutic pharmaceutical agents.

Adoption of Visual Training as a Treatment Option. As the concern of optometrists for the binocular vision status and the visual comfort and efficiency of their patients increased, one of the treatment options that came to be embraced was visual training, now known as vision therapy. Visual training, or vision therapy, is a program of treatment procedures designed to train patients to improve their visual function, including improvements in accommodative, convergence, perceptual, eye movement, and/or other visual skills. It is generally acknowledged that visual training was developed from the orthoptics for strabismus pioneered by Louis Emile Javal.[57,58,59] Griffin and Grisham[59] identified three schools of thought on binocular vision therapy: Javal and the French school, Worth and the English school, and optometric vision therapy.

Javal was a famous French ophthalmologist. He was first trained as an engineer but was interested in optics and vision science because of vision problems in his family. His father, sister, and two nephews had strabismus. Javal himself experienced discomfort doing near work because of astigmatism. While working as a mining engineer, Javal published research papers on astigmatism and binocular vision.[60] The acclaim Javal received as a result of these articles led him to enroll in the study of medicine at the University of Paris, in 1865. While a student, he published French translations of Donders' work on refraction and Helmholtz's treatise on physiological optics. Javal graduated from medical school in 1868, writing a thesis on strabismus. He made many contributions in optics and binocular vision, including improvements to the ophthalmometer and to an optometer as well as developing Javal's rule for predicting total astigmatism from corneal astigmatism. He produced many publications on astigmatism and strabismus. Javal's practice was mostly limited to refraction and strabismus, referring disease and surgery cases to other ophthalmologists.[60] In 1896, Javal published a book on strabismus, *Manuel théorique et pratique du strabisme [Manual on the Theory and Practice of Strabismus]*. In his 60s he went blind from glaucoma. In 1903, he published perhaps the first book on what blind persons experience.[60] The book was published in English in 1906 as *On Becoming Blind*.

Javal may well have been led to develop training procedures for strabismus to help his younger sister without resorting to surgery.[61] His father had been converted from esotropia into a large angle exotropia by surgery. Javal's orthoptics program for strabismus included refractive correction, occlusion for amblyopia, physiological diplopia and bar readers for suppression, training with Brewster and Wheatstone stereoscopes, and development of vergence in free space.[59,61] Javal continued the training for three to five years in many cases and is said to have often had good success, including with his sister.[59]

Before the development of orthoptics, treatments for strabismus included various potions and salves, and strabismus masks with holes placed such that the eyes had to be straight to view through them. Strabismus masks are usually attributed to Paulus Aegineta (625-690), Ambrose Paré (1510-1590), and Georg Bartisch (1535-1606).[62,63] The first suggestion of occlusion as a treatment for amblyopia came from the naturalist George Louis Leclerc Buffon in 1734.[64] Buffon also recognized the association of anisometropia with strabismus and amblyopia.[64,65]

Claud A. Worth was an English ophthalmologist who viewed defects of sensory fusion as the cause of strabismus. He believed that fusion training should be conducted as early in the patient's life as possible, and that in so doing surgery could be avoided. He felt that good sensory fusion led to a "desire for binocular vision."[59] Worth developed the amblyoscope for the purpose of training sensory fusion. He recognized that orthoptics improved binocular vision, not by strengthening the extraocular muscles but by training the neural mechanisms of binocular vision.[58] In 1903, Worth published a book on strabismus titled *Squint*. It went through many editions, with the seventh through ninth editions authored by Chavasse, Lyle, and Bridgeman. The ninth edition appeared in 1959.

Other ophthalmologists important in the early development of orthoptics were Frans Cornelis Donders (1818-1889) and Ernest Edmund Maddox (1863-1933). Donders wrote about strabismus in his noted book *On the Anomalies of Accommodation and Refraction of the Eye*, and he was the first to recognize the association of hyperopia and esotropia. E. E. Maddox wrote about strabismus in his book, *Tests and Studies of the Ocular Muscles*. He is known for the development of several tests, including the Maddox rod test. According to Revell, "News that ophthalmic opticians [optometrists] were practicing orthoptics at the London Refraction Hospital prompted Maddox to consider using lay assistance for orthoptic training."[66] He taught his daughter, Mary, orthoptics procedures. She subsequently opened her own practice and started an orthoptics school.[66] Mary Maddox is often recognized as the first orthoptist/vision therapist.

Early ophthalmological orthoptics was largely concerned with strabismus. David W. Wells, a Boston University Professor of Ophthalmology, noted in 1912 that "concerning the clinical importance of heterophoria ophthalmologists are not agreed....there has arisen a class of eminent practitioners whose members absolutely ignore the subject, and omit all tests for imbalance, unless there exists actual heterotropia."[67] It would be mostly optometrists who would adapt early orthoptics into visual training and vision therapy for non-strabismic binocular vision disorders and other vision conditions. One could identify several schools of thought within optometric vision therapy.[68] The following is a brief, roughly chronological overview of the development of optometric vision therapy.

Among the first American optometrists to be noted for work in visual training were E. LeRoy Ryer (1880-1972), Elmer E. Hotaling (1887-1950), R. M. Peckham (1876-1944), and T. J. Arneson (1883-1965).[57,69] Ryer and Hotaling were associated in practice in New York City and were heavily involved in the activities of professional optometry in the first half of the twentieth century.[70] They co-authored two books, *Optometric Procedure: Basic and Supplementary* and *Ophthalmometry*. Ryer drew up the original concept of the American Academy of Optometry.[71] He authored many papers, including a 1908 paper recommending bifocals as a new treatment method for esotropia.[69] One memoir of Ryer said that he "embodied the highest ideals of the profession."[72] The museum in the International Library, Archives, and Museum of Optometry at the American Optometric Association headquarters in St. Louis, Missouri, was named the Ryer Museum in his honor. R. M. Peckham published the first book on visual training by an optometrist in 1926, *The Modern Treatment of Ocular Imbalances*.

Important in the development of binocular visual training was the formulation of a standard examination routine including phoria measurements, fusional vergence ranges, relative accommodation measurements, and other tests. Charles Sheard (1883-1963) formulated a battery of 18 tests, which he published in his 1917 book, *Dynamic Ocular Tests*. Sheard also published *Dynamic Skiametry and Methods of Testing the Accommodation and Convergence of the Eyes* in 1920.

A significant event in the history of optometric vision therapy was the formation of the Optometric Extension Program (OEP) in 1928 by E. B. Alexander and A. M. Skeffington.[57,73] For almost 50 years, Skeffington served as the Director of Education for the OEP. Skeffington introduced a broad concept of vision into optometry and is often recognized as the father of behavioral optometry.[74,75] He emphasized that vision was the dominant sense for acquiring information and for directing movement, and that vision was integrated with other sensory, neural, and cognitive functions. He also emphasized environmental influences on visual function. Skeffington had

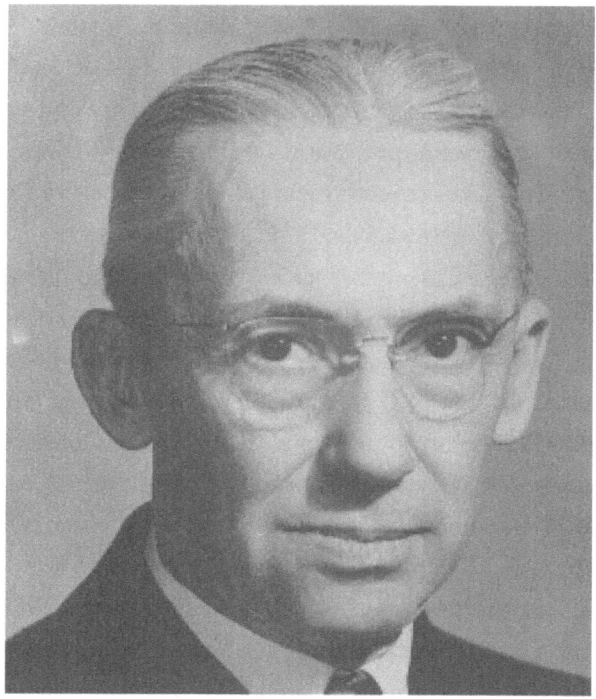

Figure 3.3. E. LeRoy Ryer (1880-1972). (Image courtesy of the Archives & Museum of Optometry and The AOA Foundation)

significant influence on the thinking of many optometrists through his extensive lecturing and writing.

Visual training has always been a frequent topic in the literature that OEP distributed to its members. Authors of material on visual training in OEP publications included George Crow and H. Fuog in the 1930s, S. K. Lesser in the 1940s, and Lawrence MacDonald, Robert Kraskin, Ralph Schrock, and Tole Greenstein in the 1960s.[57] In the mid-twentieth century, studies by pediatric physician Arnold Gesell at the Gesell Institute led to the recognition that vision plays a role in the development of general motor abilities and behavior.[76,77] This prompted an emphasis on developmental vision in visual training. The optometrists involved in the studies at the Gesell Institute, including

Continuing Twentieth-Century Challenges and Changes

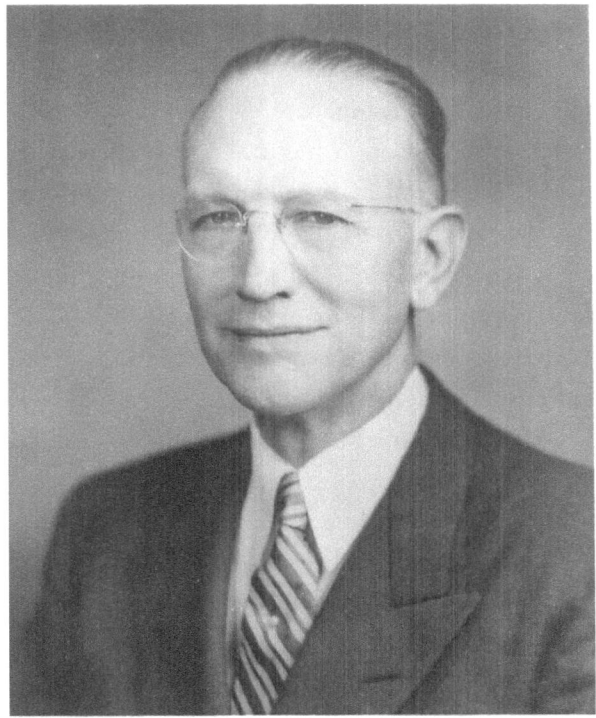

Figure 3.4. A.M. Skeffington (1890-1976), leader in the formation and activities of the Optometric Extension Program. (Photo courtesy of the Archives & Museum of Optometry and The AOA Foundation)

G. N. Getman, John Streff, and Richard Apell, authored several writings in the OEP literature in the 1950s and 1960s.

One of the optometric giants in visual training was Frederick Brock.[78,79,80,81,82] He published extensively on visual training, binocular vision, and strabismus in various journals from the late 1930s through the 1960s. Of particular note were his regular contributions in *Optometric Weekly*, extending from 1947 to 1959, which could easily constitute a textbook on visual training. He described using large training targets in strabismus to make use of peripheral fusion, and he emphasized training equipment that simulated real space. He was among the first to write about eccentric fixation. He devised many testing and training techniques; among the best known are the Brock string, the Brock Stereomotivator, and the Brock posture board.

The 1940s and 1950s were marked by significant research on fundamental aspects of accommodation and convergence function, particularly at The Ohio State University and the University of California at Berkeley. Glenn Fry, Henry Hofstetter, Meredith Morgan, Mathew Alpern, and others described accommodation and convergence relationships and the zone of clear single binocular vision, established clinical test norms, and investigated interrelationships and variability of test findings.[83,84,85] In the late 1950s and early 1960s, Merton Flom of the University of California at Berkeley studied the factors that had a bearing on prognosis in visual training for strabismus.[86]

A remarkable individual important in visual training was Bernard E. Vodnoy.[87,88] Vodnoy graduated from the Northern Illinois College of Optometry in 1938 and remained there as a faculty member until 1941. He served in the U.S. Army as an optometrist from 1941 to 1946, when he established a practice in Michigan City, Indiana. In 1948, he moved the practice to South Bend, Indiana. In 1949, he contracted polio, which severely affected both his legs. He went back to work with a special wheel chair. Vodnoy heard from optometrists at some of the many continuing education lectures he gave that a source of affordable visual training equipment was needed. As a consequence, he formed the Bernell Corporation in 1954. Vodnoy invented or developed numerous devices for vision therapy and testing that have been in common usage for many years, including vectographic and anaglyphic systems for training fusional vergence, stereoscope training systems, and aperture rule trainers. Vodnoy also authored detailed instructional materials to accompany the equipment.

Optometrists have, since the 1970s, been concerned with the effect of vision problems on reading and learning abilities. Some of the authors who have addressed this issue extensively are Nathan Flax, Ralph Garzia, John Griffin, Sidney Groffman, Jack Richman, Jerome Rosner, and Harold Solan.[89,90,91,92,93,94,95]

The later part of the twentieth century saw the extension of vision therapy into new areas, including the alleviation of vision problems associated with computer use, enhancement of visual skills used in sports, and the remediation of vision anomalies found after brain injury.[96,97,98,99,100] In the later decades of the twentieth century, there was also increased attention to research studies showing the effectiveness of vision therapy for various vision conditions.[101,102,103,104,105,106,107,108,109,110]

Contact Lenses. Contact lenses became popular in the 1950s with the introduction of the plastic corneal contact lens. Patients became very interested in using them, and optometrists then in practice clamored to learn how to fit the lenses. Contact lenses had been around for some time, but the combination of a lens resting only on the cornea (corneal contact lens) instead of covering both the cornea and part of the sclera (scleral contact lens), and the use of plastic instead of glass resulted in a lens that could be both comfortable and highly functional.

The first suggestion of a small lens that could be placed in contact with the eye to substitute for spectacles was by Leonardo da Vinci.[111,112] The margin notes that described Leonardo's concept for such a lens were recorded in one of his notebooks in about 1508. Descriptions of optical systems placed in contact with the eye were also made by René Descartes and Thomas Young.[113,114] In 1636, Descartes suggested that a water-filled tube placed in contact with the eye could be used to improve vision. In 1801, Young wrote about an experiment in which water was held in place between his eye and a botanical microscope by wax, showing that the cornea was not responsible for accommodation. In 1823, John F. W. Herschel suggested that it may be possible to place a lens on the eye to treat cases of irregular cornea.

The first actual uses of contact lenses occurred independently by Adolph Eugen Fick, Friedrich Muller, and E. Kalt in about 1888 in Europe.[113] From 1888 to 1948, most of the contact lenses that were used were scleral lenses made of glass. In 1929, Josef Dallos introduced a method of taking impressions of the anterior surface of the eye to improve scleral lens fitting. In the first two decades of the twentieth century, Carl Zeiss Optical Works of Jena, Germany made a glass corneal lens, but it was not successful because of its weight. In 1936, New York optometrist William Feinbloom developed a scleral lens with a glass optical portion and a plastic scleral band around it. In 1938, John Mullen and Theo Obrig presented methods for making scleral lenses entirely out of polymethyl methacrylate (PMMA) plastic.[113,115]

A big breakthrough in contact lenses occurred in 1947 when Kevin Tuohy, a California optician, started making corneal lenses out of plastic.[116] Because the weight of these plastic lenses was about half of the weight of comparable glass lenses and because of their fit on the cornea rather than onto the sclera, they were more successful than any previous lenses.[113] The plastic lens was, of course, also less likely to break than the glass lens. The overall diameter of the Tuohy lenses were generally 10.8 to 12.5 mm, about the same, or slightly less, than the diameter of the cornea.[113,117] In 1952 and 1953, Wilhelm Söhnges in Germany, Frank Dickinson in England, and John C. Neill in the United States developed a lens with a smaller overall diameter than the Tuohy lens.[113,118,119] There were numerous subsequent improvements and developments in PMMA corneal contact lens design, manufacturing, modification procedures, fitting procedures, and education. Some of the many people who contributed to these developments include Neal Bailey, Charles Bayshore, Norman Bier, Irvin Borish, John de Carle, Joe Goldberg, Edward Goodlaw, George Jessen, Donald Korb, Robert Mandell, Charles Shick, and Newton Wesley.[113,114,117,119,120]

The next major breakthrough in contact lenses was the production of a hydrogel material, hydroxyethyl methacrylate (HEMA), for soft contact lenses by Czech chemist Otto Wichterle.[121] Wichterle was first author on a 1959 paper in the journal *Nature* entitled "Hydrophilic Gels for Biological Use." Wichterle received patents for hydrogel contact lenses in the United States in 1962 and 1965. Wichterle collaborated with American optometrist Robert Morrison to make improvements in the design and production of the lens.[121] Bausch & Lomb gained rights to the lens and was getting ready to start selling lenses in 1968 when the United States Food and Drug Administration (FDA) ruled that the lens would be classified as a drug and would have to go through the process for drug approval.[122] Bausch & Lomb gained approval in March of 1971 and started marketing the lens as *Soflens*. By the end of 1971, the sales of *Soflens* by Bausch & Lomb had exceeded 10 million dollars, and by 1974, there were an estimated one million patients wearing *Soflens* contact lenses.[123] For a while, the Bausch & Lomb *Soflens* was the only soft contact lens on the market, but other lenses, such as American Optical's *Softcon* lens, and the Continuous Curve Contact Lens Company's *Hydrocurve* lens, were introduced in the mid-1970s.

The first rigid gas permeable contact lens was developed in 1978. By 1990, there were over 20 million soft contact lens wearers and over three million rigid gas permeable contact lens wearers.[122] By the end of the twentieth century, there were more than 25 rigid gas permeable contact lens materials.[122] By 2000, there were also more than 25 hydrogel polymers for soft contact lenses.[122] Since the 1970s, developments in contact lens materials, fitting and assessment procedures, technologies, etc., have accelerated at an amazing rate. Some of these developments include increased knowledge of corneal physiology, improvements in technology for corneal topography assessment, extended wear, disposable lenses, soft toric lenses, multifocal lenses, and orthokeratology.[120,122,124]

Low Vision Care. The term *low vision* is often used to describe situations in which patients have lower than normal visual acuity with the best spectacle correction, and/or they have a loss of visual field. Previously used terms include *partial sight, partial blindness, vision impairment,* and *subnormal vision*.[125] The field of care for patients with low vision has been referred to simply as *low vision* but also as *low vision care* or *low vision rehabilitation*. It is likely that telescopes and microscopes were used as low vision aids in the seventeenth century,[126,127] but the field of low vision didn't show much advancement until the twentieth century.

It has been noted that an 1897 invention by Charles Prentice, the typoscope, a horizontal aperture in black cardboard used to guide reading, is a simple but useful low vision device.[128] In 1918, Louis Otto Moritz von Rohr, working for Carl Zeiss of Jena, Germany, designed a telescopic lens for low vision.[129] Moritz von Rohr (1868-1940) also worked for Zeiss from 1895 to 1935, and from 1913 to 1940, he was a professor of optics at the University of Jena.[130] He worked on optical instruments, the optics of spectacle lenses, and photographic lens systems, and he wrote extensively on the history of optics.

The man often recognized as the "father of low vision" was William Feinbloom.[131] While in high school, Feinbloom worked for his father, Louis Feinbloom, a self-educated optometrist. William graduated from the optometry school at Columbia University at the age of 19, and later earned Master's and doctoral degrees in biophysics and visual psychology.[132] Starting in the 1930s, he designed telescopic and microscopic low vision aids, presented a systematic description of the optics of low vision care, and published case series from his low vision work.[129,131] He continued to develop innovative optical systems for low vision for the next 50 years. The low vision clinic at the Pennsylvania College of Optometry is known as the William Feinbloom Vision Rehabilitation Center in his honor, and in 1983, the American Academy of Optometry established the William Feinbloom award to recognize persons who have "made a distinguished and significant contribution to clinical excellence and the direct clinical advancement of visual and optometric service, and thus the visual enhancement of the public."[133]

A contributor to low vision care in the 1950s and 1960s was William W. Policoff, who designed a microscope low vision aid, developed refractive techniques for low vision patients, and emphasized the importance of multidisciplinary care in low vision.[134] Policoff was also recognized for his work in contact lenses.[135,136] Policoff was 18 when he completed a six-month course in optometry at the Pennsylvania College of Optics and Ophthalmology. He subsequently earned degrees in veterinary medicine, pharmacy, and law.[136,137] He also later received honorary degrees from LaSalle University, the University of Scranton, and the Massachusetts College of Optometry. After service in the United States Army and a short time playing the cello professionally, Policoff established an optometry practice in Wilkes-Barre, Pennsylvania, in the 1920s. He later cofounded a multidisciplinary vision rehabilitation clinic in Scranton, Pennsylvania.[134]

In the 1950s, new visual acuity test charts were introduced by Louise Sloan (1898-1982), a vision scientist at the Wilmer Institute of the Johns Hopkins University School of Medicine, who also made several other contributions in low vision as well as in color vision and perimetry.[138] In the 1970s, the logMAR chart design was originated by Ian Bailey and Jan Lovie-Kitchin. Bailey has published over 100 papers on various aspects of low vision.[139] Sam Genensky, a scientist for the Rand Corporation with a severe vision impairment himself, developed a closed-circuit television system for low vision in the 1960s and published several articles on low vision in professional journals in the 1960s and 1970s. George Woo published a number of papers on the use of contrast sensitivity testing in low vision and for various conditions in the 1970s and 1980s, and he has had a long career in low vision care and optometric education and administration.[140] Some of the other individuals who have contributed to low vision are ophthalmologists Eleanor Faye and Gerald Fonda; vision scientist Gregory Goodrich; and optometrists Vincent Ellerbrock, Paul Freeman, Allan N. Freid, Robert J. Jacobs, Randy Jose, Charles Margach, Edwin B. Mehr, Rodney Nowakowski, Eli Peli, Bruce P. Rosenthal, and Alfred A. Rosenbloom.[141,142,143,144,145,146,147]

Environmental Vision. The term *environmental vision* is often used to describe the evaluation of requirements for effective visual performance, eye protection, illumination needs, and other visual and optical aspects of the occupational, educational, or recreational environment. Some of the areas of optometric care that might be considered part of environmental vision are occupational optometry, industrial vision, computer vision, sports vision, vocational vision, and motorist's vision.[60,148,149,150,151,152,153,154] Optometric care in the area of environmental vision can also include advice on ergonomics or eye protection; prescription of specialized spectacles, contact lenses, or other optical devices; the application of vision therapy; and education on aspects of the visual environment.[155]

Kleinstein[156] noted that devices that provide for eye protection have been used for thousands of years, an example being the face shields with eye slits used by the Inuits for protection from ultraviolet light. Optometrists undoubtedly prescribed lenses for specific occupational needs of their patients throughout much of the history of optometry, but by the 1950s, it became apparent that a significant body of knowledge on industrial vision, or occupational optometry, had been accumulating.[157] Kleinstein[156] observed that interest in industrial optometry peaked just after World War II, followed by a decrease in interest and then an increase again in the 1990s. His observation appears to be supported by a search of the cumulative indexes of the *American Journal of Optometry and Archives of the American Academy of Optometry* and the *American Journal of Optometry and Physiological Optics*. From 1924 to 1943, there was one article listed under industrial and occupational vision. From 1944 to 1973, there were 48 articles, followed by no articles at all under that listing from 1974 to 1983. Using a *PubMed* search of the journal *Optometry and Vision Science* for the keywords *industrial* or *occupational*, there were 32 articles found for the years 1989 to 2005. Attention to sports vision and to vision problems associated with the use of computers increased greatly in the late part of the twentieth century.

Diagnostic and Therapeutic Pharmaceutical Agents. A significant change, beginning in the 1970s, was the expansion of the scope of optometric practice to include the use of diagnostic and therapeutic pharmaceutical agents. This was a radical departure from the centuries-long nature of optometry being concerned exclusively with optics and visual function. While one could possibly identify many reasons for this change, the major reasons may be classified into four general areas:

(1) There was a wider distribution of optometrists than ophthalmologists in small and medium-sized towns. Ophthalmologists were more concentrated in larger cities. Patients with eye diseases or injuries in small towns often had to be referred to an ophthalmologist in a large city, sometimes many miles away, or to the general practice physician (GP) in the same town. The optometrists had slit lamp biomicroscopes and other instrumentation that the GP typically did not have, and the optometrists had learned more about the eye than had the local GP. Through the fitting of contact lenses in the 1950s and 1960s, optometrists had become more comfortable with touching ocular structures. Thus, it became a matter of convenience and better care for the patient to have the local optometrist handle minor eye diseases and injuries.

(2) More optometrists became interested in the biomedical sciences. Some of the early twentieth-century optometry educational programs were associated with departments of physics. As the undergraduate pre-optometry requirements increased, pre-optometry students started taking more and more biology courses. Undergraduate majors in physics were generally not designed as a pre-professional background for applied studies like optometry. Undergraduate majors in biology were well designed for pre-professional students, such as pre-medical and pre-dental programs, and that became a common major also for pre-optometry students. As optometry students spent more time in the study of the biomedical sciences, expansion of practice into biomedical areas seemed to be a natural change.

(3) Increases in the amount of instruction in ocular disease in optometry schools were instituted, in part, due to criticism of organized ophthalmology that optometrists didn't know enough about ocular disease. The relationship of organized ophthalmology and optometry was rocky through much of the mid-twentieth century. In 1935, the American

Medical Association had passed a resolution that ophthalmologists should not lecture to optometric groups.[158] That rule was lifted in 1950, but it was reinstated in 1955, only to be lifted again in the 1960s.[159] The earlier discussion of the Cyrus Bass lawsuit against the AMA noted that in 1954, the American Optometric Association, due to concerns about lay persons doing refractions, passed a resolution that "the field of visual care is the field of optometry, and should be exclusively the field of optometry."[159] Many in ophthalmology took the resolution to mean that optometry wanted to exclude ophthalmology from refraction, and the rule against lecturing to optometrists was again put in place. In 1955, in an attempt to smooth things over with ophthalmology, the American Optometric Association passed a resolution that stated, in part, that "optometry has no desire to extend its practice to include any limited or other form of medical eye care."[159] Even as optometry was trying to mollify ophthalmology by proclaiming no desire to practice medical eye care, the fact that optometrists didn't use pharmaceutical agents was used to suggest their inferiority to medical doctors in negative descriptions of optometry.[160] Ophthalmology had adopted refractive methods pioneered by optometrists, but they used the fact optometrists didn't prescribe drugs as negative publicity.

(4) Many optometric leaders thought that if optometrists used pharmaceutical agents, they would have a stronger argument that they were the primary care practitioners for eye and vision care. The concept of primary care developed in the 1960s and 1970s, and the primary care practitioner (PCP) is the point of entry for a patient into the health care system.[161] The PCP can care for most conditions and refer to other practitioners for others. Secondary and tertiary care practitioners care for patients upon referral. Optometrists had, in fact, been functioning as PCPs for eye and vision care for many years. They handled most refractive and binocular vision conditions, and then referred cases of ocular and systemic disease to ophthalmologists and other physicians. Furthermore, their greater numbers and their wider geographical distribution than ophthalmologists made them the logical candidate for primary eye and vision

care. With the passage of various types of federal health care legislation in the 1960s and the greater involvement of the government and third parties in health care, it was thought that the recognition of optometry as a PCP was essential to the future welfare of the profession. There was also the belief that the identification of optometrists as the primary care practitioner for eye and vision care, and their ability to recognize and diagnose eye disease, would be enhanced by the incorporation of pharmaceutical agents in the scope of practice.

The discussions of the incorporation of pharmaceutical agents into optometry practice intensified in the late 1960s, but there had been previous attempts to establish drug laws. In 1937, Albert Fitch, dean of the Pennsylvania State College of Optometry, worked to have a bill introduced into the Pennsylvania Legislature that would make optometrists "permitted to practice all things taught" in recognized colleges of optometry.[162] He made the point that the Pennsylvania State College of Optometry at the time was providing over 4,000 hours of instruction in basic and ocular sciences. The bill did not pass, but it is often mentioned as an example of how it was recognized that the existence of strong education in a given area was a good argument for its inclusion in practice. In 1961, a bill to authorize the use of diagnostic pharmaceutical agents by optometrists was introduced into the Pennsylvania General Assembly.[163] It was supported by the Pennsylvania Optometric Association but opposed by the American Optometric Association. Facing opposition from organized medicine and from some Pennsylvania optometrists, the bill was not passed.

In the mid- and late-1960s, several formal and informal meetings explored the potential importance, and possible advantages for the future of optometry, of expansion of scope of practice into medical areas. The first meeting at which the American Optometric Association officially addressed the issue was the Conference on Optometric Practice held in French Lick, Indiana, in April 1966.[163] Eighteen participants were invited to the meeting, with one of the topics to be the use of drugs in optometry practice. Speaking against the use of drugs was H. Ward Ewalt, Jr., of Pittsburgh, who had been president of the American Optometric Association from 1962 to 1963. Gregg[164] noted that Ewalt "served the AOA in many important capacities for over two decades and was possibly one of the most experienced men to assume the presidency." Speaking in favor of the use of drugs in optometry practice was Harold M. Fisher of New York City, who had been president of the American Academy of Optometry from 1947 to 1948 and who was a charter member of the National Board of Examiners in Optometry.[165] Among the arguments in favor of adoption of the use of drugs were reduction of over-referral, less loss of patients to ophthalmologists to whom patients were referred, greater prestige, better use of diagnostic instrumentation, and better government recognition as a health care provider.[166] Some of the points raised against using pharmaceuticals were loss of professional identity, problems with drug side effects, need for additional equipment and training, and potential exposure to malpractice risk.[166]

An important informal meeting of a few optometric educators and practitioners was held over three days in January 1968 at the LaGuardia Airport in New York City.[163,167,168] Following the idea of Albert Fitch in previous years that optometry is what is taught in the schools, Alden Norman Haffner, who was at that time executive director of the Optometric Center of New York and later dean of the College of Optometry at the State University of New York, called the meeting. Among the attendees were William R. Baldwin, at that time dean of the Pacific University College of Optometry; Irvin M. Borish, private practitioner and part-time faculty at Indiana University; Milton J. Eger, private practitioner and editor of the *Journal of the American Optometric Association*; Spurgeon B. Eure, Southern College of Optometry; Richard Hazlett, Indiana University; Gordon G. Heath, Indiana University; Charles Seger, private practitioner and chairman of the American Optometric Association Council on Optometric Education; and Norman Wallis, University of Houston.[167,169,170] The group recognized that optometric educational requirements had expanded to the point where a logical progression would be to include the use of pharmaceutical agents. They agreed to initiate a push for the expansion of offerings in pharmacology in the optometry schools, to prepare to be able to offer necessary continuing education for practicing optometrists, and to prepare to assist in the legislative efforts to establish the necessary laws.[163,167,168,169,170,171]

An American Optometric Association-sponsored meeting that included the discussion of drug use was held February 10-12, 1969 at the Airlie House conference center in Warrenton, Virginia.[163,172,173,174] Eighteen conference participants and about 30 observers attended the Airlie House Conference to make recommendations concerning optometry's role in health care to the American Optometric Association Board of Trustees. Although there were no specific actions taken on pharmaceutical use as an immediate consequence of that meeting, it is often pointed to as an important milestone in the debate on the topic.[163] Subsequent meetings convened by the American Optometric Association to discuss topics including drug use were the National Optometric Conference held in 1972 in New Orleans, Louisiana, and the Conference on the Future of Optometric Practice held in 1975 in Tucson, Arizona.[163]

Debate raged in both optometric meetings and professional publications about adopting the use of pharmaceuticals. The major points made by those who advocated their use can be summarized as follows[160,163,166,167,168,169,170,171,175]: (1) Use of diagnostic pharmaceutical agents makes possible the use of a wider range of diagnostic tests. (2) Because of the wider geographical distribution of optometrists compared to ophthalmologists, it would be more convenient for patients if optometrists treated minor ocular diseases and injuries. (3) Optometrists had been criticized by ophthalmology for not using drugs. (4) There continued to be friction between optometry and ophthalmology, so optometry should no longer passively accept restrictions favored by ophthalmology. (5) The time required to complete an optometric education had increased greatly so that a next logical step was the inclusion of pharmacology. (6) With greater involvement of third-party systems in health care delivery, optometry's competitive position would be enhanced with adoption of drug use. Optometry could firm up its role as a primary care practitioner for eye and vision care with the addition of pharmaceutical drug use. (7) The use of pharmaceuticals could enhance collegiality and communication with GPs, dentists, and other health care providers. (8) Big drug companies were playing increasing roles in promotion of health care. They were likely to slight optometry if optometrists didn't use drugs. (9) Patients often didn't return to the optometrist after they were referred out for evaluation of possible ocular disease.

Arguments against the adoption of pharmaceutical use included the following:[166,176,177,178] (1) Optometry had taken a leadership role in areas of functional vision care, such as refraction, binocular vision, and contact lenses. The inclusion of pharmacology could threaten optometry's ability to maintain its leadership in those areas. (2) Optometry had filled an important role in health care. By emulating ophthalmology, it could lose its niche and identity. (3) There might be a greater risk of malpractice. (4) Additional equipment and training would be needed. (5) Optometry had prospered without invading the practice of medicine. Getting along with medicine is necessary in the health care field, and incursion into medicine could jeopardize that. (6) Refractive problems and binocular vision conditions are much more common than ocular disease. By excelling in its traditional areas of expertise, optometry would serve a large proportion of the population. (7) Optometrists should emphasize quality of care and cost effectiveness instead of a wider scope of practice.

While debate continued, optometric leaders in individual states were taking the initiative to push for new laws to establish optometric usage of pharmaceutical agents. The first law for the use of diagnostic pharmaceutical agents (DPAs) was passed in 1971 in Rhode Island. The optometrists who led the effort to have that law passed were Morton W. Silverman, David W. Ferris, and Richard I. Albert.[179] Silverman[160] recalled that one of their inspirations for pushing for the law was a speech by A. N. Haffner to the New England Council of Optometry in March 1968, emphasizing the role of government in the future recognition of health care providers, and that optometry should move beyond the traditional detection of ocular disease to be included in that recognition. Their first attempts to have a DPA bill passed in 1969 and 1970 failed, but they were able to get a bill passed in 1971. The next state to pass DPA legislation was Pennsylvania in 1974, followed by Tennessee, Oregon, Maine, Louisiana, and Delaware in 1975. By 1989, all 50 states and the District of Columbia had passed DPA legislation.

The first state to pass legislation for the use of therapeutic pharmaceutical agents (TPAs) was West Virginia in 1976. The optometrists leading the work in the passage of that legislation were David John Janney, John Casto, and Walter S. Ramsey.[179] Janney had been the chief of an optometry clinic in the armed services, and because there was no ophthalmologist in his clinic, had treated and co-managed many types of eye diseases and injuries.[163] The next state to pass TPA legislation was North Carolina in 1976, led by John Costabile and John Robinson.[163] Before the passage of the legislation, both West Virginia and North Carolina had contracted with the Pennsylvania College of Optometry for the education needed for TPA usage. It wasn't until 1984 that Oklahoma became the third state to pass TPA legislation, with 21 more states following from 1985 to 1989. By 1998, all 50 states and the District of Columbia had passed TPA legislation.

Many factors made it possible for optometrists to have DPA and TPA laws passed. One factor was the grassroots effort of optometrists to educate their legislators in the ways in which such laws could benefit their constituents, particularly improved access to care.[171] Other factors were the support of organizations without pecuniary interest, such as the American Public Health Association, and the fact that curricular changes appropriate for DPA and TPA use were already underway in the optometry schools.[171] Also of importance was the testimony in favor of the legislation by respected persons who had experience in medical areas. One such person was Lowell Bellin, a physician formerly on the Commission of Health in New York City, who testified on behalf of optometry in 21 states.[163] Other persons who testified for optometry included Lesley L. Walls and Sally Hegeman. After graduating from optometry school, Walls attended medical school and became a family practice physician. His experience in medical practice, academic medicine, and optometric education made his testimony helpful in many states. Sally Hegeman, holder of a doctorate in pharmacology and instructor of both medical students and optometry students at Indiana University as well as a frequent continuing education speaker, testified in many states concerning pharmacology curricula in medical schools and optometry schools. In 2000, Haffner[180] observed that as suggested by sociology studies, the next phase after the passage of legislation —"the institutionalization of the culture, habits, practice models, and professional environment of optometry resulting from both DPA and TPA authority"—was "currently now well underway."

As more and more states adopted the use of pharmaceutical agents by optometrists, concern was often expressed that optometry should incorporate such responsibilities as an expansion of scope of practice rather than a shift in scope of practice toward a medical model. A cautionary note was expressed by Irvin M. Borish, who had often been described as a visionary and one of optometry's foremost leaders.[181,182,183] Having the benefit of living in the thick of more than 70 years of optometry history, Borish often emphasized the importance of understanding history when trying to anticipate future trends.

Borish observed that because medicine did not embrace the use of spectacles in their early history, only becoming interested in prescribing them in the nineteenth and early twentieth centuries, there was plenty of time for optometry to fill that niche and develop into a flourishing profession. Borish cautioned that optometry, in broadening its scope of practice, should not leave a similar vacuum for another profession to fill.

He stated that "it is essential that optometry not lose its sharp cutting edge advantage in the field of refraction."[168] To maintain its traditional areas of strength within the context of a wider scope of practice and changing trends in the health care field, Borish recommended that optometry establish group practices, increase delegation to ancillary personnel, make more effective use of automated instrumentation, and develop more effective testing techniques.[168,184]

Chapter 3: Notes

1. Hofstetter HW. *Optometry: Professional, Economic, and Legal Aspects*. St. Louis, MO: Mosby, 1948:91.
2. Prentice CF. *Legalized Optometry and the Memoirs of its Founder*. Seattle, WA: Casperin Fletcher Press, 1926:320.
3. Prentice, 322.
4. Prentice, 378.
5. Patterson KH. Letter to the editor. *Optical J Rev Optom*. 1920;46:580.
6. Reply to letter to the editor. *Optical J Rev Optom*. 1920;46:580.
7. Simpson J. Professional use of the "doctor" title. *Optical J Rev Optom*. 1946;83(10):50,52,70.
8. Hofstetter, 95.
9. The term "doctor" in America. *Optical J Rev Optom*. 1946;83(10):36-37.
10. Fitch A. *My Fifty Years in Optometry*. Philadelphia, PA: Pennsylvania State College of Optometry, 1955;1:6.
11. Hofstetter, 93.
12. Fitch, 245.
13. Kahn LB. A little personal optometric history. *Hindsight* 2008;39:72-74.
14. Fitch, 165.
15. Gregg JR. *Origin and Development of the Southern College of Optometry, 1904-1984*. Fullerton, CA: Southern College of Optometry, 1984:163,187.
16. Moline SW. *Century of Vision: The New England College of Optometry, An Anecdotal History of the First Hundred Years*. Boston, MA: The New England College of Optometry, 1994:60.
17. Stewart CR. *The Founding Years: University of Houston College of Optometry 1952-1961*. Georgetown, TX Armadillo Publishing, 2003:65,201-202.
18. Williams CW. Education: Key to a profession's future [address given to optometrists in 1957]. *Newsletter Optom Hist Soc*. 1982;13:70-79.
19. Goss DA. History of the Indiana University Division of Optometry. *Indiana J Op-*

20 Robinson JD, Lilly B, Enoch JM. Communications concerning the O.D. degree and licensure. *Hindsight* 2008;39:75-77.
21 Gregg JR. *History of the American Academy of Optometry 1922-1986*. Washington, DC: American Academy of Optometry, 1987:4-8.
22 Gregg, 18-19.
23 Gregg, 192.
24 Gregg, 1-207.
25 Newcomb RD, Eger M. *History of the American Academy of Optometry 1987-2010*. Washington, DC: American Academy of Optometry, 2012.
26 *The Distinguished Service Foundation of Optometry: Purposes, Officers, Medalists, Fellows, Constitution and By-Laws*. Undated pamphlet. Files of the American Optometric Association Archives and Museum of Optometry.
27 Nichols AS. A tribute to the Distinguished Service Foundation of Optometry. *J Am Optom Assoc.* 1944;15:264-265.
28 The Distinguished Service Foundation's aims and purposes. *Optical J Rev Optom.* 1949;86(11):64.
29 Houghton GS. The Distinguished Service Foundation of Optometry. *J Am Optom Assoc.* 1933;4(6):5,8.
30 Part 7, Ancillary groups in optometry: the Distinguished Service Foundation of Optometry. *J Am Optom Assoc.* 1959;30:649-650.
31 Dr. George S. Houghton 1867-1933. *J Am Optom Assoc.* 1933;5(5):7.
32 Obituary: Clinton R. Padelford. *J Am Optom Assoc.* 1962;33:454.
33 Laurence P. Folsom. *J Am Optom Assoc.* 1957;28:421.
34 Obituary: Theodore A. Brombach. *J Am Optom Assoc.* 1961;32:732.
35 Fiorillo J. Berkeley *Optometry: A History*. Berkeley, CA: University of California School of Optometry, 2010:149.
36 Uglum JR. The Distinguished Service Foundation of Optometry. *J Am Optom Assoc.* 1980;51:214.
37 American Optometric Association. *Directory of the American Optometric Association*. St. Louis, MO: Author, 1972:365.
38 Goss DA. A history of the Distinguished Service Foundation of Optometry. *Hindsight* 2015;46:2-9.
39 Dablemont M. Letter to Eger MJ. December 25, 1979. Files of the American Optometric Association Archives and Museum of Optometry.
40 American Optometric Association. Directory of the American Optometric Association. St. Louis, MO: Author, 1972:96.
41 American Academy of Optometry Foundation. Ezell Fellows: A Historical Listing. 2018. www.aaopt.org/home/aaof/programs/programs-for-graduate-students/programs-graduates/ezell-fellows-historical-listing
42 Hirsch MJ, Wick RE. *The Optometric Profession*. Philadelphia, PA: Chilton, 1968:155-156.

43 Gregg JR. American Optometric Association: A History. St. Louis, MO: American Optometric Association, 1972:72-74.
44 Riis RW. Optometry on trial. Readers Digest 1937; 31(184):77-85; 31(186):89-96.
45 Hofstetter, 122.
46 Kiekenapp EH. Editorials. J Am Optom Assoc. 1937;9:12-14,54-58.
47 Koetting RA. The American Optometric Association's First Century. St. Louis, MO: American Optometric Association, 1997:22.
48 Alden K. Battle for your eyes. Coronet 1963;1(1):48-52.
49 Classé JG. Legal Aspects of Optometry. Boston, MA: Butterworth, 1989:17-18.
50 Classé, 24.
51 Gregg JR. History of the American Academy of Optometry 1922-1986. Washington, DC: American Academy of Optometry, 1987:123-124.
52 Bennett I. The 1954 American Optometric Association Seattle Resolution and medical reaction to it. Hindsight 2011;42:102-105.
53 Bennett I. The lawsuit of optometrist Cyrus Bass versus the AMA. Hindsight 2012;43:2-4.
54 Mizener FD, Bennett I. The lawsuit of optometrist Cyrus Bass versus the AMA: More data and reader comments. Hindsight 2012;43:75-81.
55 Bennett I. More on the Cyrus bass lawsuit: Correcting an error and adding more information. Hindsight 2013;44:3-4.
56 Wolfberg MD, Eichhorst TE. American Optometric Association complaint to the U.S. Department of Justice regarding activities of organized medicine in the field of vision care which hinder and restrain the profession of optometry. Hindsight 2012;43:47-57.
57 Birnbaum MH. Behavioral optometry: A historical perspective. J Am Optom Assoc. 1994;65:255-264.
58 Press LJ. The evolution of vision therapy. In: Press LJ, ed. Applied Concepts in Vision Therapy. St. Louis, MO: Mosby, 1997:2-8.
59 Griffin JR, Grisham JD. Binocular Anomalies: Diagnosis and Vision Therapy, 4th ed. Amsterdam, the Netherlands: Butterworth-Heinemann, 2002:263-268.
60 Leeds J. Javal's blindness. Hindsight 1992;23:19-22.
61 Revell MJ. Strabismus: A History of Orthoptic Techniques. London, UK: Barrie & Jenkins, 1971:15-18.
62 Gregg JR. The Story of Optometry. New York, NY: Ronald Press, 1965:237-238.
63 Wade NJ. A Natural History of Vision. Cambridge, MA: MIT Press, 1998:293-294.
64 Gregg, 238-239.
65 Wade, 293,296.
66 Revell, 41.
67 Wells DW. The Stereoscope in Ophthalmology with Special Reference to the Treatment of Heterophoria and Heterotropia, 4th ed. Boston, MA: E. F. Mahady, 1928:i.
68 Birnbaum MH. Optometric Management of Nearpoint Vision Disorders. Boston, MA:

Butterworth-Heinemann, 1993:283-286.
69   Gregg, 246-248.
70   Fisher HM. Recollections of Dr. LeRoy Ryer. *J Am Optom Assoc.* 1974;45:1424-1428.
71   Hofstetter HW. E. LeRoy Ryer. *Am J Optom Arch Am Acad Optom.* 1973;50:593-594.
72   Dablemont M. Ryer and the ILAMO. *Newsletter Optom Hist Soc.* 1976;7:1-3.
73   MacDonald LW. Optometric Visual Training: Its History and Development. In: Schwartz I, Shapiro A, eds. *The Collected Works of Lawrence W. MacDonald.* Santa Ana, CA: Optometric Extension Program, 1993;2:38-51.
74   Cox JL. A.M. Skeffington, O.D.: The man. *J Behav Optom.* 1997;8:3-6.
75   Maples WC. A.M. Skeffington: The father of behavioral optometry—His contributions. *Proc SPIE.* 1998;3579:17-23.
76   Gesell A, Ilg FL, Bullis GE. *Vision: Its Development in Infant and Child.* New York, NY: Paul B. Hoeber, 1950.
77   Ilg FL, Ames LB. *School Readiness: Behavior Tests Used at the Gesell Institute.* New York, NY: Harper & Row, 1972.
78   Brock FW. A chronicle of orthoptic history covering 25 years of practice. *Optom Weekly.* 1966;57(5):25-31;57(6):31-35;57(7):23-27.
79   Wittenberg S. Brock's research in stereopsis. *Am J Optom Physiol Opt.* 1981;58:663-666.
80   Birnbaum MH. Perspectives on the contributions of Frederick Brock. *Am J Optom Physiol Opt.* 1981;58:667-670.
81   Greenwald I. Frederick Brock: An optometric giant. *J Optom Vis Dev.* 1993;24:4-7.
82   Goss DA. Biographical sketch: Frederick W. Brock (1899-1972). *Hindsight* 2008;39:120-123.
83   Alpern M. Types of movement. In: Davson H, ed. *Muscular Mechanisms*, 2nd ed. Volume 3 of *The Eye.* New York, NY: Academic Press, 1969:65-174.
84   Fry GA. Basic concepts underlying graphical analysis. In: Schor CM, Ciuffreda KJ, eds. *Vergence Eye Movements: Basic and Clinical Aspects.* Boston, MA: Butterworths, 1983:403-437.
85   Hofstetter HW. Graphical analysis. In: Schor CM, Ciuffreda KJ, eds. *Vergence Eye Movements: Basic and Clinical Aspects.* Boston, MA: Butterworths, 1983:439-464.
86   Flom MC. Treatment of binocular anomalies of vision. In: Hirsch MJ, Wick RE, eds. *Vision of Children: An Optometric Symposium.* Philadelphia, PA: Chilton, 1963:197-228.
87   Vodnoy BE. *The Practice of Vision Care, Orthoptics, and Corneal Contact Lens Fitting*, 4th ed. South Bend, IN: Bernell Corporation, 1972.
88   Andrews C. [biography of Bernard Vodnoy]. Bernell catalog, 2004:75.
89   Rosner J. *Helping Children Overcome Learning Difficulties*, 3rd ed. New York, NY: Walker, 1993.
90   Garzia RP, ed. *Vision and Reading.* St. Louis, MO: Mosby, 1996.

91 Griffin JR, Christensen GN, Wesson MD, Erickson GB. *Optometric Management of Reading Dysfunction*. Boston, MA: Butterworth-Heinemann, 1997.
92 Flax N. Vision and learning: Optometry and the Academy's early role —An historical overview. *J Optom Vis Dev*. 1999;30:105-110.
93 Rosner J. Symposium on Vision and Learning: Optometry's role. *J Optom Vis Dev*. 1999;30:116-121.
94 Scheiman MM, Rouse MW, eds. *Optometric Management of Learning-Related Vision Problems*, 2nd ed. St. Louis, MO: Mosby Elsevier, 2006.
95 Flax N. Selected Works of Nathan Flax. Santa Ana, CA: Optometric Extension Program, 2007;1:43-152.
96 Sheedy JE, Shaw-McMinn PG. *Diagnosing and Treating Computer-Related Vision Problems*. Amsterdam, the Netherlands: Butterworth-Heinemann, 2003.
97 Scheiman M, Wick B. *Clinical Management of Binocular Vision: Heterophoric, Accommodative, and Eye Movement Disorders*, 2nd ed. Philadelphia, PA: Lippincott Williams & Wilkins, 2002:550-595.
98 Kirscher DW. Sports vision training procedures. In: Classé JG, ed. *Sports Vision. Optom Clinics*. 1993;3(1):171-182.
99 Coffey B, Reichow AW. Visual performance enhancement in sports optometry. In: Loran DFC, MacEwen CJ, eds. *Sports Vision*. Oxford, UK: Butterworth-Heinemann, 1995:158-177.
100 Suchoff IB, Ciuffreda KJ, Kapoor N, eds. *Visual & Vestibular Consequences of Acquired Brain Injury*. Santa Ana, CA: Optometric Extension Program, 2001.
101 Wold RM, Pierce JR, Keddington J. Effectiveness of optometric vision therapy. *J Am Optom Assoc*. 1978;49:1047-1054.
102 Liu JS, Lee M, Jang J, Ciuffreda KJ, Wong JH, Grisham JD, Stark L. Objective assessment of accommodation orthoptics: Dynamic insufficiency. *Am J Optom Physiol Opt*. 1979;56:285-294.
103 Suchoff IB, Petito GT. The efficacy of vision therapy. *J Am Optom Assoc*. 1986;57:119-125.
104 Griffin JR. Efficacy of vision therapy for non-strabismic vergence anomalies. *Am J Optom Physiol Opt*. 1987;64:411-414.
105 Rouse MW. Management of binocular anomalies: Efficacy of vision therapy in the treatment of accommodative disorders. *Am J Optom Physiol Opt*. 1987;64:415-420.
106 Grisham JD. Vision therapy results for convergence insufficiency: A literature review. *Am J Optom Physiol Opt*. 1988;65:448-454.
107 Grisham JD. Vergence orthoptics: Validity and persistence of the training effect. *Am J Optom Physiol Opt*. 1991;68:441-451.
108 Birnbaum MH. *Optometric Management of Nearpoint Vision Disorders*. Boston, MA: Butterworth-Heinemann, 1993:381-393.
109 Ciuffreda KJ. The scientific basis for and efficacy of optometric vision therapy in nonstrabismic accommodative and vergence disorders. *J Am Optom Assoc*.

2002;73:735-762.
110 Scheiman M, Mitchell GL, Cotter S, et al. A randomized clinical trial of treatments for convergence insufficiency in children. *Arch Ophthalmol.* 2005;123:14-24.
111 Hofstetter HW, Graham R. Leonardo and contact lenses. *Am J Optom Arch Am Acad Optom.* 1953;30:41-44.
112 Hofstetter HW. Leonardo's contact concept. *Contact Lens Forum* 1984;9(12):15-17.
113 Graham R. Historical development. In: Mandell RB, ed. *Contact Lens Practice: Basic and Advanced.* Springfield, IL: Charles C. Thomas, 1965:3-14.
114 Filderman IP, White PF. *Contact Lens Practice and Patient Management.* Philadelphia, PA: Chilton, 1969:417-418.
115 Obrig TE. *Modern Ophthalmic Lenses and Optical Glass*, 3rd ed. New York, NY: Chilton, 1944:131-142.
116 Tuohy KM. The birth of an idea. *Optom World.* 1963;50(22):14,16,20.
117 Gregg JR. *The Story of Optometry.* New York, NY: Ronald Press, 1965:256-258.
118 Graham R. The evolution of the corneal contact lens. *Am J Optom Arch Am Acad Optom.* 1959;36:55-72.
119 Baldwin WR. *Borish.* Springfield, MA: Bassette, 2006:154-167.
120 Schaeffer J, Beiting J. Contact lens pioneers: Key developments in contact lens materials and design, 1975-2000. *Rev Optom.* 2007;144(8):34-42.
121 Schaeffer J, Beiting J. Contact lens pioneers: The early history of contact lenses. *Rev Optom.* 2007;144(7):28-30,32,34.
122 McMahon TT, Zadnik K. Twenty-five years of contact lenses: The impact on the cornea and ophthalmic practice. *Cornea* 2000;19:730-740.
123 Sullivan L. *Bausch & Lomb: Perfecting Vision, Enhancing Life for 150 Years: A Brief History of Bausch & Lomb's First 150 Years.* Rochester, NY: Bausch & Lomb, 2004:52-53.
124 Barr JT. 20 years of contact lenses. *Contact Lens Spectrum* 2006;21:28-38.
125 Grosvenor T. *Primary Care Optometry*, 5th ed. St. Louis, MO: Elsevier Butterworth Heinemann, 2007:435.
126 Rosenbloom AA. Low vision aids. In: Borish IM, ed. *Clinical Refraction*, 3rd ed. New York, NY: Professional Press, 1975:1007-1035.
127 Levene JR. *Clinical Refraction and Visual Science.* London, UK: Butterworths, 1977:75-76.
128 Mehr EB. The typoscope by Charles F. Prentice. *Am J Optom Arch Am Acad Optom.* 1969;46:885-887.
129 Mogk L, Goodrich G. The history and future of low vision services in the United States. *J Vis Impairment Blindness.* 2004;98:585-600.
130 Duke-Elder S, Abrams D. Ophthalmic optics and refraction. In: Duke-Elder S, ed. *System of Ophthalmology.* St. Louis, MO: Mosby, 1970;5:657-658.
131 A salute to the "father" of low vision. *Rev Optom.* 1991;128(4):10.
132 William Feinbloom, O.D., Ph.D. 1904-1985. *Am J Optom Physiol Opt.* 1985;62:359.
133 Gregg JR. *History of the American Academy of Optometry 1922-1986.* Washington, DC:

American Academy of Optometry, 1987:186.
134 Rosenbloom AA Jr. William Policoff's contribution to low vision. *Am J Optom Physiol Opt.* 1977;54:517-518.
135 Borish IM. William Policoff's contribution to optometry. *Am J Optom Physiol Opt.* 1977;54:514-516.
136 Personal Profile: William W. Policoff, O.D. *Optical J Rev Optom.* 1976;113(12):29-32.
137 Hirsch MJ, Morgan MW. A videotaped interview of Dr. William Policoff. *Am J Optom Physiol Opt.* 1977;54:509-513.
138 Bailey IL. Louise L. Sloan, Ph.D. (1898-1982). *Am J Optom Physiol Opt.* 1982;59:694.
139 Adams AJ, Lovie-Kitchin J. Ian L. Bailey: Leader in low vision and father of the LogMAR system. *Clin Exp Optom.* 2004;87:37-41.
140 Strong JG. George C Woo. *Clin Exp Optom.* 2002;85:392-396.
141 Ellerbrock VJ. Partial vision and optical aids. In: Hirsch MJ, Wick RE, eds. *Vision of the Aging Patient: An Optometric Symposium.* Philadelphia, PA: Chilton, 1960:174-201.
142 In memoriam: Vincent J. Ellerbrock. *Am J Optom Arch Am Acad Optom.* 1966;43:67-69.
143 Fonda G. *Management of the Patient with Subnormal Vision.* St. Louis, MO: Mosby, 1970.
144 Mehr EB, Freid AN. *Low Vision Care.* New York, NY: Professional Press, 1975.
145 Rosenbloom AA Jr. Care of the visually impaired elderly patient. In: Rosenbloom AA Jr, Morgan MW, eds. *Vision and Aging: General and Clinical Perspectives.* New York, NY: Professional Press, 1986:337-348.
146 Nowakowski RW. *Primary Low Vision Care.* Norwalk, CT: Appleton & Lange, 1994.
147 Grosvenor T. *Primary Care Optometry*, 5th ed. St. Louis, MO: Elsevier Butterworth Heinemann, 2007:435-455.
148 Hofstetter HW. *Industrial Vision.* Philadelphia, PA: Chilton, 1956.
149 Holmes C, Jolliffe H, Gregg J, Cameron IS, Blyth R. *Guide to Occupational and Other Visual Needs.* Los Angeles, CA: Silverlake Lithographers, 1958.
150 Allen MJ. *Vision and Highway Safety.* Philadelphia, PA: Chilton, 1970.
151 Gregg JR. *Vision and Sports: An Introduction.* Boston, MA: Butterworths, 1987.
152 Sheedy JE, London R, eds. Environmental Optics. *Prob Optom.* 1990;2(1).
153 Classé JG, ed. Sports Vision. *Optom Clinics.* 1993;3(1).
154 Loran DFC, MacEwen CJ, eds. *Sports Vision.* Oxford, UK: Butterworth-Heinemann, 1995.
155 Pitts DG, Kleinstein RN, eds. *Environmental Vision: Interactions of the Eye, Vision, and the Environment.* Boston, MA: Butterworth-Heinemann, 1993.
156 Kleinstein RN. Occupational optometry and primary care. In: Pitts DG, Kleinstein RN, eds. *Environmental Vision: Interactions of the Eye, Vision, and the Environment.* Boston, MA: Butterworth-Heinemann, 1993:3-50.
157 Gregg JR. *The Story of Optometry.* New York, NY: Ronald Press, 1965:280-282.
158 Hofstetter HW. *Optometry: Professional, Economic, and Legal Aspects.* St. Louis, MO:

Mosby, 1948:358.
159 Gregg JR. *American Optometric Association: A History*. St. Louis, MO: American Optometric Association, 1972:223-224, 251-254.
160 Silverman MW. Optometry's first drug law: A personal memoir. *J Am Optom Assoc.* 1998;69:188-198.
161 Grosvenor T. *Primary Care Optometry*, 5th ed. St. Louis, MO: Elsevier Butterworth Heinemann, 2007:456.
162 Fitch, 337-351.
163 Wolfberg MD. A profession's commitment to increased public service: Optometry's remarkable story. *J Am Optom Assoc.* 1999;70:145-170.
164 Gregg, 296.
165 Gregg, 309.
166 Report of the Conference on Optometric Practice, French Lick, Indiana, April 20-21, 1966.
167 Eger MJ. Now it can and should be told. *J Am Optom Assoc.* 1989;60:323-326.
168 Borish IM. Optometry: Its heritage and its future. *Indiana J Optom.* 2001;4:23-31. http://www.opt.indiana.edu/IndJOpt/PDF/ijofall01.pdf
169 Haffner AN. The LaGuardia Conference: The meeting that changed the profession. *Hindsight* 2010;41:17-20.
170 Bennett I. The meeting that changed the profession. *Hindsight* 2010;41:21-23.
171 Wallis N, Wedding D. The battle for the use of drugs for therapeutic purposes in optometry: Lessons for clinical psychology. *Prof Psych: Res Pract.* 2004;35:323-328.
172 Robinson JD. General Statement for the Conference on Optometry's Role in Health Care, Airlie House, Warrenton, Virginia, February 10-12, 1969, American Optometric Association.
173 Eger MJ. The Airlie House Conference. *J Am Optom Assoc.* 1969;40:429-431.
174 Hopping RL. Facing the issues. *J Am Optom Assoc.* 1969;40:506-509.
175 Warnock S. The optometrist's rise to power in the health care market, or "It's optometric physician, to you." *Sci Communication.* 2005;27:100-126.
176 Ball RJ. Should we be first class ODs or second class MDs? *Optom Weekly.* 1976;67:874,875,894,895.
177 Buchner EL. ...and con. *Optical J Rev Optom.* 1976;113(5):8.
178 Peters HB. The dog and the bone. *Am J Optom Physiol Opt.* 1976;53:276-277.
179 Classé JG. *Legal Aspects of Optometry*. Boston, MA: Butterworths, 1989:22-24.
180 Haffner AN. What has changed? *Optom Vis Sci.* 2000;77:165-167.
181 Baldwin WR. *Borish*. Springfield, MA: Bassette, 2006.
182 Herrin S. The idea man: Irvin M. Borish, optometry's architect. *Rev Optom.* 1982;119:18,19,21,22,24.
183 Kirkner R. The most influential optometrist of our time. *Rev Optom.* 1999;136:22-24.
184 Borish IM. Don't leave a vacuum. *Optom Economics.* 1991;1(7):19-22.

Chapter 4
The Profession Advances and Gains in Recognition

Additional changes in optometry have continued, extending from the twentieth century into the early twenty-first century. Some of the most visible of these trends include increasing numbers of women optometrists, solidification of optometry's status as a scholarly profession, and greater recognition and standing within the health care system. Just as optometry had to struggle for licensure laws in the early twentieth century, it has had to continue to strive for acceptance and recognition in various agencies, systems, and services, justifying its inclusion by its preparation and by providing quality care.

CHANGING DEMOGRAPHICS AND EMPLOYMENT PATTERNS

The number of licensed optometrists in the United States increased through the second half of the twentieth century. In 1930, there were about 18,000 licensed optometrists in the U.S. compared to about 34,000 in 1997, and about 40,000 in 2013 (see Table 4.1). That is nearly a doubling in number from 1930 to the beginning of the twenty-first century, but the population of the U.S. more than doubled in that same period of time. In 2019, there were more than 39,000 optometrists employed in the United States. It is thought likely that as many as one-fourth of those optometrists in 1930 actually divided their time between optometric work and selling jewelry.[1] And it is also likely that many of the 1930 optometrists were practicing opticianry in addition to optometry, by filling the glasses prescriptions of other refractionists.[1]

Table 4.1. Numbers of optometrists in the United States.

Year	Number of Optometrists	Source
1928	18,079	Blue Book of Optometrists[1]
1930	17,931	Blue Book of Optometrists[1]
1944	17,264	Blue Book of Optometrists[1]
1966	20,610	Directories and U.S. Census[2]
1990	29,000	American Optometric Association[3]
1992	30,500	American Optometric Association[4]
1997	34,000	American Optometric Association[5]
2013	40,000	American Optometric Association[6]
2019	39,420	U.S. Bureau of Labor Statistics[7]

Note. Criteria for inclusion vary depending on the source of the data.

The number of students attending optometry school decreased greatly during World War II. After the war, the optometry schools swelled with large numbers of veterans attending on the G.I. Bill (see Appendix 2). Because of the aging of the large number of optometrists who graduated in the years immediately following World War II, the median age of optometrists in the United States hit a high of 50 in 1977.[5] As they began to retire and their ranks were filled by new optometry graduates, the median age of practicing optometrists started to drop, falling below 40 in 1995.[5]

In 1944, there were 17,264 licensed optometrists in the United States. Also providing eye care in 1944 were 1,819 ophthalmologists and 4,363 eye, ear, nose, and throat specialists.[1] An American Optometric

Association survey indicated that of the 17,264 optometrists licensed in 1944, less than 13,000 were actually practicing optometry.[1] A 1995 study, which took into account estimates of numbers of persons not practicing and persons practicing part-time, suggested that at the time there were 27,646 full-time-equivalent optometrists and 14,091 full-time-equivalent ophthalmologists.[8]

A trend since the 1970s has been an increase in the number of women in optometry. In 1944, only 3% of practicing optometrists were women.[1] Until the mid-1970s it was still common for many optometry school classes to have no female members. For example, although Pacific University had some female graduates before 1970, they had an all-male class as late as the class graduating in 1974. At Indiana University, females made up fewer than 10% of graduates every year from 1956 to 1973. After 1973, the proportion of female graduates at Indiana University increased steadily, topping 50% for the first time in 1993 and exceeding 60% in 2002.[9,10] As a result of the increases in numbers of female graduates at all schools, the percentages of women among practicing optometrists increased to 15% in 1990, to 26% in 1997, and to 43% in 2016.[3,6,11] Data on the percentages of women among entering optometry students can be found in Appendix 2.

The average net income of optometrists is given in Table 4.2.

Table 4.2. Income of optometrists.

Year	Mean	Median	Source
1929		$3,750	American Optometric Association[12]
1944		$5,950	American Optometric Association[12]
1949		$4,343	1950 United States census[13]
1951		$7,740	Elmstrom[14]
1958		$9,970	American Optometric Association[12]

1959		$8,772	1960 United States census[13]
1968		$20,926	American Optometric Association[12]
1977		$37,403	American Optometric Association[12]
1982	$46,786		American Optometric Association[6]
1987	$57,190		American Optometric Association[6]
1988	$66,110	$60,000	American Optometric Association[15]
1990	$74,845	$68,000	American Optometric Association[15]
1992	$81,571	$75,000	American Optometric Association[15]
1994	$88,690	$80,000	American Optometric Association[15]
1996	$92,637	$85,000	American Optometric Association[15]
1998	$108,262	$90,000	American Optometric Association[15]
2000	$138,846	$115,000	American Optometric Association[15]
2014	$129,692		American Optometric Association[16]
2016	$139,469		American Optometric Association[17]

The increase from 1988 to 2000, in nominal terms a doubling, represents an increase of 31.7% in 1988 dollars.[15] A 1945 survey showed optometrists' net income increasing over the first 10 years in practice.[18] In 1968, Hirsch and Wick[13] observed that the income of optometrists in private practice tended to remain low the first five years, increase gradually the next 10 years, and reach a peak in the fourteenth to eighteenth years of practice, with a decline beginning in about the twenty-eighth year. They noted that optometry practice income could remain at a fairly high level into the fortieth and even fiftieth years of practice. A 1997 survey asked graduates of Indiana University what percentages of their income were derived from various aspects of patient care.[19,20] The results, in average percentages, were as follows: from examination and follow-up care for spectacles, 57%; from examination and follow-up for contact lenses, 34%; from treatment of eye diseases, 7%; from vision therapy, 1%; from low vision care, 1%. Four of the 733 survey respondents derived 30% or more of their income from vision therapy. Of the 733 respondents, 136 worked in offices that included both optometrists and ophthalmologists. Of these 136, 45 (or 6% of the total survey sample) obtained the majority of their income from the treatment of eye diseases.

Surveys by the American Optometric Association in the last decade of the twentieth century indicated the highest net average incomes were found among optometrists in group practice, followed by optometrists in solo practice, with optometrists who were in the employment of someone else lower than those in solo practice.[5,6,15,21] Those trends were also found in a 2018 income survey conducted by the *Review of Optometry*.[22] Although the largest incomes could be obtained in private practice, the proportion of optometrists in private practice declined from 71% in 1990 to 65% in 1998 and to 58% in 2017.[3,17,21] There were corresponding increases in the percentages of optometrists in the employ of optical chains, ophthalmologists, HMOs, and clinics.

The first optometry residency programs were a residency in orthoptics and vision training at the Optometric Center of New York begun in 1963 and a residency in vision and child development begun in 1967 also at the Optometric Center of New York.[23] These were 15-week to 18-week programs. The first 12-month optometry residency program was started in 1974, with four residents in vision therapy at the State University of New York.[24,25] The first residency program to receive accreditation by the Council on Optometric Education was at the Kansas City Veterans Administration Medical Center, which began in 1975.[26] By 1979, there were 18 residency programs, and by 1984, there were 46 residency programs with 80 available positions.[23,26] In 1992, there were 56 accredited residency programs with 85 positions,[27] and in 2019, there were more than 250 accredited residency programs with more than 460 positions.[28] Residencies have increasingly become an important route to developing a practice specialty, to preparing for a career as a clinical educator, and to establishing credentials for employment.

FOUNDING OF ADDITIONAL NATIONAL ORGANIZATIONS

In previous chapters, the beginnings of the American Optometric Association (AOA), the American Academy of Optometry, and the Optometric Extension Program were discussed. The last four decades of the twentieth century saw the formation of additional significant national optometric organizations to provide community for specific groups or interests.

The American Optometric Student Association (AOSA) was formed in 1968 with the cooperation of the AOA. Students considered the AOSA co-founders were Ellis J. Hoffman of the Pennsylvania College of Optometry, Raymond I. Myers of Indiana University, and Burton E. Worrell of University of California at Berkeley.[29] Myers served as the first president. By 1972, all American optometry schools had AOSA chapters and 80% of students were members.[30] By 2017, AOSA had more than 7,100 members at 24 optometry schools in the United States, Canada, and Puerto Rico.[31]

The National Optometric Association (NOA) was founded at a meeting in 1969 called by C. Clayton Powell of Atlanta, Georgia, and John L. Howlette of Richmond, Virginia, to "establish a nationally recognized optometric organization comprised of black doctors."[32] Co-founders Powell and Howlette assured the original members that they did not intend to compete with the AOA, but rather to give black optometrists a strong voice, whether within or outside the AOA.[32] At the time, they were especially concerned about the recruitment of minority optometry students and optometry practice in minority communities. Powell served as NOA president from 1969 to 1974. At its convention in 2019, the NOA celebrated not only its 50th anniversary and the fact that it remained the largest organization representing minority optometrists, but it also celebrated several service projects, including the awarding of over three-quarters of a million dollars in scholarships and student travel grants.

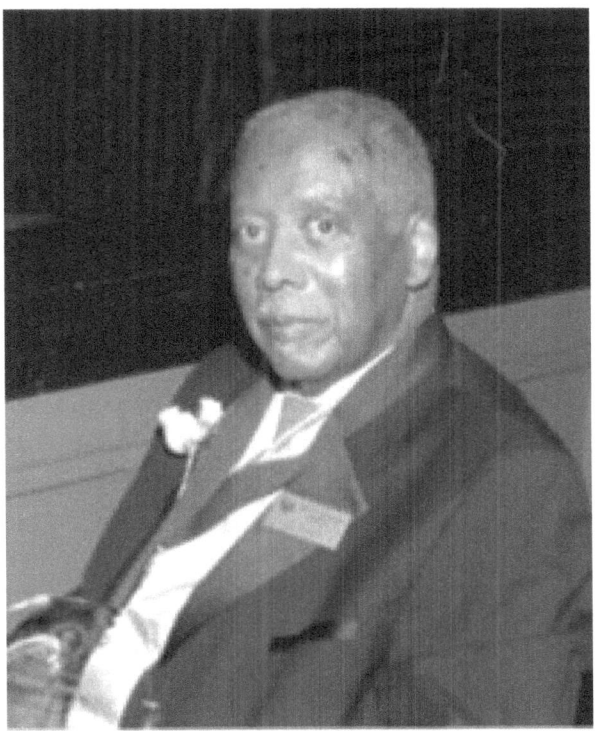

Figure 4.1 C. Clayton Powell (1927-2020), co-founder of the National Optometric Association. (Image courtesy of the Archives and Museum of Optometry and the AOA Foundation)

The Optometric Historical Society (OHS) began in 1969, with Maria Dablemont, the AOA librarian and archivist, and Henry Hofstetter, the past president of the AOA, as co-founders.[33] Thirty-four persons sent in $5 checks for membership dues to become founding members.[34] The OHS was formed as an independent organization to study, preserve, and promote optometry history. Hofstetter served as president from 1970 to 1974, and Dablemont was secretary-treasurer from 1970 to 1987. The OHS has produced a quarterly publication since 1970. In 2009, OHS president Irving Bennett signed a memorandum of understanding that the OHS would become a program of Optometry Cares, the AOA Foundation, and by the late 2010s, that merger was complete.

The Armed Forces Optometric Society (AFOS) was formed in 1970 with Frederick van Nus as the first president.[35] In 1982, AFOS was granted affiliate status in the AOA, comparable to the status of state associations. In 1986, AFOS expanded membership to include Veterans Administration and Civil Service optometrists.[36]

The College of Optometrists in Vision Development (COVD) was formed in 1971 through the merger of three organizations of optometrists doing work in vision therapy and developmental vision. Leonard Press wrote that COVD was ahead of its time, at its beginning, in developing board certification, promoting maintenance of competency, and showing diversity in its initial governing board, with two women officers, Amorita Treganza as president and Joyce Adema as treasurer.[37] COVD started giving its Fellowship certification examinations in 1972.[38]

Volunteer Optometric Services to Humanity (VOSH) was founded in 1972 in Kansas.[39] VOSH/International was incorporated in the state of Indiana in 1979. The first student chapter of VOSH was formed at the New England College of Optometry in 1984. By 2019, there were more than 80 VOSH chapters, providing professional volunteer eyecare worldwide to people in need.[39]

The National Association of Veterans Administration Optometrists (NAVAO) was founded in 1977. The goals of the NAVAO are "to encourage and promote the best possible primary eye and vision care for our nation's Veterans and to promote the education, training, professional growth, and welfare of optometrists, staff, research/clinical fellows, residents, and students."[40] The first president of NAVAO was Robert Newcomb, who served in that position from 1977 to 1983.

The Neuro-Optometric Rehabilitation Association (NORA) was formed in 1990 with William Padula as president.[41] NORA held its first symposium in Atlanta, Georgia, in 1992. NORA encourages an interdisciplinary approach to the rehabilitation of vision problems associated with traumatic brain injury and other neurological insults.[41]

INTRODUCTION OF COMPULSORY CONTINUING EDUCATION

From the early decades of the twentieth century, national organizations, such as the American Optometric Association, the American Academy of Optometry, and the Optometric Extension Program, offered opportunities for practicing optometrists to expand their knowledge and skills.[42,43,44,45] Regional organizations have also provided continuing education for many years. For example, the Southern Council of Optometrists held its first meeting in Greenville, South Carolina, in 1924, the Heart of America Congress first met in Kansas City in 1962, and in 1966, the North Central States Optometric Council had its first educational conference.[46,47,48] But for much of the twentieth century, there was no requirement of continuing education for maintenance of licensure.

The first state to require optometrists to attend continuing education was Iowa, where a law passed in 1938 established the requirement of two days or 12 hours of continuing education per year.[49] Kansas was the second state, with a law passed in 1940.

It is thought that a 1971 report of the Department of Health, Education, and Welfare (HEW) to Congress on the licensure of health manpower may have led to efforts toward mandatory continuing education of health professionals.[50] HEW acknowledged that optometry led all health professionals in requiring continuing education attendance for license renewal.[51] By 1985, optometrists in 46 states had requirements for continuing education compared to nine states for dentists, 20 states for doctors of medicine, and 21 states for pharmacists.[52]

INCREASED USE OF OPTOMETRIC TECHNICIANS

For the first half of the twentieth century it was quite common for optometrists to not have employees, even for receptionist or secretarial duties. A 1958 survey in a large (unidentified) state found that the percentages of optometrists who did not have an assistant were 75% among those who had been in practice less than three years, 40% of those in practice for 10 to 12 years, and 30% of those in practice for more than 19 years.[53] In the 1960s, there was a perceived shortage of optometrists for the U.S. population.[54,55] One of the suggestions for addressing the shortage was increased efficiency of optometry practices through the employment of ancillary personnel.

In 1967, the *Journal of the American Optometric Association* published papers debating whether optometric technicians should assist optometrists by performing some portion of examination testing. Ralph Wick of Rapid City, South Dakota, argued for the affirmative, and E. C. Nurock of Trenton, New Jersey, argued for the negative. Wick put forth that freeing optometrists from time spent on routine duties would allow them to practice at the level of their training, resulting in better vision care.[56] However, he did caution that "optometry has continued to exist because of the completeness of its vision care by one individual. That service can be degraded if too many tests are delegated to technicians." Wick emphasized that technicians should be well trained.

Nurock argued that testing should be performed by the optometrist because it takes an experienced clinician to recognize the information gained from the way patients answer questions during testing as well as from the numerical results of those tests. Nurock stated that "nothing that requires professional judgment should be delegated to anyone except a person licensed in that field."[56]

Consideration of the nature and training of paraoptometric personnel in the 1970s led to the identification and definition of three levels of personnel.[57] (1) *Optometric assistants* did not require formal university training of a technical nature and typically worked in reception and secretarial functions. (2) *Optometric technicians* had training at the Associate of Arts level or the equivalent. They could also be considered optometric technicians by gaining technical experience. In the 1970s, it was widely recognized that optometric technicians could be delegated to tasks such as frame selection, dispensing and adjustment of spectacles, maintenance of patient records, patient instruction on contact lens care, and the performance of tests such as visual acuity, color vision testing, stereopsis, and visual fields screening.[56,58,59] (3) The *optometric technologist* would have training at the Bachelor's level or higher and would have specialty functions more suited to optometric education or industry than to private practice.[57]

The first academic program for optometric assistants was started in 1966 at Merritt College in Oakland, California.[57] Training programs increased in number over the next decade but subsequently decreased. There were 23 two-year Associate's degree programs for paraoptometric training in 1977, 14 in 1986, and only seven in 1992.[60] There were eight two-year optometric technician educational programs offered by, or associated with, optometry schools in 1981, but by 1992 there were only two.[57,60] Although the graduates of optometric technician programs at optometry schools readily found employment, these programs closed because of relatively low enrollments and the expense of maintaining the programs.[60,61]

By the end of the twentieth century, optometric technicians, many of whom were trained by the doctors for whom they worked, had become fixtures in optometric practice. The first educational program at the American Optometric Association annual congress, specifically for paraoptometric personnel, was given in 1974; and in 1978, the AOA formed the Paraoptometric Section.[62] In 2000, the AOA established the Commission on Paraoptometric Certification (CPC).[63] By 2011, more than 5,000 paraoptometrics had achieved certification at one of three levels.[63]

IMPROVED STANDING OF OPTOMETRISTS IN THE MILITARY

At the entry of the United States into World War II in 1941, optometry had no standing in the Army or Navy, and optometrists who were drafted were treated the same as other draftees.[64] Some optometrists applied to Officer Candidate School and became officers, but they served in capacities other than practicing optometry.[65] Some enlisted optometrists were placed in the Army Medical Department to perform refractions, but with the rank of private, they didn't get the cooperation and respect they would have had they been officers.[66,67,68]

In 1942, the American Optometric Association started pressing for officer status for optometrists and hired Washington attorney William P. MacCracken to assist in those efforts. The commissioning of optometrists was opposed by organized ophthalmology and the American Medical Association.[66] However, the Navy became convinced to commission some optometrists as ensigns in the Hospital Specialists Corps during World War II, and by the end of the war about 120 were on active duty. A few optometrists served as Aviation Specialists in Recognition (AVSIR) to teach gunners how to quickly and correctly visually identify enemy aircraft. The training they provided was highly successful in helping gunners reduce the number of friendly aircraft they shot down.[64] P.N. DeVere, who later was president of the AOA in 1959-60, was one of those who served as an AVSIR.

Late in World War II, in 1945, the AOA worked to have a bill introduced into Congress that would create an Optometry Corps of 60 officers. The House and the Senate both passed the bill, but the Army Surgeon General convinced President Truman to veto it.[64]

The Military Reorganization Act of 1947 did help optometry gain some recognition. Upon entrance into the military, Army and Air Force optometrists would be commissioned as second lieutenants (the Air Force became a separate branch of the U.S. military in 1947), and Navy optometrists would be commissioned as ensigns. The Army created a Medical Service Corps with an Optometry Section in 1947, and John W. Sheridan became the first optometrist commissioned as an officer in the U. S. Army.[68] The Air Force Medical Service was formed in 1949, and optometrists began to be commissioned as Air Force officers that year.[69]

The commissioning of optometrists in the Army started slowly, and with the onset of the Korean War in 1950, there was a shortage of optometrists. The AOA complained that the Army reverted to "old habits" when it drafted optometrists and used them as enlisted soldiers to work as optometrists.[68] The Army's use of enlisted optometrists finally ended in 1957, well after the end of the Korean War, and subsequently the Army employed only commissioned optometrists.[68]

With the involvement of the United States in the Vietnam War in the 1960s, demand for optometrists once again escalated. In 1968, the Army started including optometrists in combat divisions, with two optometrists and two optical technicians per division.[64] There were 28 optometrists in Vietnam by 1969, and a total of about 150 served there during that conflict.[64,68] Many of the optometrists in Vietnam found themselves called upon out of necessity to use therapeutic pharmaceutical agents, not yet authorized in civilian optometric practice to treat various ocular conditions. Some of those optometrists became active in working for the passage of optometric TPA laws in their home states upon their return to civilian life.

A sore spot for military optometrists in the 1970s was that unlike physicians and dentists, they were not commissioned as captains. That was rectified with the passage of the Defense Officer Personnel Management Act of 1980.[68]

The Uniformed Services Health Professions Revitalization Act of 1972 established the Health Professions Scholarship Program that has helped with optometry school expenses for many students in exchange for service as commissioned officers.[70,71] Except for being briefly discontinued from 1985 to 1991, this program has operated through most of the last five decades. Optometry student externships began to be available at Armed Forces bases in the late 1970s. By 1995, the Air Force, for example, had optometry student externships at 29 bases affiliated with 13 optometry schools.[70] After optometry residencies became well established, some residencies with the Armed Forces were organized. For example, the United States Air Force optometry residency began in 1989.[72]

In summarizing the history of Army optometry through the end of the twentieth century, Ginn noted that optometry's story in gaining recognition and acceptance "was not a straight line development, but rather an up and down saga of gains and losses."[68] Ultimately, optometry was successful because "time and again, the United States found that the support of soldiers in combat necessitated a medical team that included officers skilled in administrative and scientific specialties, such as optometry."[68]

OPTOMETRY IN THE DEPARTMENT OF VETERANS AFFAIRS

In 1946, Veterans Administration (VA) hospitals established affiliations with medical schools and dental schools,[73,74,75] and a few optometrists were appointed to VA staffs in 1947. A federal law passed in 1957 established authority for the employment of more optometrists, but as late as 1976, there were still only eight full-time optometrists in the entire VA system. The underutilization of optometry was due, in large part, to the opposition of organized ophthalmology and medical schools, who viewed the VA hospitals as their domain.[73] It didn't help that optometry at that time had little experience in hospital settings.

In about 1970, Henry B. Peters, dean of the University of Alabama, Birmingham (UAB), School of Optometry, entered into discussions with the VA concerning a program for clinical training of optometry students.

In 1972, it was announced that such a program would begin through the affiliation between the UAB School of Optometry, the UAB Medical Center, and the Birmingham VA Hospital.[76] The Optometry Service in the Birmingham VA Hospital started seeing patients in January 1973, with Jeffrey T. Keller as its chief.[77]

In 1975, an optometric residency program was begun at the Kansas City VA Medical Center through the work of David M. Amos, OD, and Albert N. Lemoine, MD. The first optometrist to complete the program was Thomas J. Stelmack. This became the first optometric residency program accredited by the Council on Optometric Education.[78]

In 1976, federal legislation mandated appointment of optometrists to the VA and establishment of optometric educational programs affiliated with schools of optometry, but progress was slow. In 1977, a joint report of the American Optometric Association and the Association of Schools and Colleges of Optometry urged the incorporation of optometric care and educational programs into the VA system. Also in 1977, the Southern California College of Optometry received a training grant, which, in part, made possible documentation of how optometry was being used in the VA system and of the unmet eye care needs. In 1978, the U.S. General Accounting Office issued a report titled "Role and Utilization of Optometry in the VA Need Improvement." Later in 1978, Congress stressed its expectation that optometry be fully integrated into the VA system, leading to funding for appointment of optometrists and affiliations with optometry schools.[73]

In the 1980s, the number of optometric residencies in the VA system increased, so that by 1987, there were 46 positions,[79] 70 percent of which were hospital-based. By 2009, there were 600 optometrists, more than 1,000 optometry students, and 145 optometry residents providing care and learning in VA facilities.[75]

OPTOMETRY IN THE INDIAN HEALTH SERVICE

The Indian Health Service (IHS) is a bureau of the United States Public Health Service and provides care to American Indians and Alaska Natives. It was founded in 1955, when health services were transferred from the Department of the Interior's Bureau of Indian Affairs.[80] Initially, the IHS eye program emphasized the elimination of trachoma, with care provided by an IHS ophthalmologist, and a few private optometrists and ophthalmologists.[81,82] The campaign against trachoma was successful, and in the 1970s, program emphasis shifted to student examinations, with examinations of smaller children and adults given when possible.

The first IHS optometrist was hired in 1966, and by 1968, there were five IHS optometrists. By 1990, there were more than 60 IHS optometry clinics across the continental western United States and Alaska. Optometry has been well accepted by the IHS administration and patients. An optometry school clinic was established in conjunction with the IHS and the Cherokee Nation, soon after the start of the College of Optometry at Northeastern State University in Tahlequah, Oklahoma, in 1979.[83] Since then, externship and residency programs have been set up at IHS clinics in affiliation with several optometry schools. IHS optometrists made extensive early use of therapeutic pharmaceutical agents and were among the first optometrists to attain hospital privileges.[84]

OPTOMETRY'S INVOLVEMENT IN PUBLIC HEALTH

The field of public health had its origin in efforts to control epidemics, and it evolved into more comprehensive consideration for the health and well-being of populations, encompassing areas such as health care administration, epidemiology, health manpower, health economics, health care planning, environmental health, and occupational health.[85] As projects such as the development of procedures for vision screening of elementary school children and studies of visual factors in industrial performance were conducted in the 1950s, it became obvious that optometry had an obligation to engage with the public health arena, not only for the sake of the standing of the profession but also for the visual welfare of society.[86]

In the 1950s, the American Optometric Association formed its Committee on Social and Health Care Trends through the leadership of A. N. Haffner and Felix Koetting; in 1958, it changed the name of that group to the Committee on Public Health and Optometric Care.[87,88,89] In 1963, the AOA became an agency member of the American Public Health Association (APHA).[90] In the 1960s and 1970s, optometry schools started adding courses on public health to their curricula, and optometrists started completing graduate programs for the Master of Public Health (MPH) degree.[86,89]

In 1974, the AOA Committee on Public Health and Optometric Care asked the APHA to establish an Optometric Health Section, but the APHA board deferred action on the request. In 1979, through efforts of optometrist members of the APHA, the Vision Care Section was created.[89] Burton H. Skuza, OD, was the first to chair the Vision Care Section.[90] At about the same time, the American Academy of Optometry created a Section on Public Health and Environmental Vision.[91]

Between 1979 and 1997, the Vision Care Section of the APHA sponsored 16 resolutions that were approved by the APHA Governing Council. Among these were resolutions that optometry should be included in Medicare and that state legislatures should be encouraged to update optometry laws to allow use of therapeutic pharmaceutical agents by optometrists who had completed the appropriate training.[89,92]

By 1999, there were more than 150 optometrists with MPH degrees. As an indication of the respect that optometry has gained within the public health field, in 2011, an optometrist, Melvin D. Shipp, was elected president of the APHA.[93] By 2000, A. N. Haffner could state: "That optometry is now more centrally placed in the mainstream of health care services is evident in a host of daily circumstances and, indeed, by its work and by its institutional focus as a public health profession in the public service."[91]

OPTOMETRIC PARITY IN MEDICARE

Medicare was established in 1965, but examination services by optometrists were originally excluded. Initially, the only optometric service covered by Medicare was the fitting and provision of lenses for aphakic patients.[94] Medicare did reimburse ophthalmologists, or other doctors of medicine or osteopathy, for examinations for symptoms of eye disease or injury.[95] The American Optometric Association worked to try to achieve inclusion in Medicare but for many years met with little success.[96] Legislation passed in 1980 expanded coverage for optometric service to include examination procedures, other than the refraction, for aphakic patients.

Starting in April 1987, optometry finally achieved parity under Medicare. Optometrists could then be reimbursed for services they were authorized to perform in the state they practiced.[95] The turning point came when Congresswoman Barbara Mikulski, who knew of the abilities of optometrists from her friend and AOA Board of Trustees member, Egon Werthamer, negotiated the addition of a provision to the 1986 Budget Reconciliation Bill that optometrists be included as physicians for the purposes of Medicare.[67,96] This achievement of recognition of optometrists as physicians with Medicare parity is often seen as one of optometry's most significant milestones.[67]

Medicare became a significant part of many optometry practices. In 2004, optometrists received 611 million dollars from Medicare, and in 2011, optometrists served 5.7 million Medicare patients.[7]

THE COMANAGEMENT MOVEMENT

For much of the twentieth century, it was necessary for optometrists to refer all cases of ocular disease to ophthalmologists for diagnosis and treatment. Some optometrists were able to form trusting relationships with ophthalmologists; in these relationships, reports and communications between the referring optometrist and the ophthalmologist moved in both directions in a respectful manner. However, many optometrists found that referred patients did not return to them.

The concern over loss of patients and the confusion, inconvenience, and expense experienced by patients led some members of the Board of Trustees and alumni association of the Southern College of Optometry to form the Vision Educational Foundation (VEF) for comanagement of patients.[97] VEF was formed as a nonprofit, independent organization in 1972 and was granted tax-exempt status in 1974. VEF opened an Eye Center in Atlanta, Georgia, in 1980 and another in Oklahoma City, Oklahoma, in 1985.

The VEF centers were directed by an optometric board and an on-site optometrist. Ophthalmologists were hired for secondary and tertiary level care. Referring optometrists would have their patients returned to them for post-surgical care and all primary care.[98]

The VEF disbanded in 1997, but the VEF system provided a useful model for interprofessional cooperation, encouraging both optometrists and ophthalmologists to practice at the full extent of their training and to continue to enhance their skills. By 2014, more than 18 similar centers had opened across the country.[98] Some ophthalmologists also embraced an analogous model in opening clinics where they employ optometrists to handle all non-surgical cases so that they can concentrate on doing surgeries. This became an increasingly popular form of employment for graduating optometrists.

INCREASE IN OPTOMETRIC RESEARCH

The research output of optometry has increased steadily since the 1920s and 1930s. One metric to illustrate this is the number of papers in the journal published by the American Academy of Optometry (variously titled the *American Journal of Optometry and Archives of the American Academy of Optometry*, the *American Journal of Optometry and Physiological Optics*, and *Optometry and Vision Science*). In the 10-year span of the 1930s and again in the 1940s, it published fewer than 500 papers.[99] In the 1970s, it published almost 1,500 papers, and in the 1980s, the count was well over 2,000. Beginning in the 1940s and 1950s, optometry has been the leader in research on refractive errors, accommodation and convergence function, vision therapy, and contact lenses.

In the late 1980s and early 1990s, there were calls for increased research in optometry. Sivak[100] acknowledged that research was being done at all optometry schools, but he suggested that "a primary care profession consisting of over 30,000 North American practitioners should be capable of doing more." The American Optometric Association created its Council on Research in 1986, and a few years later, it polled representatives from state optometric associations, optometry schools, and various optometric organizations about research objectives for optometry. The respondents gave the highest priorities to research in pediatrics and developmental vision, binocular vision and vision therapy, the aging eye, and preventive eye care, but they also recognized the need for research on refractive anomalies, contact lenses, environmental vision, ocular disease, and low vision.[101]

Myers[102] suggested that optometry should concentrate its resources on clinical research rather than basic biological science studies. In contrast, Jennings[103] argued that optometry should do research in basic medical sciences because optometrists had started prescribing medications for the treatment of eye diseases. Flom[104] advised that "we need to recognize the importance of both basic and applied research in the overall scientific enterprise." Zadnik[105] argued that "fields advance the fastest and achieve the most when the basic scientist and the patient-based researcher work on parallel tracks and eventually converge, when the clinician feeds patient-based observations or hypotheses to both areas for testing and examination."

Another source of concern in the late 1980s was that optometry was not obtaining as much funding as it should from the National Eye Institute (NEI), the largest funding source for eye and vision research. However, optometry was relatively successful in receiving funding from the applications that were submitted. Myers[106] reported that from 1982 to 1987, 68% of optometry applications to NEI were funded, better than the 46% for all NEI applications. But only about 3% of the grant awards went to optometry during that time period. Myers suggested that optometry actually was doing well because there were only 16 optometry schools compared to over 100 departments of ophthalmology and hundreds of departments of anatomy, biology, psychology, and other fields that do eye research. Optometry has continued to be successful in obtaining funding from NEI: for example, designing and participating in large multicenter studies on various topics, such as keratoconus, myopia, refractive development, vision in preschoolers, low vision, and convergence insufficiency,[107,108,109,110,111,112] each of which resulted in multiple publications. Optometry's research output continued to increase in the late twentieth century and into the twenty-first. The number of pages in the American Academy of Optometry's journal, over 10-year periods, increased from 9,850 in the 1980s to 13,459 pages in the 2010s. Optometrists and researchers at optometric institutions also increasingly published in ophthalmology and basic science journals.

Since the passage of laws allowing optometrists to use pharmaceutical agents, optometry has increased research in ocular disease and the underlying basic sciences. For example, a perusal of the annual indexes of the American Academy of Optometry's journal shows that in 1969, there were fewer than 10 papers on ocular disease, physiology, and pharmacology, but in 2004, there were more than 30. This trend continued as evidenced by the fact that between 2011 and 2015, *Optometry and Vision Science* published feature issues, each of which included 20 or more papers, on glaucoma, age-related macular degeneration, and dry eye disease, in addition to other disease-related papers published regularly. Optometry has also continued to publish papers on refractive anomalies, binocular vision, and contact lenses in a number of different journals.

EXPANSION OF PRE-OPTOMETRY AND OPTOMETRY CURRICULA

By 1967, all optometry schools had increased their requirements to two years of pre-optometry study and four years of optometry school. By the late 1990s, the standard for pre-optometry work had become four years. In 2000, A. N. Haffner, writing about the evolution of optometry in the twentieth century, could state that "the major progenitor of change was undoubtedly the establishment and enhancement of the structured system of formal professional and scientific education of the optometrist….Today, all schools and colleges of optometry are professional programs of 4 years duration, constructed upon prior baccalaureate undergraduate experience with appropriate concentration in advanced sciences and mathematics."[91]

In the late twentieth century, optometry school curricula bulged with increased coverage of ocular disease and pharmacology as well as greater time spent in clinic.[113,114] Decreases in coverage of optical science were minimal because of the recognition that optical treatments remained the core of optometric care and because of the advent of new technologies in clinical observation, measurement, and treatment.[115,116,117,118] The responsiveness and leadership of optometry schools in modifying and enhancing their curricula has been, as Haffner noted, a key element in the advancement of optometry. The history of optometric education is discussed further in Chapter 6.

CONTINUING EXPANSION OF SCOPE OF PRACTICE

The previous chapter noted that the first state to pass legislation granting optometrists the privilege of using diagnostic pharmaceutical agents (DPAs) was Rhode Island in 1971, the first therapeutic pharmaceutical agent (TPA) legislation was passed in West Virginia in 1976, and the second TPA legislation was passed in North Carolina in 1977. It wasn't until 1989 that all states and the District of Columbia had DPA laws, and it was 1998 when all states and D.C. had TPA laws.[119] The agents that could be used varied considerably according to the laws passed in the different states. The 1977 North Carolina TPA law, for example, included glaucoma medications, oral drugs, and injectable agents[120] while the West Virgina TPA law included glaucoma medications but did not include oral drugs or injectable agents.[120] It was not until 2004 that 49 of 50 states had glaucoma treatment authority.[121] By 2018, there was authority for injectable agents in 38 of 50 states.[121] The first legislation to provide specific authorization for removal of superficial foreign bodies from the eye and adnexa was passed in 1985 in Iowa.[120] In 1998, Oklahoma became the first state to have a law authorizing optometrists to use lasers for certain treatment purposes, and in 2011, Kentucky became the second state where optometrists had privileges to use lasers for certain surgical procedures.[119,121] Between 1971 and 2011, there were more than 180 legislative expansions of optometric scope of practice into medical eye care, some of them small incremental changes.[120]

Borish wrote that optometrists "should be quite pleased with the expansion of the scope of optometry" but "must be careful not to leave a vacuum in the leadership role in refractive care."[122] Similarly an author of a much later generation, Benjamin Casella, recently wrote that we should not "lose sight of the foundation from whence we came. Vision science is—and has traditionally been—a defining attribute of optometry which separates us and makes us exceptionally special to health care. Let us also not lose sight of the fact that optometry would have never come into existence without…glasses."[123] Like Borish's exhortation that an expansion of scope of practice is better than a shift in scope away from optometry's traditional strengths, Casella advocates focus on vision care as well as on disease.[123]

In considering the effects of optometry's expansion of scope as well as its greater integration into the health care system, increased research output, and other changes in the late twentieth century and into more recent years, it is interesting to note the perspective of Irving Bennett, who practiced optometry from 1946 to 1992. Bennett was editor of the *Journal of the American Optometric Association* and of *Optometric Management* magazine, co-founder of OptiFair, and president of the Optometric Historical Society, among many other optometric leadership positions. Writing in 2016, he said that the biggest change in optometry that he had observed since he had started practice was improvement in image.[67] He noted that early in his career, most city newspapers followed the guidelines of the national *AP Stylebook* in not referring to an optometrist as doctor. He contrasted that with the fact that *U.S. News and World Report* has more recently included optometry in its list of the 25 best jobs.[124] Bennett also pointed to the inclusion of optometrists in the definition of physician for Medicare reimbursementas as a major milestone for optometry.

Despite optometry's underdog status in the health care system at times in its history, it must be acknowledged that optometrists have always had a very important role in society in guarding and improving people's vision. Recognition of that role, as well as a perspective from the long view of a study of optometry history, led Henry Hofstetter to proclaim his appreciation for "optometry's centuries-long existence and emergence from a prestigious and sophisticated handicraft to its present academic stature, a truly proud history."[125]

Chapter 4: Notes

1. Hofstetter HW. *Optometry: Professional, Economic, and Legal Aspects*. St. Louis, MO: Mosby, 1948:313-314.
2. Hirsch MJ, Wick RE. *The Optometric Profession*. Philadelphia, PA: Chilton, 1968:347.
3. Bennett I, Barresi BJ, Edlow RC, Nussenblatt H, Aron F. *Caring for the Eyes of America: A Profile of the Optometric Profession 1991*. St. Louis, MO: American Optometric Association, 1991:4-7.
4. Bennett I, Edlow RC, Stuckey C Jr, Aron F. *Caring for the Eyes of America: A Profile of the Optometric Profession 1992*. St. Louis, MO: American Optometric Association, 1992:5-9.
5. Bennett I, Aron F. *Caring for the Eyes of America: A Profile of the Optometric Profession 1998*. St. Louis, MO: American Optometric Association, 1998:7-16.
6. American Optometric Association. *The State of the Optometric Profession: 2013*. www.aoa.org/Documents/news/state_of_optometry.pdf
7. U.S. Bureau of Labor Statistics. *Occupational Statistics: Optometrists*. www.bls.gov/oes/current/oes291041.htm
8. White AJ, White C, Doksum T. *Workforce Study of Optometrists: Final Report*. Cambridge, MA: Abt Associates, 2000:A-3.
9. Goss DA. History of the Indiana University Division of Optometry. *Indiana J Optom*. 2003;6:28-74.
10. Kovacich S. The changing student body at the IU School of Optometry. *Indiana J Optom*. 2004;7:36.
11. American Optometric Association. The future is female. *Inside Optometry News*, 2019. www.aoa.org/news/inside-optometry/the-future-is-female
12. Classé JG. *Legal Aspects of Optometry*. Boston, MA: Butterworths, 1989:21.
13. Hirsch & Wick, 228-229.
14. Elmstrom GP. *Optometric Practice Management*. Radnor, PA: Chilton, 1963:263.
15. Edlow RC, Brost KE, Edmonds SA, Hoppe ES, Kowalczyk B, Markus GR. *Caring for the Eyes of America: A Profile of the Optometric Profession 2002*. St. Louis, MO: American Optometric Association, 2002:14-17.
16. American Optometric Association. *2015 AOA Survey of Optometric Practice*. 2016. www.aoa.org/Documents/ric/2015IncomeFromOptometryExecutiveSummary_FINAL.pdf
17. American Optometric Association. *2017 AOA Survey of Optometric Practice*. 2018. www.aoa.org/Documents/2017_Practicing_ExecutiveSummary.pdf
18. Hofstetter, 156-157.
19. Grosvenor TP, Goss DA. The traditional examination: Still an important source of optometric income. *Optom Economics*. 1997;7(1):40-43.
20. Grosvenor T, Goss DA. A survey of Indiana University School of Optometry alumni. *Optom Ed*. 1998;23:114-120.

21. Edlow RC, Elliott LE, Ferrucci RR, Hoppe ES, Bennett I, Kowalczyk B, Markus GR. *Caring for the Eyes of America: A Profile of the Optometric Profession 2000.* St. Louis, MO: American Optometric Association, 2000:10-20.
22. Mantorp C. 2018 income survey: Where do you stand? *Rev Optom.* Dec. 15, 2018. www.reviewofoptometry.com/article/2018-income-survey-where-do-you-stand
23. Bleything WB. The optometric residency: Its bloom. *J Optom Ed.* 1979;5:16-21.
24. Suchoff I. The first year-long optometric residency education program. *Hindsight* 2010;41:122-125.
25. Estren H. Recollections of participation in the first year-long optometric residency program. *Hindsight* 2010;41:126-128.
26. Amos JF. A brief history of optometric residency education. *J Am Optom Assoc.* 1987;58:374-376.
27. Amos JF. What role will residency education take in the profession by the year 2000? *J Am Optom Assoc.* 1992;63:787-789.
28. Association of Schools and Colleges of Optometry. *FAQs about Residencies. 2019.* www.optometriceducation.org/students-future-students/residency-programs/faqs-about-residencies/
29. Myers RI. The origins of the American Optometric Student Association. *Hindsight* 2017;48:90-95.
30. Ferrucci RR. AOSA: The formative years and beyond: A capsule summary of the years 1971-74. *Hindsight* 2017;48:96-102.
31. Quint JM. The American Optometric Student Association in the 2010s. *Hindsight* 2017;48:114-115.
32. National Optometric Association. *Our history.* https://nationaloptometricassociation.com/about-us/our-history
33. Hofstetter HW. How and when we began. *Newsletter Optom Hist Soc.* 1997;8:55-57.
34. Goss DA. 20/20 hindsight: A history of the Optometric Historical Society as chronicled in its newsletter and journal. *Hindsight* 2019;50:4-12.
35. American Optometric Association. *History of Optometry.* https://fs.aoa.org/optometry-archives/optometry-timeline.html
36. Armed Forces Optometric Society. *History. 2020.* www.afos2020.org/aws/AFOS/pt/sp/history
37. Press L. COVD: Recapitulating 40 years of excellence. *Optom Vis Dev.* 2010;41:137-142.
38. Wold RM. COVD: The first 25 years. *J Optom Vis Dev.* 1995;26:177-189.
39. VOSH International. *Milestones in VOSH history. 2019.* www.vosh.org/milestones-in-vosh-history/?lang=en
40. NAVAO. *About us.* www.navao.org/about-us
41. Neuro-Optometric Rehabiliation Association. *About NORA. 2020.* www.noravisionrehab.org/about-nora

42 Hébert K. A century of continuing education: The American Optometric Association's distance learning program at 100. *Hindsight* 2019;50:103-109.
43 Gregg JR. *History of the American Academy of Optometry 1922-1986*. Washington, DC: American Academy of Optometry, 1987.
44 Hoare AE. The Duncan Diary. Part I, The Optometric Extension Program. The first forty years. *Optom World*. 1967;54(5):10,12,15,16,20.
45 Milkie GM. Optometric Extension Program: An established model for continuing education. *J Am Optom Assoc*. 1978;49:617-622.
46 Hofstetter HW. Fifty years of continuing education. *Newsletter Optom Hist Soc*. 1983;14:87.
47 Heart of America Eye Care Congress. HOAECC History. 2019. www.hoaecc.org/our_history.cfm
48 North Central States Optometric Council. *History*. www.ncsoc.org/history/
49 Robinson JD. [Untitled] Pre-conference paper, Williamsburg Conference of Continuing Education, American Optometric Association, Williamsburg, Virginia. November 27-29, 1972.
50 Shimberg B. Assuring the continued competence of licensed optometrists: A modest proposal. *J Am Optom Assoc*. 1984;55:786-788.
51 Cohen HS. The HEW view. *Am J Optom Physiol Opt*. 1980;57:336-338.
52 Classé JG. *Legal Aspects of Optometry*. Boston, MA: Butterworths, 1989:165-167.
53 Elmstrom, 78-79.
54 Morgret F. Optometric education in the United States. *J Am Optom Assoc*. 1963;34:785-795.
55 Baldwin WR. Do we need more schools of optometry? *J Am Optom Assoc*. 1967;38:293-296.
56 Wick RE, Nurock EC. Debate – Resolved: The optometric profession approved the use of the optometric assistant (technologist) and that these personnel be formally trained in the performance of ancillary optometric duties. *J Am Optom Assoc*. 1967;38:27-38.
57 Scott M. Education of the paraoptometric. *J Am Optom Assoc*. 1981;52:31-34.
58 Grosvenor T. The role of the technician in optometric practice. *J Am Optom Assoc*. 1975;46:1265-1272.
59 Muhr CE. The technician in optometric practice. *J Am Optom Assoc*. 1977;48:69-74.
60 Pickel SC. What is and what will be the need for formally educated optometric technicians? *J Am Optom Assoc*. 1992;63:870-872.
61 Saladin JJ, Carter RL. *Vision Realized: A History of the MCO*. Big Rapids, MI: Ferris State University Michigan College of Optometry, 2012:62.
62 AOA Paraoptometric Section. The bridge between the AOA Paraoptometric Section and you! (undated PowerPoint slide presentation) www.pdfs.semanticscholar.org/
63 Luebbert J. A new option for paraoptometrics. *Optom*. 2011;82:5-6.

64 Lang GL, Jr. Recollections of 60 years of the history of optometry. *J Am Optom Assoc.* 1989;60:391-404.
65 Mahlman HE. Optometry in the military. *Newsletter Optom Hist Soc.* 1982;13:17-18.
66 Osborn M, Riggs J. *Mr. Mac: William P. MacCracken Jr. on Aviation Law Optometry.* Memphis, TN: Southern College of Optometry, 1970:193-195.
67 Bennett I. A witness to history. *Rev Optom.* July 21, 2016. www.reviewofoptometry.com/article/a-witness-to-history
68 Ginn RVN. *Army Optometrists: From World War I through the Cold War.* Office of Medical History, Office of the Surgeon General, Department of the Army, 2003.
69 Sloan AM. Letter to the Editor: Air Force optometry. *J Am Optom Assoc.* 1995;68:668-669.
70 Wong D. Two military programs available to the optometry student: The Armed Forces Health Professions Scholarship Program and the Optometry Externship Program. *J Am Optom Assoc.* 1995;66:214-217.
71 Sem SR. Air Force optometry: An overview. *J Am Optom Assoc.* 1995;66:204-205.
72 Kent JF. The United States Air Force optometry residency program. *J Am Optom Assoc.* 1995;66:206-207.
73 Myers KJ. Public health and the Department of Veterans Affairs. In: Hatch S, Whitener JC, McAlister WH, Block S, eds. *Optometric Care within the Public Health Community.* Cadyville, NY: Old Post Publishing, 2010:1-34.
74 Interview: From the Inside: VA's Myers on the growth of optometry. *J Optom Ed.* 1977;3(1):9-12.
75 Newcomb RD. History of optometry in the VA. *Hindsight* 2010;41:6-8.
76 Amos JF. The genesis of the optometry training program in the Birmingham Veterans Affairs Hospital. *Hindsight* 2013;44:50-70.
77 Keller JT. Optometry training in a Veterans Administration hospital. *Am J Optom Physiol Opt.* 1974;51:425-428.
78 Amos JF. A brief history of optometric residency education. *J Am Optom Assoc.* 1987;58:374-376.
79 Maino JH, Messer TI, Messer DH. Veterans Administration residency programs: An overview. *J Am Optom Assoc.* 1987;58:378-380.
80 Rhoades ER, Reyes LL, Buzzard GD. The organization of health services for Indian people. *Public Health Rep.* 1987;102:352-356.
81 Caplan L. The American Indian: The long road to eye care. *J Am Optom Assoc.* 1978;49:203-205.
82 Ashby E. Indian Health Service eye care manpower and services. In: Goss DA, Edmondson LL, eds. *Eye and Vision Conditions in the American Indian.* Yukon, OK: Pueblo Publishing Press, 1990:167-172.
83 Schmitt EP. Vision care to Indian people in Northeastern Oklahoma: History and development of Northeastern State University College of Optometry vision ser-

vices. In: Goss DA, Edmondson LL, eds. *Eye and Vision Conditions in the American Indian.* Yukon, OK: Pueblo Publishing Press, 1990:191-203.

84 Caplan L. "I" to eye: 66 years of optometry through the eyes of a clinician, educator, administrator, consultant, and public health optometrist. *Hindsight* 2016;48:5-24,74-75.

85 Marshall EC. The optometrist's role in public health. *J Am Optom Assoc.* 1982;53:371-378.

86 Peters HB. Public health and the practicing optometrist: In: Newcomb RD, Jolley JL, eds. *Public Health and Community Optometry.* Springfield, IL: Charles C. Thomas, 1980:12-18.

87 Haffner AN. Optometric milestones in the public health movement. In: Newcomb RD, Jolley JL, eds. *Public Health and Community Optometry.* Springfield, IL: Charles C. Thomas, 1980:5-11.

88 Whitener JC. A link to the future for community/public health programs. *J Am Optom Assoc.* 1982;53:829-831.

89 Caplan L. Optometry and the American Public Health Association. *J Am Optom Assoc.* 1999;70:703-714.

90 Silverman MW. An historic overview of the American Public Health Association and optometric establishment of the Vision Care Section. *J Am Optom Assoc.* 1994;65:94-97.

91 Haffner AN. What has changed? *Optom Vis Sci.* 2000;77:165-167.

92 Wolfberg MD. A profession's commitment to increased public service: Optometry's remarkable story. *J Am Optom Assoc.* 1999;70:145-170.

93 Newcomb RD. *Our History in Focus: The First 100 Years of The Ohio State University College of Optometry.* Columbus, OH: The Ohio State University, 2014:168.

94 Jolley JL. Review of federal law and regulations: Reimbursement under Medicare. *J Am Optom Assoc.* 1983;54:743-750.

95 Garland N. Optometric parity legislation under Medicare. *J Am Optom Assoc.* 1987;58:518-519.

96 Bennett I. My recollections of how optometry got into Medicare. *Hindsight* 2016;47:49-51.

97 Bucar AA. Our ophthalmic heritage: The beginning of ophthalmic comanagement. *J Am Optom Assoc.* 1995;66:10-11.

98 Bucar AA. Ophthalmic comanagement and optometry. *Hindsight* 2014;45:59-61.

99 Lyle WM, Williams TD, Chase WW. A six-decade topical survey of journal articles. *Optom Vis Sci.* 1992;69:745-746.

100 Sivak JG. Invited editorial: Optometry and vision science. *Optom Vis Sci.* 1989;66:2-3.

101 Bleything WB. Establishing national research objectives in optometry: A report of the Council on Research, American Optometric Association. *J Am Optom Assoc.* 1989;60:348-350.

102 Myers KJ. Optometry research. Part 1: Funding sources. *Optom Vis Sci.* 1992;69:728-738.

103 Jennings BJ. Basic science research in optometry: Are we adequately prepared? *J Am Optom Assoc.* 1992;63:844-846.

104 Flom MC. Comparing basic and clinical research: A dilemma. *Optom Vis Sci.* 1998;75:384-387.

105 Zadnik K. Guest editorial: Research vs. research. *Optom Vis Sci.* 1998;75:375.

106 Myers KJ. More research, yes! But what kind? *J Am Optom Assoc.* 1989;60:815-819.

107 Wagner H, Barr JT, Zadnik K. Collaborative Longitudinal Evaluation of Keratoconus (CLEK) Study: Methods and findings to date. *Contact Lens Anterior Eye* 2007;30:223-232.

108 Gwiazda J, Marsh-Tootle WL, Hyman L, et al. Baseline refractive and ocular component measures of children enrolled in the correction of myopia evaluation trail (COMET). *Invest Ophthalmol Vis Sci.* 2002;43:314-321.

109 Jones-Jordan LA, Sinnott LT, Graham ND, et al. The contributions of near work and outdoor activity to the correlation between siblings in the Collaborative Longitudinal Evaluation of Ethnicity and Refractive Error (CLEERE) Study. *Invest Ophthalmol Vis Sci.* 2014;55:6333-6339.

110 Kulp MT, Ying GS, Huang J, et al. Associations between hyperopia and other vision and refractive error characteristics. *Optom Vis Sci.* 2014;91:383-389.

111 Stelmack JA, Tang C, Wei Y, et al. Veterans Affairs Low-vision Intervention Trial II: One-year follow-up. *Optom Vis Sci.* 2019;96:718-725.

112 Barnhardt C, Cotter SA, Mitchell GL, et al. Symptoms in children with convergence insufficiency: Before and after treatment. *Optom Vis Sci.* 2012; 89:1512-1520.

113 Bamberg HM, Grenier EM, Harris MG. An evaluation of U.S. optometry school curricula. *Optom Ed.* 1998;23:41-47.

114 Maier H, Smith A, Coffey B. A curriculum comparison of U.S. optometry schools: Looking back over the decade. *Optom Ed.* 2005;30:39-55.

115 Goss DA, Penisten DK. The subordination of refraction. *J Am Optom Assoc.* 1996;67:560-562.

116 Sheedy JE. What is the role of glasses in optometry? *Optom Ed.* 1996;21:111-113. 117.

117 Atchison DA. Who needs optics? *Clin Exp Optom.* 2003;86:1-2.

118 Lakshminarayanan V. Teaching optics in a multi-disciplinary curriculum: Experience from optometry programs. In: *Education and Training in Optics and Photonics.* Optical Society of America Technical Digest Series, 2007, paper ETA4.

119 American Optometric Association. *History of Optometry.* https://fs.aoa.org/optometry-archives/optometry-timeline.html

120 Cooper SL. 1971-2011: Forty-year history of scope expansion into medical eye care. *Optometry* 2012;83:64-73. www.newsfromaoa.wordpress.com/2012/03/23/1971-2011-forty-year-history-of-scope-expansion-into-medial-eye-care/

121 Kekevian B. Expanding scope of practice: Lessons and leverage. *Rev Optom.* October 15, 2018. www.reviewofoptometry.com/article/expanding-scope-of-practice-lessnons-and-leverage
122 Borish IM. Optometry: Its heritage and its future. *Indiana J Optom.* 2001;4:23-31.
123 Casella BP. Sights are set on perfect vision in 2020. *Optometry Times,* Jan. 21, 2020;12(1). www.optometrytimes.com/editorials/sights-are-set-perfect-vision-2020....
124 Wyckoff WB. The 25 best jobs of 2020. https://money.usnews.com/money/careers/slideshows/the-25-best-jobs.
125 Hofstetter HW. The OHS mission. *Hindsight* 1996;27:17-18.

PART II
Some Elements of the Development of Optometry as a Scholarly Profession

Trying to plan for the future without a sense of the past is like trying to plant cut flowers. —Daniel Boorstin[1]

Understanding the past helps broaden one's viewpoint, enriches one's perspective, and provides counterbalance to the idea that only what solves today's problem is worth knowing. —Lucretia McClure[2]

If we don't look to our past and see an example where the bar has been set, how are we going to know what to reach for? —Mark Abbott[3]

In Part I, we saw how among the elements of the transition from trade to scholarly profession were the capacity to provide a unique and valuable service and a body of knowledge learned through formalized educational programs. Three particular aspects of passage to profession are important for our discussion now with an emphasis on developments in the United States: the maturation of optometric testing procedures, the development of optometric education, and optometric publications.

The maturation of optometric testing procedures made possible the provision of a unique and valuable service. After schools of various types started appearing in the late nineteenth century, optometric education showed remarkable changes in the twentieth century, gradually becoming more rigorous and more standardized. In addition, optometric periodical literature and optometry books served a role in the dissemination and advancement of the body of optometric knowledge.

Part II: Notes

1. Boorstin D. Quoted in: McCullough D. *The American Spirit: Who We Are and What We Stand For*. New York: Simon & Shuster, 2017:105.
2. McClure L. Who needs history? *Academic Medicine* 1995;70:461-462.
3. Abbott M. In: Red-Horse V, Hurd GA, producers. *Choctaw Code Talkers*. Video from Native American Public Telecommunications, aired on PBS, 2010.

Chapter 5

Maturation of the Optometric Examination

In the early days of spectacle making for presbyopia, the lens power was based on age. Later an individual could try on several pairs of spectacles to find what he or she thought to be most appropriate. The transition from self-selection of spectacles to a system in which the spectacle maker did testing to determine the proper power was significant, not only in itself but also because it marked the transition from a business transaction by a spectacle seller to a service by a spectacle prescriber and health care provider. This transition was gradual and was not complete until the twentieth century. The transition involved not only increased sophistication in refractive testing but also the addition of procedures for evaluating binocular vision, ocular accommodation, and ocular health.

By the beginning of the twentieth century, most of the basic elements of today's eye and vision examination had been developed to some extent. Procedures and equipment for retinoscopy, ophthalmoscopy, keratometry, visual acuity testing, subjective refraction, and dissociated phoria measurement had become available. Looking at the tests presented in a popular 1895 optometry correspondence course gives some idea of the nature of the optometric examination at that time. That year, Dr. H. A. Thomson of the South Bend [Indiana] College of Optics authored 20 lessons that could be taken for $25. The lessons covered geometrical optics, basic physiological optics, examination methods, and diagnosis and management of refractive and binocular vision conditions. The examination procedures covered in the course included visual acuity testing, amplitude of accommodation, prism vergence ranges, bichrome test, subjective refraction by maximum plus (or minimum minus) to best visual acuity, the clock dial test for astigmatism, retinoscopy, and ophthalmoscopy.

Thomson was opposed to the use of optometers to determine refractive error. His words in this regard are interesting, not only for his reasons for not liking them but also for his description of optometers in use at the time:

> Although I hope none of my pupils will ever be so unscientific as to use an optometer, it is desirable to understand the principles upon which it is constructed. The common optometer consists of a convex lens through which the patient looks at a card attached to a slide. The card is moved until seen most distinctly, when we have the focus of that eye. If it stopped at the principal focus of the lens, we know that the rays emerged parallel and that he is emmetropic. If beyond the principal focus they [the rays] emerged converging showing him to be hypermetropic; if nearer than the focus, diverging, and he is myopic. By marking the slide at different distances we have only to look where the card stands and the number tells the glass required. Other more complicated optometers are on the market but are based on the same principle. The objection is that accommodation, convergence, astigmatism, etc., are not considered, thus rendering the instruments inaccurate.[1]

Because the level and type of education of optometrists varied greatly at the beginning of the twentieth century, the breadth and depth of the vision examinations they performed varied greatly as well. Recognizing the need for standardization of the optometric examination, Charles Sheard in 1917 published a book titled *Dynamic Ocular Tests*. At the time he was director of the optometry school at The Ohio State University. Sheard recommended that "full and accurate data should be preserved for every

Maturation of the Optometric Examination 149

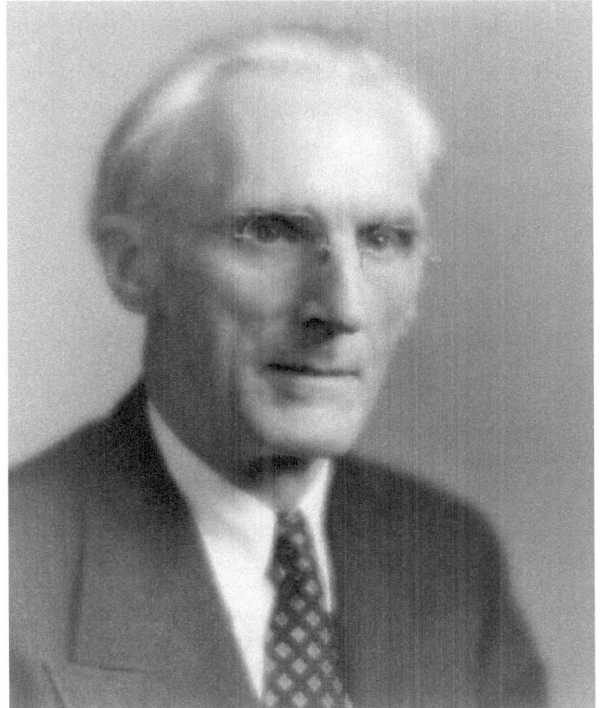

Figure 5.1. Charles Sheard (1883-1963). (Photo courtesy of the Archives & Museum of Optometry and The AOA Foundation)

patient examined."[2] He stated that he recorded the results of his routine examination of 18 tests on a plain white 5x8-inch card. The 18 tests included case history, ophthalmoscopy, ophthalmometry (keratometry), static and dynamic retinoscopy, subjective refraction with binocular balance by equalization of visual acuity, version tests, dissociated phoria tests, amplitude of accommodation, and fusional vergence ranges.[3]

In 1931, A. M. Skeffington published *Differential Diagnosis in Ocular Examination*, in which he also recommended an examination of 18 tests. Skeffington was instrumental, with E. B. Alexander, in forming the Optometric Extension Program in 1928 to help upgrade the clinical education of optometrists then in practice. Skeffington, S. K. Lesser, and their colleagues in the Optometric Extension Program further elaborated on the series of tests, expanding it to 21; this routine of tests came to be known as the 21 points.[4,5] This system of numbering tests became very popular, and many optometrists throughout the twentieth century had examination forms with blanks numbered from 1 to 21 for the tests in the 21-point examination. Those tests are shown in Table 5.1.

Table 5.1. Tests in the 21-point examination from the Optometric Extension Program

Test #	Test Description
1	Ophthalmoscopy
2	Ophthalmometry (keratometry)
3	Habitual lateral dissociated phoria at distance
13A	Habitual lateral dissociated phoria at near
4	Static retinoscopy
5	Dynamic retinoscopy at 20 inches (50 cm)
6	Dynamic retinoscopy at 40 inches (1 m)
7	Subjective refraction: maximum plus to 20/20 minus visual acuity
7A	Subjective refraction: maximum plus to best visual acuity
8	Lateral dissociated phoria at distance through #7 finding
9	Base-out to first blur fusional vergence range at distance
10	Base-out to break and recovery fusional vergence range at distance
11	Base-in to break and recovery fusional vergence range at distance
12	Vertical dissociated phoria and fusional vergence ranges at distance
13B	Lateral dissociated phoria at near through the #7 finding
14A	Unfused (monocular) cross cylinder

15A	Lateral dissociated phoria at near through the #14A finding
14B	Fused (binocular) cross cylinder
15B	Lateral dissociated phoria at near through the #14B finding
16A	Base-out to blur out fusional vergence range at near
16B	Base-out to break and recovery fusional vergence range at near
17A	Base-in to blur out fusional vergence range at near
17B	Base-in to break and recovery fusional vergence range at near
18	Vertical dissociated phoria and fusional vergence ranges at near
19	Analytical amplitude (minus to blur with card at 13 inches)
20	Minus to blur out with card at 16 inches
21	Plus to blur out with card at 16 inches

Source: Birnbaum MH. *Optometric Management of Nearpoint Vision Disorders*. Boston, MA: Butterworth-Heinemann, 1993:128-133.

THE DIOPTER

From the invention of spectacles through most of the nineteenth century, there was no one agreed-upon unit to describe spectacle lens power. Francesco Maurolyco in the mid-sixteenth century noted that spectacle makers "exercised such care that they indicated by small marks—one for each year—the age for which the spectacles were suited."[6] The English optician Edward Scarlett, optician to King George II, may have been the first to use focal length for numbering lenses. Scarlett advertised that he marked "the focus of the glass upon the frame."[6] Focal length in inches was commonly used for lens power for many years, but the length of an inch varied from country to country. For example, in his 1864 book, Donders used the Parisian inch, which is equal to about 27 mm.

In 1867, the German ophthalmologist Albrecht Nagel recommended a lens power unit based on the reciprocal of one meter.[7] In 1868, Frenchman F. Monoyer, a professor of medical physics, published a paper supporting Nagel's idea. A competing idea proposed by French ophthalmologist Emile Javal based the measuring unit on the reciprocal of 240 cm.[7]

In 1872, Monoyer published another paper strongly backing the "dioptrie," as he named it. (Johannes Kepler is usually given credit for coining the term *dioptric* based on his classic 1611 optics book *Dioptrice*.) The lens power unit was a topic of discussion at an ophthalmology congress in Heidelberg, Germany, in 1875. Due to the strengths of Monoyer's arguments, the diopter was backed by Nagel, Javal, Donders, and John Soelberg Wells, and its use as the international standard was promoted by the attendees of the ophthalmology congress.[6,8] However, focal length in inches continued to be stamped on frames in some locations into the twentieth century. The diopter has been the universal unit for lens power since about 1920.[9]

DISTANCE TEST CHARTS AND PROJECTORS

The first distance vision test charts were designed for evaluation of visual acuity. The first studies of visual resolution grew from interest in astronomy. The earliest experimental investigations of visual acuity may have been conducted by an English scientist, Robert Hooke, in the 17th century.[10] German mathematician and astronomer Tobias Mayer experimented with grid and checkerboard patterns in the 18th century.[9] It is unclear when the first letter charts were used in eye examination. In 1807, Thomas Young wrote about a letter chart attachment to an optometer, and in 1823, Purkinje wrote of an acuity apparatus designed by a Leipzig optician named Tauber.[11]

In 1843, Heinrich Küchler produced test charts with Gothic script letters of descending size. In 1854, Viennese ophthalmologist Eduard von Jaeger produced a similar chart with several lines of letters smaller than those of Küchler.[9] In 1862, Herman Snellen introduced a letter chart with letter design and sizes that became widely used for many years.[12]

The progression of letter sizes on the Küchler and Jaeger charts was based on availability of typefaces rather than an orderly system. Snellen's system had seven lines.[11] The letter sizes in what is now known as the Snellen fraction, which actually was proposed by Donders, were 20/20, 20/30, 20/40, 20/50, 20/70, 20/100, and 20/200. Today, a logarithmic progression of letter sizes, such as in the Bailey-Lovie chart, is preferred by most vision scientists.[13] It is interesting to note that in 1906, the French ophthalmologist Henri Armaignac empirically derived a progression of letter sizes very close to a logarithmic progression.[14,15]

The first transparent vision test charts were developed in 1893 by Cohn, who had optotypes painted on glass plates that were placed in front of a window.[16] Transparent test charts backlit by electrical lights followed soon after that.[16] A significant development in distance vision testing was the invention of electronic projector systems designed specifically for vision examination. While targets in addition to letters, such as clock dials, were available on some paper charts and backlit systems, projectors allowed the incorporation of targets for a wider variety of test procedures.

It appears that the first projector for vision examination, or at least the first commercially successful projector in the United States, was the Clason Visual Acuity Meter, which was marketed for many years by Bausch & Lomb. It was based on a 1916 patent by Milo B. Clason,[17] an optometrist who was born in Iowa and moved to Columbus, Georgia, when he was about 20.[18] The headstone on his grave in Georgia says he was a "scientist and inventor of national optical fame—all who came to him were benefited through his skill and kindly understanding."[19]

With the Clason projector, the examiner could choose between one large letter, a block of mid-sized letters in three lines with three letters in each line, and a block of small letters in five lines with five letters in each line. A zoom system varied the size of the letters. When examiners ordered a Clason projector, they specified the distance between the projector screen and where the projector was to be placed. Based on that distance, a scale was placed on the projector indicating the decimal visual acuity of the small letters.[20] Letters could be presented in a block or masked to form a horizontal row or vertical column. Rotating T and sunburst targets for astigmatism testing were also available. A photo of an early Clason projector is shown in Figure 5.2, and the slides used in a later Clason projector are shown in Figure 5.3. The Clason Visual Acuity Meter was included in the 1948 edition of the *Bausch & Lomb Ophthalmic Reference Book*, so it would appear that Bausch & Lomb was producing the Clason projector at least as late as 1948.[20] Bausch & Lomb had a later design projector, the Compact Acuity Projector, that they were also making in 1948.[21]

In 1932, Arthur P. Wheelock filed a patent for the projector system that would become the American Optical Project-O-Chart.[22] A November 1933 advertisement said that the Project-O-Chart was "radically new, scientifically correct" and that it "offers new versatility and convenience in the subjective examination."[23] Various versions of the Project-O-Chart have been available from American Optical and its successor company Reichert into the twentieth-first century.

Wheelock was an Iowa optometrist who, from 1941 to 1944, was president of the American Academy of Optometry.[24] He was presiding over the American Academy of Optometry meeting in Chicago on December 7, 1941, when someone entered the room and whispered to him. He had to announce that Pearl Harbor had been attacked. He called for a recess but then resumed the meeting some minutes later.[25] In 1970, Wheelock was awarded an honorary life fellowship in the Academy.[26]

Among four papers that Wheelock published in the *American Journal of Optometry and Archives of the American Academy of Optometry* was a 1933 paper on visual requirements for railroad employees.[27] That fact becomes more interesting when it is noted that Wheelock owned a profitable rail-

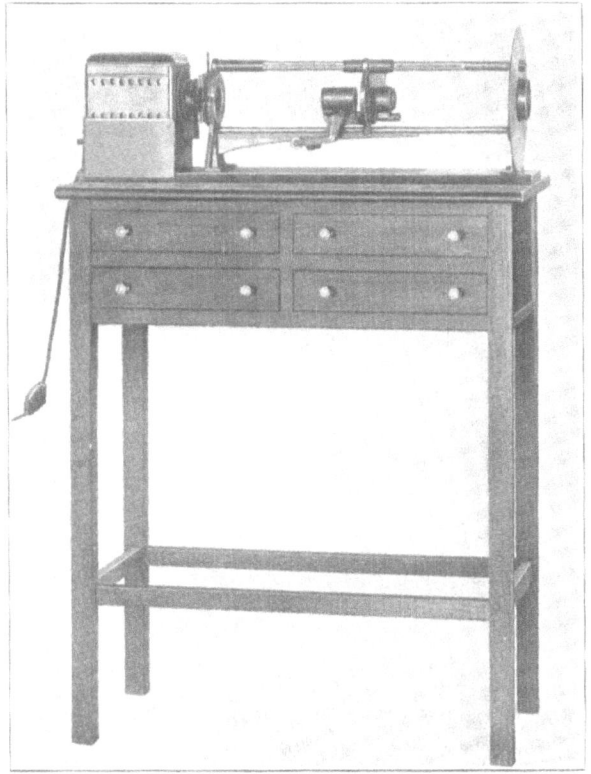

Clason Visual Acuity Meter on Mahogany Table

Figure 5.2. An early Clason projector. The lens projection system was mounted to slide on the two horizontal rods, resulting in enlarged or reduced size of the projected test targets. (Image from *The Clason Visual Acuity Meter: A Manual of Information for Users*, Bausch & Lomb Optical Co., undated)

road line in Iowa, which, though only seven miles long, connected two major lines.[24]

In the late 1950s, Don Frantz introduced what he called *natural color stereoscopic refraction*.[28,29] In his office, examination rooms were in an L-shaped configuration. An approximately six-foot-wide projection screen covered the wall at the top of the L. Dual projectors produced a color stereoscopic picture that filled the screen. The center of that picture was

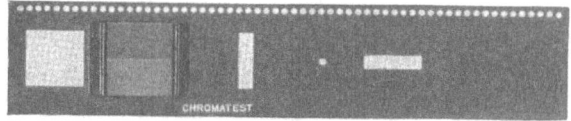

Chroma-Test Slide.

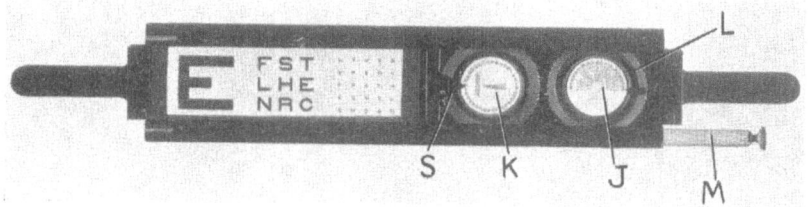

Hamilton Slide.
Figure 2

J—*Sunburst Dial; Fan Dial.*   L—*Index for Sunburst Dial.*
K—*"T" Chart.*   M—*Rod.*
     S—*Index for "T" Chart.*

Figure 5.3. Test slides from a later Clason projector. The sunburst dial and rotatable T chart were used for testing astigmatism. (Photo from *The Clason Acuity Meter with Hamilton Slides: Directions for Use*, Bausch & Lomb Optical, undated)

blanked out so that a third projector could present a standard test chart. It was thought that this helped to minimize accommodation when a refraction was done with a standard test chart in the center of, for instance, a distant mountain scene. Even though the appearance was quite striking, this technique was not widely adopted.

Frantz was born in Iola, Kansas, and worked in his father's optometry office when he was in high school.[30] He received a bachelor's degree from Northwestern University and graduated from optometry school at the Northern Illinois College of Optometry in Chicago. In 1942, he established a practice in DeKalb, Illinois, which grew into a professional corporation with five optometrists, three opticians, and 10 assistants in a two-story building. He served the American Optometric Association for many years in various capacities, including the presidency from 1961 to 1962.[31] He lectured and wrote for the Optometric Extension Program on practice management and other topics, and he taught practice management at the Illinois College of Optometry. He was well known for the inspiring stories in his lectures and writings.[32] He received DOS honorary degrees from Southern College of Optometry and Illinois College of Optometry.[33]

The use of polarization to allow monocular testing without occlusion was investigated as early as 1939.[34] This technique became widely available in the late 1960s, when Bernard Grolman developed adult and child vectographic slides that could be used in the American Optical projector for binocular refraction.[35]

Grolman was born and raised in Brooklyn, New York. He graduated from Brooklyn Polytechnic Institute in 1942 and worked for General Electric as a draftsman before serving as a radarman from 1944 to 1946 in the U.S. Navy.[36] Grolman attended Hofstra University and graduated from optometry school at Columbia University in 1952. He earned BS and MO degrees from Columbia.[37] From 1952 to 1955, he was a development engineer at Burroughs Business Machines Corporation, designing and testing optical telescopic missile tracking systems.[36] From 1955 to 1985, he was a research scientist at the American Optical Corporation/Reichert. He received more than 50 patents for various optical and ophthalmic instruments.[36] He is probably best known for his invention of the non-contact tonometer. He was awarded honorary doctoral degrees by the Illinois College of Optometry and the New England College of Optometry, and the William Feinbloom Award from the American Academy of Optometry.[38]

A relatively recent development in projectors for eye and vision examination is that of automated remote-controlled projectors. In 2014, one website listed remote-controlled projectors made by eight different companies.[39] These projectors offer a wide array of features, including randomization of letters presented; horizontal, vertical, or single letter masking; vectographic targets; red-green targets; binocular vision tests; children's targets; a clockdial test; stereopsis tests; etc.

KERATOMETERS

The use of the keratometer allows measurement of curvature of the anterior surface of the cornea. Because the anterior corneal surface is the greatest source of variability in astigmatism, the measurement provides a clue as to how much astigmatism the eye may have. Keratometers are based on the principle that the size of a reflected image is proportional to the curvature of the reflecting surface.

Keratometers found wide usage in the twentieth century as devices to predict the total astigmatism of the eye and as aids in the fitting of contact lenses. The first instrument that could be recognized as a keratometer was constructed in the late eighteenth century by Jesse Ramsden, an English optician and instrument maker. It was designed for an experiment to test whether the cornea changed during accommodation.[40] The experiment was conducted with Everard Home, an English anatomist and surgeon.

After leaving an apprenticeship with a clothworker, Ramsden apprenticed with an instrument maker. Then, after working for well-known opticians Jeremiah Sissons, George Adams, Sr., and Peter Dollond, he opened his own shop in 1762 marked by a sign of "Golden Spectacles." Ramsden created a numbering system for powers of convex and concave spectacle lenses, and he was among the first opticians known to use sequential sets of lenses for vision testing.[41] He classified convex lenses by focal length in English inches. His set of 13 convex lenses had powers with a range of about +1.0 to +6.7 D. His set of 22 concave lenses covered a much wider range of powers. An employee of Ramsden named Samuel Pierce may have made Benjamin Franklin's bifocals.[42]

Ramsden was considered by many to be the best scientific instrument maker of the eighteenth century, and he was particularly well known for his telescopes.[43] Among the other instruments made in his shop were astronomical instruments, electrical machines, portable barometers, thermometers, theodolites (a surveying instrument), surveying levels, micrometers, dynameters (a device to measure the magnifying power of telescopes), precision balances, microtomes, and dividing engines (a device used to mark gradations on measuring instruments).[44] Ramsden was well known for his ability to improve existing scientific instruments or to devise new ones. He published about 15 pamphlets and papers describing the design and/or usage of various scientific instruments.[45] He was elected to the Royal Society in 1786.[46]

In Ramsden's instrument for examination of corneal curvature, a telescope was used to view the doubled image reflected from the cornea.[47] Home and Ramsden could not discern a change in corneal curvature with accommodation and they concluded that the cornea was not its primary source.

Decades later, in 1853, Hermann von Helmholtz created a keratometer in which two images reflected from the cornea were observed, after reflection from two movable glass plates. The amount of movement of the glass plates needed to make the edges of the images touch represented the size of the images, and thus, the curvature of the cornea.[48] Helmholtz's keratometer was primarily a laboratory instrument.

Credit for adapting Helmholtz's design into a clinically useful instrument goes to Louis Emile Javal and Hjalmar August Schiotz. In 1881, they built a keratometer that could be rotated to measure separate meridians.[48] It had a fixed doubling system in which the separation of the mires was adjusted to take measurements. The Javal-Schiotz type of keratometer was produced by many companies, perhaps most notably by the Haag-Streit Company.[49]

In 1899, the Chambers-Inskeep Ophthalmometer (Figure 5.4) was announced.[50] It was the first keratometer with self-illuminated mires. The separation of the mires was constant and the position of doubling prisms was varied to take corneal measurements. The Chambers-Inskeep Company was a partnership of David Chambers, Charles Inskeep, E. A. Chambers, and Carey Inskeep. It was originally known as the Ottumwa Optical Company when it was founded in 1887 in Ottumwa, Iowa, in David Chambers' drug store.[51] Chambers and his prescriptionist nephew,

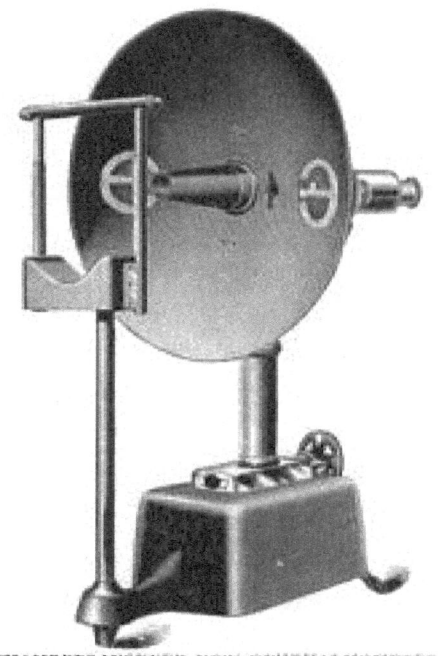

Figure 5.4. Chambers-Inskeep Ophthalmometer used to measure curvature of the anterior surface of the cornea. (Photo from *Jewelers Review*, May 24, 1899;32:652)

Charles Inskeep, taught themselves optics and started selling spectacles. The company moved to Chicago in 1888, and a year later the name of the company was changed to the Chambers-Inskeep Company. The company also developed a self-illuminating retinoscope and ophthalmoscope, and one of the first lensometers. The company was purchased by the F. A. Hardy Company in 1903, which in turn was later taken over by the American Optical Company.[51] The Chambers-Inskeep Ophthalmometer was the basic design for the American Optical ophthalmometer that was produced for many years.

The Javal-Schiotz and Chambers-Inskeep instruments were rotated to take readings in one principal meridian and then rotated again to align for measurement of the other principal meridian. Those keratometers are often referred to as *two-position keratometers*. In 1906, John Sutcliffe designed a one-position keratometer, where only one rotation was needed to align with both perpendicular principal meridians. This keratometer also incorporated a focusing system based on the Scheiner disc principle.[48]

Sutcliffe was a British ophthalmic optician (optometrist).[52] His father, Robert Sutcliffe, founded the British Optical Association in 1895. The son served as secretary of that association from 1896 to 1940; he also served as a president of the International Optical League. He founded the British Optical Association Museum in 1901 and built it up by soliciting donations and making purchases. In 1932 Sutcliffe edited the *British Optical Association Library and Museum Catalogue*. He was also the long-time editor of the British Optical Association's journal, the *Dioptric Review*. In addition to his keratometer, he designed a trial frame and a bifocal lens.

The well-known and widely used Bausch & Lomb keratometer was introduced in 1932.[52] It is a one-position keratometer with variable doubling produced by movable prisms that are oriented perpendicular to each other.[53] Its basic design has been copied by several different manufacturers.

In 1981, the first autokeratometer, the Humphrey Autokeratometer, was introduced.[54,55] The first combination autokeratometer and autorefractor was introduced by Canon in 1987.[55]

Although the index of refraction of the cornea is about 1.376, the index used to calculate a keratometer power from the measured radius of curvature of the anterior surface of the cornea is 1.3375 for most keratometers. It has been reported that Javal selected this value because a radius of curvature of 7.5 mm resulted in a convenient power value of 45 D.[48] With such powers, Javal composed a formula for the prediction of total astigmatism of the eye, which has come to be known as Javal's rule:

Total astigmatism = 1.25 (keratometer astigmatism) + 0.50 D against-the-rule astigmatism

In the twentieth century, several authors offered modifications of Javal's rule, which may have yielded marginal improvements in predicted astigmatism, but they also complicated it.[56] Grosvenor and colleagues fit mean data into a regression of refractive astigmatism on keratometer astigmatism and suggested that a simplification of Javal's rule provided a better fit of the data.[57] In the simplified formula, sometimes referred to as *Grosvenor's rule*, the 1.25 is dropped from Javal's formula so that the predicted total astigmatism becomes simply the keratometer astigmatism plus 0.50 D against-the-rule astigmatism.

Related in principle to keratometry, keratoscopy is a procedure used to assess the contour of the cornea over most of its anterior surface. The first keratoscopes were simply some form of pattern, usually concentric circles, which could be reflected from the cornea, with the reflections then viewed by the examiner. Levene[58] credited English physician Henry Goode as the first to report observations with a keratoscope in 1847. Portuguese oculist Antonio Plácido was the first to develop a photokeratoscope. Zeiss, in the 1930s, was the first company to produce a commercially available photokeratoscope.[59] The first photokeratoscope to achieve wide usage was the Wesley-Jessen Photo-Electronic Keratoscope, or PEK, which was developed in the 1950s and first marketed in the 1960s.[60,61,62] The next photokeratoscopes to be developed commercially were the Corneascope and the Nidek Photokeratoscope.[63,64] In the 1980s and 1990s, video technology was combined with computer scanning and analysis, with the first commercially produced videokeratoscope being the Corneal Modeling System developed by Computed Anatomy.[65] Videokeratoscopes quickly became common in optometry offices for evaluating corneal topography in contact lens care, orthokeratology monitoring, keratoconus management, corneal disease diagnosis, and refractive surgery comanagement.

RETINOSCOPY

The introduction of retinoscopy was a significant step in the history of clinical refraction in that it provided a relatively accurate objective method for estimating refractive error. Arthur Bennett[66] described retinoscopy as "an offshoot from ophthalmoscopy" because British ophthalmologist Sir William Bowman reported in 1859 that he was able to detect slight degrees of keratoconus by observing shadow movements obtained by rotating his ophthalmoscope mirror. Donders[67] stated that Bowman also was able to use the technique to detect astigmatism and identify the principal meridians.

Credit for the development of retinoscopy is generally given to the French ophthalmologist, Ferdinand Cuignet.[67,68,69] He described the shadows he saw when rotating his ophthalmoscope mirror in a series of papers published from 1873 to 1887 in the journal *Recueil d'Ophthalmologie*.[69]

Cuignet was a military physician who served in Algeria and was decorated in 1870. He later taught ophthalmology at the medical school in Lille, France.[70] He was coeditor of the journal *Recueil d'Ophthalmologie*. According to Hirschberg,[70] he published only a few papers in addition to his work on retinoscopy and a 271-page book, *Ophthalmie d'Algerie* (1872).

Cuignet used the term *keratoscopie* for the technique that we know today as *retinoscopy* because he thought the phenomenon was due to the cornea. Other terms suggested for retinoscopy included *dioptroscopie, optometrie scotoscopique, shadow test, pupilloskopie,* and *koreskopie*.[69,70,71] *Skiascopy* and *skiametry* were commonly used terms for retinoscopy extending well into the twentieth century.

Popularization of retinoscopy in the late nineteenth century came through the efforts of European ophthalmologists Mengin, Chibret, Parent, and Landolt.[67,69] By the turn of the twentieth century, retinoscopy was popular enough that books were being devoted to the topic. Early books on retinoscopy by ophthalmologists were *Skiascopy and Its Practical*

Application to the Study of Refraction by Edward Jackson, 1895 (112 pages) and *Retinoscopy (or Shadow Test) in the Determination of Refraction*, by James Thorington, 1897 (66 pages). Some of the first books on retinoscopy by optometrists were *Skiascopy: A Treatise on the Shadow Test in Its Practical Application to the Work of Refraction* by George A. Rogers, 1899 (221 pages); *Skiametry, Static and Dynamic* by William B. Needles, 1900 (56 pages); *A System of Ocular Skiametry* by Andrew Jay Cross, 1903 (181 pages); and *Skiascopy Without the Use of Drugs* by Robert M. Lockwood, 1906 (112 pages).

The first retinoscopes were perforated mirrors on a handle with illumination from a candle or from a lamp separate from the retinoscope mirror. Figure 5.5, taken from Rogers' 1899 book, shows retinoscopy being performed.[72] The examiner held the retinoscope mirror and reflected light from a lamp into the patient's eye. The lamp here appears to be mounted on a wall, and a trial lens set can be seen on the table between the examiner and the patient. The first retinoscope with an electric light source incorporated into the retinoscope itself was made in 1901 by Wolff.[71] An early prominent electric self-luminous retinoscope was the De Zeng retinoscope.[72]

The first electric retinoscopes projected a spot of light. The streak retinoscope, which facilitated the observation of astigmatism, was patented by Jack C. Copeland in 1927.[73] Copeland graduated from the Northern Illinois College of Optometry in 1922. He started work at Bausch & Lomb as a technical consultant in optics in 1927. He held more than 35 patents,[74] and from 1931 to 1956, he was editor of the monthly periodical *Optical Developments*. From 1965 until his death in 1973, Copeland taught in the Department of Ophthalmology at the Marquette University School of Medicine, now the Medical College of Wisconsin. Copeland did much to popularize streak retinoscopy through his publications, lectures, and demonstrations.[75]

The initial application of retinoscopy was in the measurement of refractive error, a procedure that has come to be known as *static retinoscopy*.

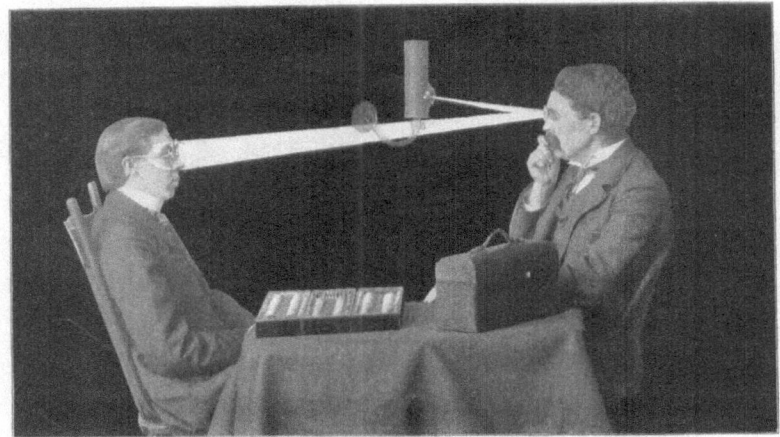

SKIASCOPIC EXAMINATION AT ONE METER.
Light, by way of mirror, at 1½ meters. Testing the horizontal meridian.

Figure 5.5. Illustration of the performance of retinoscopy in 1899 showing how light from a lamp on the wall was reflected from the retinoscope and directed toward the patient. (Photo from Rogers GA. *Skiascopy, A Treatise on the Shadow Test in its Practical Application to the Work of Refraction.* Philadelphia: Keystone, 1899:12)

The early development of the use of retinoscopy to assess accommodative function, known as *dynamic retinoscopy*, is usually credited to American optometrist Andrew Jay Cross. Sheard made a statement that Cross devised his system of dynamic retinoscopy in the early 1880s.[76] Cross devoted a significant portion of his 1903 book on retinoscopy, *A System of Ocular Skiametry*, to dynamic retinoscopy. In 1911, Cross published a tome on dynamic retinoscopy, *Dynamic Retinoscopy in Theory and Practice*.

Pascal[77] mentioned an early use of dynamic retinoscopy in 1895 by R. Greef to show that accommodation in the blind eye of a young boy occurred when accommodation was stimulated in the other eye. Retinoscopy was mentioned by Edward Jackson in 1895 as a potential objective method for determining amplitude of accommodation.[78]

Cross devised an attachment for retinoscopy with letters and dots. He asked the patient to read letters or count dots as retinoscopy was performed. Cross advocated adding plus lenses to reversal. In today's dynamic retinoscopy, this most resembles low neutral retinoscopy: when a lag of accommodation is observed, plus is added to the first observed neutral. Canadian optometrist Ivan Nott described a dynamic retinoscopy procedure in which the nearpoint target remained at a fixed distance, while the retinoscope was moved separately back behind the target until neutral was observed.[79] This procedure, in which the distance of the retinoscope from the patient yields an accommodative response measurement, is known as Nott retinoscopy.

Probably the most commonly used dynamic retinoscopy procedure today is the monocular estimation method (MEM). In 1960, Pacific University College of Optometry faculty member, Harold Haynes, detailed a method for finding lag of accommodation by estimating in diopters how far the retinoscopic reflex was from neutral, and using lenses "interposed only momentarily to check the examiner's estimates."[80] Various authors have thus credited Haynes with devising MEM retinoscopy.[81,82,83] Several other dynamic retinoscopy procedures, such as bell retinoscopy, book retinoscopy, and stresspoint retinoscopy, have also been described.[84]

SUBJECTIVE REFRACTION, THE TRIAL LENS SET, AND THE PHOROPTER

As we have seen, for many years after the invention of spectacles in the late thirteenth century, the lenses available were plus lenses for presbyopia. Spectacles were initially ordered on the basis of the buyer's age.[84] The first documented use of spectacles for myopia was in the fifteenth century.[86] Included in the 1623 book, *The Use of Eyeglasses*, by Daza de Valdes, there is a diagram with which individuals could find their punctum remotum and from that determine the power of concave lenses they needed for myopia.[85] For presbyopia, Daza de Valdes recommended convex lens powers based on age.[87]

As spectacles came to be mass-produced, buyers could visit a shop and pick from a supply of spectacles those that seemed to work best for them, or they could buy from the stock carried by a traveling spectacle peddler. Gregg[86] referred to this as the "do-it-yourself fitting of glasses." Obviously, this allowed neither careful determination of refractive error nor individualized correction of conditions such as anisometropia or astigmatism.

The availability of equipment such as trial lens sets—and later phoropters—made it possible to perform a subjective refraction testing procedure. This allowed the making of individualized lens prescriptions, and of particular significance, it advanced the process of obtaining spectacles from an interchange between buyer and seller to the provision of a service.

Arthur Bennett[37] credits a German monk named Johann Zahn with describing the first rudiments of a subjective refraction procedure. Zahn made a plano-convex polyspherical lens and a plano-concave polyspherical lens. Each consisted of a single piece of glass with six concentric zones of different powers. The zones could be sequentially brought in front of the eye to estimate spherical refractive error. Zahn was also aware that the distance of the punctum remotum from a myopic eye could be used to determine the focal length of the correcting lens.[89]

Credit for the development of a trial lens case generally goes to a Bavarian physician, Georg Fronmüller, because in 1843, he published the first account of designing one.[89,90] However, it is known that English opticians Jesse Ramsden and William Cary had ranges of different lens powers they used for refractive testing before then.[88] Even though trial lens sets made it possible for some opticians to make glasses to order as early as the eighteenth century, spectacle shops with do-it-yourself fitting and spectacle peddlers persisted for many more years.

An appreciation of the development of refractive procedure would not be complete without some consideration of the contemporary knowledge of refractive errors. For many years, hyperopia was not distinguished from presbyopia. Levene[89] suggested that the writings of physicians

William Charles Wells and James Ware were the first to recognize the difference, but it wasn't until the work of Donders that hyperopia "was treated adequately, both clinically and on a sound scientific basis."

An understanding of refractive methods in the late nineteenth century can be gained from the 1896 book *The Human Eye: How to Correct Its Defects by Properly Fitting Glasses*, published by Queen and Company as authors. They noted the test for hyperopia was that the eye can see "as distinctly, or more distinctly, through a convex lens." To determine the amount of hyperopia, they recommended covering one eye and then placing in the trial frame "successively stronger and stronger convex lenses, until they become so strong that the distant vision is less distinct," with the lens correction being "the strongest lens that left the vision clear."[90] The authors also said that if distance visual acuity was reduced and near visual acuity was better than distance visual acuity, it could be deduced that myopia was present. They advised that the selection of minus lens power for each eye could be guided by the level of distance visual acuity in that eye and that the weakest concave lens that resulted in the best distance visual acuity was the amount of the myopia.[91] For presbyopia, Queen and Company recommended lens powers based on the near point of accommodation and the habitual near point working distance. In a table of dioptric lens powers, they presented columns with working distances of 30, 20, 15, 12, 10, 9, and 8 inches; and rows with near points of accommodation of 8, 9, 10, 12, 15, 20, 30, and more than 40 inches. For example, for a working distance of 15 inches and a near point of accommodation of 20 inches, the table indicates a recommendation of +1.25 D. Parenthetically, the fact that they repeated the table with lens powers in focal length inches[92] illustrates that the diopter still hadn't achieved universal acceptance.

To test for astigmatism, Queen and Company advised using a distance astigmatic test card with "sets of parallel black and white lines of uniform size, running in different directions."[93] These could be in the form of "astigmatic letters" in which the letters are made up of parallel stripes with varying orientation from letter to letter or in the form of lines radiating from a common center, as in a clock dial.[95] In his 1895 book, Bohne[94] stated that he found striped letters, designed by a Dr. Pray and a Dr. John S. Owens to be more "convenient" for finding the axis of astigmatism than a "fan or a dial" target.

In the early twentieth century, common tests for astigmatism were clock dial-like targets, which some optometrists mounted with a pin in the center so that finer gradations of axis other than the separations of the lines could be obtained, and the "swinging cylinder" method in which a cylinder lens was rotated back and forth in a trial frame until the patient reported that visual acuity was best.[95] Irish mathematician and physicist George Gabriel Stokes had designed a lens system that acted as a variable power cross cylinder in the 1840s, for the measurement of astigmatism, but it never achieved common usage.[96] In papers published between 1887 and 1907, American ophthalmologist Edward Jackson described testing procedures for astigmatism that have come to be known as the *Jackson cross cylinder test*.[89] Slowly, over the first three or four decades of the twentieth century, it became the preferred subjective method of astigmatism measurement that it is today.

A significant development in the field of refraction was the invention of the phoropter. Bennett[89] credits French ophthalmologist Marc Antoine Girard-Teulon with producing a prototype of what might be considered a phoropter. However, it was Henry L. De Zeng, Jr. who made the phoropter we think of today: an instrument useful for both distance and near testing, with accessories such as rotary prisms, cross cylinders, and Maddox rods.

In 1885, De Zeng started working for an optical company. Later he attended Hobart College, studied medicine in Chicago, and took refraction and optics courses.[97,98] Between 1895 and 1915, De Zeng patented 41 inventions, including a refractometer, a phorometer (a device with rotary prisms and other accessories for measuring phorias and vergences), an electric ophthalmoscope, the first battery handle ophthalmoscope, and other diagnostic equipment.[99,100] De Zeng's first phoropter was patented in 1909, which was then produced in a somewhat altered form by the De Zeng Standard Company.[99] In 1917, De Zeng published a 68-page manual titled *The Modern Phorometer, Including the Phorometer-Trial Frame, Phoro-Optometer, and the Rotary Cross Cylinder*, and five years later, he published a 120-page book, *The Phoroptor*. In 1925, De Zeng sold his company to the American Optical Company,[100] which produced phoropters similar to the De Zeng phoropter into the 1940s. A competing phoropter was the Bausch & Lomb Greens' Refractor, developed in the 1930s, by Clyde L. Hunsicker, Aaron S. Green, Louis D. Green, and M. I. Green.[101]

Optometers have sometimes served as an adjunct or even a replacement for subjective refraction. Optometers can be as simple as a single convex lens with a scale or they can incorporate elaborate optical systems. Scottish physician William Porterfield was the first to describe an optometer in a 1737 paper, and in his 1759 two-volume *Treatise on the Eye, the Manner and Phaenomena of Vision*.[102] Porterfield's optometer made use of the Scheiner double aperture principle.[104] Later Thomas Young used an improved version of Porterfield's optometer to discover his own astigmatism.

The late nineteenth century and early twentieth century saw the development of several optometers that went by names such as *punctumeter, refractometer, ophthalmometroscope, stigmatometer, ametropometer, ametrometer, autophoro-optimeter,* and *refractionometer*.[103,104] Problems with alignment and instrument accommodation limited their usefulness. A significant development in the automation of optometers was the introduction of the Bausch & Lomb Ophthalmetron in 1971. Since then, many more autorefractors have appeared on the market.[104,105] It has been argued that retinoscopy by an experienced clinician is a better starting point for the subjective refraction than autorefraction.[105,106] However, factors such as time-savings for the doctor by delegation of autorefraction to a technician, and the favorable impression of tech-

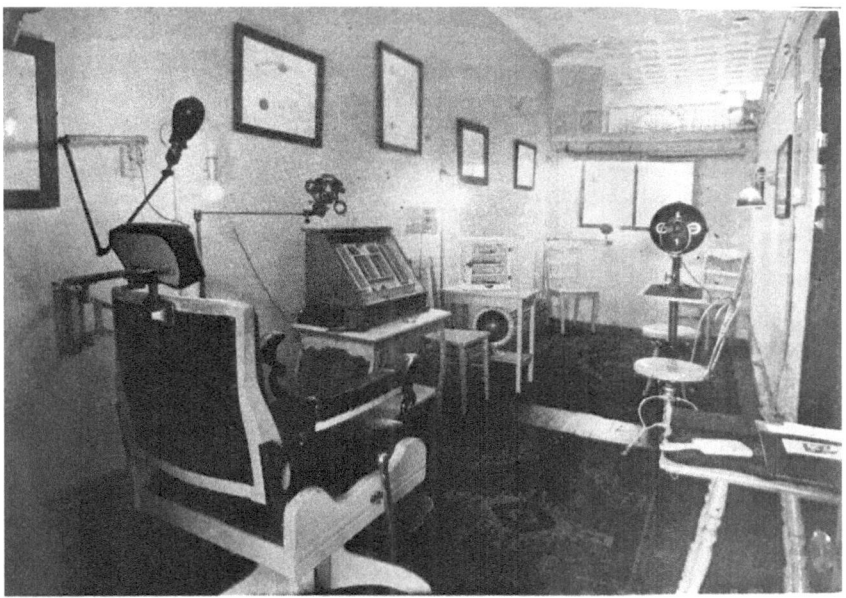

Figure 5.6. A 1921 photograph of an optometry examining room. An ophthalmometer can be seen on the right side of the photograph. A trial lens set is on the table just to the left of the center of the picture, and a phorometer is suspended just above and in front of the patient's chair. (Photo from Wiseman EG. *Building Optometry*. Philadelphia: Keystone, 1921:250)

nology on patients, have led to much wider use of autorefraction in optometry practices.[107] With autorefraction, just as with retinoscopy, the interpretation and professional judgment of the practitioner are necessary.[108]

DISSOCIATED PHORIA AND FUSIONAL VERGENCE RANGE TESTING

A dissociated phoria test measures the magnitude of misalignment of the ocular lines of sight with the object of regard when binocular fusion has been disrupted. The design of dissociated phoria tests must, thus, have some method of preventing binocular fusion, and they use either a scale or prisms to measure the ocular misalignment.

It appears that the first subjective dissociated phoria test was the von Graefe prism diplopia test. A German ophthalmologist, Albrecht von Graefe, described the test in 1861.[109,110] As with the procedure as it is practiced today, for lateral phorias, von Graefe used a vertical prism to eliminate fusion and found the amount of lateral prism that aligned the diplopic images. The test target that von Graefe used for lateral phorias was a dot with a vertical line passing through it. Later it was recognized that control of accommodation during the test was important, so today, letter targets are used for the test.

The Maddox rod test was originated by a British ophthalmologist, Ernest Edmund Maddox.[111,112] In this test, fusion is prevented by the distortion produced over one eye by the Maddox rod. The initial form of the Maddox rod was a short glass rod mounted on a metal disc; later, it was several pieces of glass rod laid side by side and sealed together.[113] Maddox described the performance of the test as follows:

> On looking at a distant flame with this before one eye, it appears converted into a long streak of light, which there is no desire to regard as a false image of the flame, from its dissimilarity, especially if red glass be used. If the streak pass through the flame, equilibrium is perfect, but if otherwise, its distance indicates the amount of latent deviation. The prism that is able to bring the line and the flame together is the measure of it.[114]

In the test that is commonly known today as the *modified Thorington test*, a Maddox rod is held over one eye while the other eye views a tangent scale calibrated for use at a particular distance. A light is shined from the zero point on the tangent scale. The patient reports where the line produced by the Maddox rod appears on the tangent scale. When the tangent scale is at the correct distance from the patient, the location of the line on the scale indicates the amount of the phoria. Although the test typically is eponymous to James Thorington, it appears that priority should go to E. E. Maddox or Charles Prentice. Maddox described the test in an 1890 paper,[115] Maddox later noted that this test could be used to measure lateral and vertical phorias at distance and at near.[116] Charles Prentice may have independently designed a test like this one at about the same time although he used a +12 D cylindrical lens instead of a Maddox rod.[117] When Thorington described this test in a 1913 book, he made no claim for priority and he referred to the tangent scale as the "tangent scale of Prentice."[118] The origin of this test being known as the *modified Thorington test* may have come from a 1948 paper by Hirsch and Bing.[119] Maddox may have gotten the idea for this phoria test from tangent scales of Landolt and Hirschberg (1875), who used them with diplopia tests to determine the angle of deviation in strabismus,[120] although it is interesting to note that von Noorden referred to a tangent scale for that purpose as a "Maddox cross."[121]

Another test for lateral phorias is one popularized by Australian optometrist Edwin Howell.[122] This test makes use of a scale arranged along a horizontal line with an arrow directed vertically at the zero point on the scale. A vertical prism is used to double the scale and the patient reports the number on the doubled scale to which the arrow points, as well as whether the arrow is to the right or the left of the zero on the doubled scale. Some publications have attributed this test to Charles Prentice,[122,123] but it appears that priority might belong to E. E. Maddox, who described the test in 1889.[124]

Prisms used for phoria measurements have included loose prisms, prism bars, Stevens phorometers (1888), and Risley rotary prisms (1889).[125,126] The first phoropter, patented by De Zeng in 1909, included a Stevens phorometer, rotary prisms, and Maddox rods.[127] Another early instrument that could be used to test phoria status was the Hazen kratometer, an instrument that could be clamped to a table. In the

Hazen kratometer, a "prism battery," a slide with a series of different prisms, could be used to vary prism power in front of one of the patient's viewing ports.[128,129]

By the beginning of the twentieth century, phoria testing was part of the repertoire of many optometrists. The 1895 correspondence course of the South Bend College of Optics included "muscle insufficiencies" as one of its 20 lessons.[130] A 1911 article in *Optical Journal and Review of Optometry* declared, "Many optometrists now consider a test of the muscle balance as much a part of every examination, as is the record of visual acuity."[131]

Fusional vergence range testing involves determining the range of prism powers, base-in and base-out, through which the patient can see clearly and/or singly. It is unclear who originated fusional vergence range testing. In the 1860s, Donders[132] implied ranges of relative convergence in his studies of the zone of clear single binocular vision. In the 1880s, Edmond Landolt[133] noted that the divergence limit is seldom located at a finite distance but rather the eyes can diverge beyond parallelism of the lines of sight, therefore making it necessary to use base-in prism to measure the vergence far point. For the convergence limit, Landolt[134] used a device he called an *ophthalmo-dynamometer* (not to be confused with the instrument with the same name, used for measuring blood pressure in the retinal vessels). This consisted of a black cylinder with a vertical slit and an attached tape measure. A candle was placed inside the cylinder, and the illuminated vertical slit served as a target for a near point of convergence determination. The distance at which the patient noted that the slit doubled was measured with the tape measure.

In 1889, Maddox[135] described measurement of the "relative range of convergence" by using base-in prism for negative vergence and base-out prism for positive vergence. Maddox suggested that "this test would probably be the most valuable of any, if the best ratio between the negative and positive parts were well worked out for different distances."[136] Maddox recommended using pairs of prisms rather than a single prism over one eye.

Maturation of the Optometric Examination

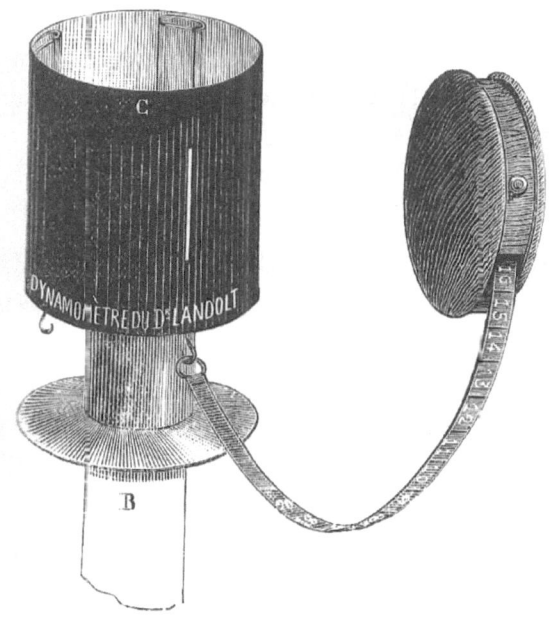

Figure 5.7. Landolt's device for the measurement of near point of convergence. (Image from Landolt E. *The Refraction and Accommodation of the Eye and Their Anomalies.* Translated by: Culver CM. Edinburgh: Pentland, 1886:283)

The British astronomer John Herschel showed that when two prisms were placed in opposition and rotated in opposite directions, the resultant effect would be that of a single increasing prism.[137] That principle was used by S. D. Risley in 1889 to make a rotary prism system with a smooth increase in prism power for clinical use.[138] Risley rotary prisms have been incorporated in phoropters for many years.

The unit used for dissociated phorias and fusional vergence ranges is the prism diopter. As noted earlier, the prism diopter was first suggested by Charles Prentice in 1890. By the early twentieth century, dissociated phorias and fusional vergence ranges had become a part of the standard examination of many optometrists. Charles Sheard included them in his 1917 list of tests that should be performed by the optometrist.[139,140] They were then included in the 21-point examination introduced by the Optometric Extension Program in the early 1930s and saw wide usage for several decades.[141,142,143] They continue to be an essential part of binocular vision analysis.

CHANGES IN THE STRUCTURE OF THE OPTOMETRIC EXAMINATION IN THE 1970S AND LATER

Through the first part of the twentieth century, many optometrists came to see that optometric care involved not only an accurate refraction but also an evaluation of accommodation, binocular vision, ocular health, and visual function. There were substantial improvements in the knowledge of clinical vision science and technology in the mid-twentieth century, but the basic structure of the standard optometric examination was largely unchanged from the 1930s to the early 1970s. For example, the standard optometric examination in the early 1970s included, as taught at the Pacific University College of Optometry, distance and near visual acuity, distance and near cover test, versions, near point of convergence, amplitude of accommodation, pupillary reflexes, and the tests in the OEP 21-point examination (see Table 5.1). Slit lamp biomicroscopy was taught as part of contact lens fitting or for evaluation of the anterior segment when indicated. Students were taught as auxiliary procedures, to be used when indicated, Keystone stereoscope visual skills, the Hirschberg test, accommodative facility, dynamic retinoscopy, various binocular vision tests, selected developmental and visual perception tests, tangent screen visual fields, and color vision tests. McKay-Marg tonometry was to be performed on patients over 40. Students were also informed of other tests such as binocular indirect ophthalmoscopy, gonioscopy, Goldmann tonometry, cycloplegic refraction, visual evoked response, and contrast sensitivity, but no hands-on instruction was given as part of the required curriculum.

With the passage of legislation allowing optometrists to use diagnostic and therapeutic pharmaceutical agents in the later 1970s, tests such as binocular indirect ophthalmoscopy, Goldmann tonometry, and cycloplegic refraction became part of optometry school curricula, and practicing optometrists learned the procedures through intensive continuing education programs. Emphasis on the concept of the optometrist as a primary care provider in the broad health care system led to the inclusion of blood pressure testing by many practitioners.

Another development beginning in the 1970s was the concept of the problem-oriented examination, wherein the tests to be performed are indicated by the complaint(s) presented by the patient.[144,145] With this philosophy, emphasis shifted from a complete database of test results to a limited database that would meet legal requirements and address the problems of the individual patient. Although this concept had largely been accepted by the end of the twentieth century, Elliott[146] noted a lack of agreement among practitioners on what constituted an adequately thorough optometric examination.

The last part of the twentieth century and the beginning of the twenty-first saw increased automation and technological development in several areas of optometric instrumentation, perhaps most notably in perimetry, corneal topography, and ocular imaging procedures, such as fundus photography and optical coherence tomography.[147,148,149,150,151,152,153,154,155] Table 5.2[156,157] summarizes the results of surveys conducted by the American Optometric Association on the percentages of optometrists using new technologies.

Notable for its absence from the surveys summarized in Table 5.2 is the computer-assisted videokeratoscope, which has become very common for its use in assessing corneal topography. The data in the table show steady adoption of instrumentation that would have been very uncom-

Table 5.2. Percentages of optometrists using new technologies, based on surveys conducted by the American Optometric Association

	2003	2012	2017
Automated perimeter	91%	90%	91%
Autorefractor/ Autokeratometer	68%	79%	89%
Fundus photography	58%	73%	81%
Pachymeter	38%	66%	71%
Scanning laser ophthalmoscope	6%	48%	--
Automated refracting lane	12%	18%	--
A/B scan ultrasound/IOL Master	10%	17%	--
Optical coherence tomography	--	--	61%
Electronic health records	--	49%	72%

mon—or not available at all—in optometric offices 50 years before. Even with these advances in instrumentation, core elements of examination, such as the subjective refraction, remained as important as they were at the beginning of the twentieth century.

Chapter 5: Notes

1. *Dr. Thompson's 1895 Correspondence Course in Optics, With Historical Commentary by Monroe J. Hirsch*. Chicago, IL: Professional Press, 1975:82.
2. Sheard C. Dynamic ocular tests, 1917. In: Sheard C., *The Sheard Volume: Selected Writings in Visual and Ophthalmic Optics*. Philadelphia, PA: Chilton, 1957:42.
3. Sheard, 43.
4. Birnbaum MH. *Optometric Management of Nearpoint Vision Disorders*. Boston, MA: Butterworth-Heinemann, 1993:121-160.
5. Schmitt EP. *The Skeffington Perspective of the Behavioral Model of Optometric Data Analysis and Vision Care*. Bloomington, IN: AuthorHouse, 2006:59-227.
6. Levene JR. *Clinical Refraction and Visual Science*. London, UK: Butterworths,

1977:44-45.
7 Bennett AG. A commentary on the "history of spectacles." *Optician* 1989;198(5225):11-13.
8 Albert DM. Ocular refraction and the development of spectacles. In: Albert DM, Edwards DD, eds. *The History of Ophthalmology*. Cambridge, MA: Blackwell Science, 1996:107-123.
9 Levene, 42-43.
10 Wade NJ. *A Natural History of Vision*. Cambridge, MA: MIT Press, 1998:325-327.
11 Bennett AG. An historical review of optometric principles and techniques. *Ophthal Physiol Opt*. 1986;6:3-21.
12 Davidson DW. Visual acuity. In: Eskridge JB, Amos JF, Bartlett JD, eds. *Clinical Procedures in Optometry*. Philadelphia, PA: Lippincott Williams & Wilkins, 1991:17-29.
13 Bailey IL. Visual acuity. In: Benjamin WJ, ed. *Borish's Clinical Refraction*, 2nd ed. St. Louis, MO: Butterworth Heinemann Elsevier, 2006:217-246.
14 Armaignac H. De la nécessité d'adopter une échelle optométrique décimale universelle : Présentation d'un type, 1906. Translated by Goss DA, Carr RA. *Hindsight* 1998;29:5-12.
15 Goss DA. Armaignac's 1906 paper on the recording of visual acuity and the progression of letter sizes on visual acuity charts. *J Am Optom Assoc*. 1998;69:304-306.
16 von Haugwitz T. The history of optical instruments for the examination of the eye. Translated by FC Blodi. In: *Hirschberg's History of Ophthalmology*, Volume 11 (Part 2). Bonn, Germany: Wayenborgh, 1986:A99.
17 Clason MB. Method of and apparatus for testing visual acuity. U.S. patent no. 1174547 A. Filed Oct. 18, 1915; patented March 7, 1916.
18 M.B. Clason. *J Am Optom Assoc*. 1947;18:498.
19 Find A Grave Index. Milo Black Clason. www.findagrave.com/memorial/33743476/milo-black-clason
20 Bausch & Lomb. *Bausch & Lomb Ophthalmic Reference Book*. Rochester, NY: Author, 1948:253-267.
21 Bausch & Lomb, 237-252.
22 Wheelock AP et al. Apparatus for testing vision. U.S. patent no. 1949067 A. Filed Nov. 28, 1932; patented Feb. 27, 1934.
23 [Advertisement] *J Am Optom Assoc*. 1933;5(4):8-9.
24 Gregg JR. *History of the American Academy of Optometry 1922-1986*. Washington, DC: American Academy of Optometry, 1987:57-58.
25 Koch CC. Wheelock to be honored at Miami Beach. *Am J Optom Arch Am Acad Optom*. 1970;47:408-409.
26 Gregg, 187.
27 Weiner G, ed. *The American Journal of Optometry and Archives of the American Academy of Optometry: Forty-Four Year Cumulative Index, Volume 1 (1924) – Volume 44

(1967). Chicago, IL: Professional Press, 1968:77.
28. Frantz DA. Natural color stereoscopic refraction. *J Am Optom Assoc.* 1959;30:471-476.
29. Frantz DA. A review of three-dimensional refraction. *Optom Weekly.* 1966;57(1):23-30.
30. Profiles of personalities in optometry: Dr. Don A. Frantz, AOA President-Elect. *J Am Optom Assoc.* 1960;32:314.
31. Goss DA. Past American Optometric Association presidents remembered. *Hindsight* 2008;39:99-101.
32. Frantz DA. Thorough refraction makes blind woman see: A human interest story. *J Am Optom Assoc.* 1960;32:318-319.
33. American Optometric Association. *Directory of the American Optometric Association.* St. Louis, MO: Author, 1972:108.
34. Borish IM. *Clinical Refraction*, 3rd ed. Chicago, IL: Professional Press, 1970:765-771.
35. Grolman B. Binocular refraction: A new system. *New Eng J Optom.* 1966;17:118-129.
36. Taylor D. Obituary: Bernard Grolman, D.O.S.: Inventor of the non-contact tonometer. www.dickwhitney.net/GrolmanObituaryByDavidTaylor.html
37. American Optometric Association, 34.
38. Myers K. Thank you, Dr. Grolman. www.dickwhitney.net/GrolmanThankYoubyDrKenMyers.html
39. MedicalExpo. Products. www.medicalexpo.com/medical-manufacturer/remote-controlled-ophthalmic-chart-projector-53373.html
40. Levene, 128-131.
41. Fryer C. Jesse Ramsden F.R.S. *Ophthalmic Antiques* 2009;107:14-15.
42. Levene, 148-150.
43. Del Vecchio M, ed. *In View: The Telescopes of the Luxottica Museum.* Milan, Italy: Luxottica, 1995:30.
44. McConnell A. *Jesse Ramsden (1735-1800): London's Leading Scientific Instrument Maker.* Aldershot, England: Ashgate, 2007:157-189.
45. McConnell, 279-280.
46. McConnell, 72.
47. Mandell RB. Jesse Ramsden: Inventor of the ophthalmometer. *Am J Optom Arch Am Acad Optom.* 1960;37:633-638.
48. Gutmark R, Guyton DL. Origins of the keratometer and its evolving role in ophthalmology. *Surv Ophthalmol.* 2010;55:481-497.
49. von Haugwitz, A42-A44.
50. A new ophthalmometer. *Jeweler's Review* 1899;32:652.
51. Bruneni JL. *Looking Back: An Illustrated History of the American Ophthalmic Industry.* Torrance, CA: Optical Laboratories Association, 1994:53-54.
52. Bennett AG, Rabbetts RB. *Clinical Visual Optics*, 2nd ed. London, UK: Butterworths,

1989:466.
53 Goss DA, Eskridge JB. Keratometry. In: Eskridge JB, Amos JF, Bartlett JD, eds. *Clinical Procedures in Optometry*. Philadelphia, PA: Lippincott, 1991:135-154.
54 Grosvenor T. *Primary Care Optometry*, 5th ed. St. Louis, MO: Butterworth Heinemann Elsevier, 2007:201-204.
55 Henson DB. *Optometric Instrumentation*. London, UK: Butterworths, 1983:113-114.
56 Borish, 639-641.
57 Grosvenor, 186-187.
58 Levene JR. The true inventors of the keratoscope and photo-keratoscope. *Brit J Hist Sci*. 1965;2:324-342.
59 Emsley HH. Optics of vision, Volume 1. In: *Visual Optics*, 5th ed. London, UK: Butterworths, 1953:330-331.
60 Reynolds AE, Kratt HJ. The photo-electronic keratoscope. *Contacto* 1959;3:53-59.
61 Goss DA, Gerstman D. The optical science underlying the quantification of corneal contour: A short history of keratoscopy and Indiana University contributions. *Indiana J Optom*. 2000;3:13-16.
62 Bowden TJ. *Contact Lenses: The Story, A history of the development of contact lenses*. Gravesend, Kent, UK: Bower House, 2009:232-234.
63 Rowsey JJ, Reynolds AE, Brown R. Corneal topography: Corneascope. *Arch Ophthalmol*. 1981;99:1093-1100.
64 Goss DA. Keratoscopy. In: Eskridge JB, Amos JF, Bartlett JD, eds. *Clinical Procedures in Optometry*. Philadelphia, PA: Lippincott Williams & Wilkins, 1991:379-385.
65 Horner DG, Salmon TO, Soni PS. Corneal topography. In: Benjamin WJ, ed. *Borish's Clinical Refraction*, 2nd ed. St. Louis, MO: Butterworth Heinemann Elsevier, 2006:645-681.
66 Bennett AG. An historical review of optometric principles and techniques. *Ophthal Physiol Opt*. 1986;6:3-21.
67 Donders FC. *On the Anomalies of Accommodation and Refraction of the Eye*. London, UK: New Sydenham Society, 1864:490.
68 Millodot M. A centenary of retinoscopy. *J Am Optom Assoc*. 1973;44:1057-1059.
69 Hirschberg J. *The History of Ophthalmology*. Volume 11 (Part 1-c). Translated by FC Blodi. Bonn, Germany: Wayenborgh, 1992:687-688.
70 Rogers GA. *Skiascopy: A Treatise on the Shadow Test in Its Practical Application to the Work of Refraction*. Philadelphia, PA: Keystone, 1899.
71 von Haugwitz, A39.
72 Cross AJ. *A System of Ocular Skiametry*. New York, NY: Frederick Boger, 1903:36-37.

73 The College of Optometrists. Retinoscopy. http://www.college-optometrists.org/en/knowledge-centre/museyeum/online_exhibitions/optical_instruments/retinoscopes.cfm
74 Wayenborgh J-P, Mishima S, Keeler CR. International bio-bibliography of ophthalmologists. Volume 7 (Part 1). In: *History of Ophthalmology: The Monographs.* Oostende, Belgium: Wayenborgh, 2001:150.
75 Copeland JC. *A Simplified Method of Streak Retinoscopy.* Chicago, IL: Copeland Refractoscope Co., 1936.
76 Sheard C. *Dynamic Skiametry and Methods of Testing the Accommodation and Convergence of the Eyes.* Chicago, IL: Cleveland Press, 1920:5.
77 Pascal JI. *Studies in Visual Optics.* St. Louis, MO: C.V. Mosby, 1952:175.
78 Jackson E. *Skiascopy and Its Practical Application to the Study of Refraction.* Philadelphia, PA: Edwards & Docker, 1895:86-88.
79 Nott IS. Dynamic skiametry: Accommodation and convergence. *Am J Physiol Opt.* 1925;6:490-503.
80 Haynes HM. Clinical observations with dynamic retinoscopy. *Optom Weekly.* 1960;51:2243-2246, 2306-2309.
81 Rouse MW, Hutter RF, Shiftlett R. A normative study of the accommodative lag in elementary school children. *Am J Optom Physiol Opt.* 1984;61:693-697.
82 Valenti CA. *The Full Scope of Retinoscopy*, rev. ed. Santa Ana, CA: Optometric Extension Program, 1990:8.
83 Birnbaum MH. *Optometric Management of Nearpoint Vision Disorders.* Boston, MA: Butterworth-Heinemann, 1993:169.
84 Ilardi V. *Renaissance Vision from Spectacles to Telescopes.* Philadelphia, PA: American Philosophical Society, 2007:82-95.
85 Daza de Valdes B. *The Use of Eyeglasses*, English translation edited by Paul E. Runge. Oostende, Belgium: J. P. Wayenborgh, 2004:115-118.
86 Gregg, 141-158.
87 Bennett AG. An historical review of optometric principles and techniques. *Ophthal Physiol Opt.* 1986-6:3-21.
88 Levene, 43-44.
89 Levene, 38-40.
90 Queen and Company. *The Human Eye: How to Correct Its Defects by Properly Fitting Glasses.* Philadelphia, PA: Author, 1896:48-49.
91 Queen and Company, 57-58.
92 Queen and Company, 39-41.
93 Queen and Company, 65-66.
94 Bohne W. *Handbook for Opticians: A Treatise on the Optical Trade and Its Mechanical Manipulations*, 3rd ed. New Orleans, LA: A. B. Griswold, 1895:138.
95 One advantage of line charts. *Optical J Rev Optom.* 1914;33:258.
96 Levene, 242-246.
97 Keeler R, Singh AD, Dua HS. Reducing errors in measuring refractive errors: De

Zeng refractometer. *Br J Ophthalmol.* 2012;96:311.
98   Campbell GL. *Phoroptors: Early American Instruments of Refraction and Those Who Used Them.* Wheaton, IL: Author, 2008:57-58.
99   Campbell, 65-66.
100 Campbell, 69.
101 Campbell, 85-87.
102 Levene, 3-15.
103 Campbell, 41-53.
104 Guyton DL. Automated clinical refraction. In: Safir A, ed. *Refraction and Clinical Optics.* Hagerstown, MD: Harper & Row, 1980:505-533.
105 Grosvenor, 200-206.
106 Jorge J, Queirós A, Almeida JB, Parafita MA. Retinoscopy/autorefraction: Which is the best starting point for a noncycloplegic refraction? *Optom Vis Sci.* 2005;82:64-68.
107 Borish IM, Catania LJ. Traditional versus computer-assisted refraction: Which is better? *J Am Optom Assoc.* 1997;68:749-756.
108 Werner DL, Press LJ. *Clinical Pearls in Refractive Care.* Boston, MA: Butterworth-Heinemann, 2002:13-36.
109 Remky H. Albrecht von Graefe: Facets of his work on the occasion of the 125th anniversary of his death (20 July 1870). *Graefe's Arch Clin Exp Ophthalmol.* 1995;233:537-548
110 Von Graefe A. Uber die muscular Asthenopie. [About muscular asthenopia]. *Archiv für Ophthalmol.* 1861;8:314-367.
111 Cooper JB. Obituary: Dr. Ernest E. Maddox. *Br J Ophthalmol.* 1934;18:55-58.
112 Duke-Elder S, Wybar K. Ocular motility and strabismus. Vol. 6. In: Duke-Elder S, ed. *System of Ophthalmology.* St. Louis, OR: Mosby, 1973:245.
113 Maddox EE. *The Clinical Use of Prisms and the Decentering of Lenses,* 2nd ed. Bristol, UK: John Wright, 1893:126-127.
114 Maddox, 127.
115 Maddox EE. The investigation by the rod-test of pareses and paralyses of the ocular muscles. *Ophthal Rev.* 1890;9:287-290.
116 Maddox EE. *The Clinical Use of Prisms and the Decentering of Lenses,* 2nd ed. Bristol, UK: John Wright, 1893:127-131.
117 Prentice CF. *Ophthalmic Lenses: Dioptric Formulae for Combined Cylindrical Lenses, the Prism Dioptry, and Other Optical Papers,* 2nd ed. Philadelphia, PA: Keystone, 1907:121.
118 Thorington J. *Prisms: Their Use and Equivalents.* Philadelphia, PA: Blakiston, 1913:98-99.
119 Hirsch MJ, Bing LB. The effect of testing method on values obtained for phoria at forty centimeters. *Am J Optom Arch Am Acad Optom.* 1948;25:407-416.
120 Maddox EE. *Tests and Studies of the Ocular Muscles.* Philadelphia, PA: Keystone, 1907:224.

121 von Noorden GK. *Burian-von Noorden's Binocular Vision and Ocular Motility: Theory and Management of Strabismus*, 2nd ed. St. Louis, MO: Mosby, 1980:193.
122 Wong EP, Fricke TR, Dinardo C. Interexaminer repeatability of a new, modified Prentice card compared with established phoria tests. *Optom Vis Sci.* 2002;79:370-375.
123 Dwyer PS. The Portsea Lord Mayor's Children's Camp vision screening: A rationale and protocol for optometric screening. *Aust J Optom.* 1983;66:178-185.
124 Maddox EE. *The Clinical Use of Prisms and the Decentering of Lenses.* Bristol. UK: John Wright, 1889:86-87.
125 Duke-Elder & Wybar, 278.
126 Campbell, 55-57.
127 Campbell, 65.
128 Talbot CW. The ocular muscles. *Optical J Rev Optom.* 1910;26:939-940.
129 *Blue Book of Optometrists and Opticians.* Chicago, IL: The Optometrist and Optician, 1912:22.
130 *Dr. Thomson's 1895 Correspondence Course in Optics with Historical Commentary by Monroe J. Hirsch.* Chicago, IL: Professional Press, 1975:165-172.
131 Ward SP. Instruments for muscle tests. *Optical J Rev Optom.* 1911;28:849.
132 Donders, 110-111.
133 Landolt E. *The Refraction and Accommodation of the Eye and Their Anomalies.* Translated by CM Culver. Edinburgh, Scotland: Pentland, 1886:192.
134 Landolt, 283-284.
135 Maddox, 80-82.
136 Maddox, 81.
137 Maddox, 47.
138 Risley SD. A new rotary prism. *Trans Am Ophthalmol Soc.* 1889;5:412-413.
139 Sheard, 42-43.
140 Borish IM. Borish on "21 points." *Newsletter Optom Hist Soc.* 1987;18:23-24.
141 Lesser SK. *Fundamentals of Procedure and Analysis in Optometric Examination*, 3rd ed. Fort Worth, TX: S. K. Lesser, 1933.
142 Lesser SK. *Introduction to Modern Analytical Optometry*, rev. ed. Duncan, OK: Optometric Extension Program Foundation, 1969.
143 Hendrickson H. 21 points and more. *Newsletter Optom Hist Soc.* 1987;18:55-56.
144 Amos JF. The problem-solving approach to patient care. In: Amos JF, ed. *Diagnosis and Management in Vision Care.* Boston, MA: Butterworths, 1987:1-7.
145 Grosvenor, 99-100.
146 Elliott DB. The problem-oriented examination's case history. In: Zadnik K, ed. *The Ocular Examination: Measurements and Findings.* Philadelphia, PA: Saunders, 1997:1-18.
147 Johnson CA. The role of automation in new instrumentation. *Optom Vis Sci.* 1993;70:288-298.
148 Henson DB. *Optometric Instrumentation*, 2nd ed. Oxford, UK: Butterworth-Heinemann, 1996.

149 Reynolds AE. Introduction: History of corneal measurement. In: Schanzlin DJ, Robin JB, eds. *Corneal Topography: Measuring and Modifying the Cornea.* New York, NY: Springer-Verlag, 1992:vii-x.

150 Brody J, Waller S, Wagoner M. Corneal topography: History, technique, and clinical uses. *Int Ophthalmol Clin.* 1994;34(3):197-207.

151 Swartz T, Marten L, Wang M. Measuring the cornea: The latest developments in corneal topography. *Curr Opin Ophthalmol.* 2007;18:325-333.

152 Johnson CA, Wall M, Thompson HS. A history of perimetry and visual field testing. *Optom Vis Sci.* 2011;88:8-15.

153 Gabriele ML, Wollstein G, Ishikawa H, et al. Optical coherence tomography: History, current status, and laboratory work. *Invest Ophthalmol Vis Sci.* 2011;52:2425-2436.

154 Wojtkowski M, Kaluzny B, Zawadzki RJ. New directions in ophthalmic optical coherence tomography. *Optom Vis Sci.* 2012;89:524-542.

155 Nadler ML, Wollstein G, Ishikawa H, Schuman JS. Clinical application of ocular imaging. *Optom Vis Sci.* 2012;89:543-553.

156 American Optometric Association. *The State of the Optometric Profession: 2013.* www.aoa.org/Documents/news/state-of-optometry.pdf

157 American Optometric Association. *2017 AOA New Technology & HER Survey.* www.aoa.org/Documents/ric/2017EHR_ExecutiveSummary.pdf

Chapter 6

Optometric Education

Spectacle making and optometric procedures were taught for many years by apprenticeship. The first of what might be considered optometry schools were organized in the late nineteenth century. There was no standardization of content, methods of instruction, nor length of study at the first schools. Some involved instruction provided by companies in how to use the ophthalmic equipment they sold, thus creating demand for their wares. Some were "mom and pop" schools, run by medical or optometric practitioners, sometimes conducted with the help of their families and operated for a profit. Some were schools organized to teach ophthalmologists how to refract, which could also be attended by persons wanting to be optometrists or vice versa. Some schools offered personalized instruction based on previous optometric experience, and some offered a program of instruction by correspondence.

The early schools were often known by the name of the owners, as for example, the Klein School of Optics, which started in Boston in 1894. The word *optics* often appeared in the name of the early schools because at that time, the profession was known as optics as the word *optometry* had not yet come into common usage. The Klein School of Optics changed its name to the Massachusetts School of Optometry in 1901, becoming perhaps the first school to use the word *optometry* in its name. Another one of the first schools to use *optometry* in its name was the Needles Institute of Optometry founded in Kansas City, Missouri, in 1907, by William B. Needles.[1]

In the years between 1872 and 1901, about 60 optometry schools operated for varying periods of time.[2] Training programs varied from about two weeks to a few months. As stated by James Gregg:

> Back in 1890, a prospective optometrist could take a two-week course in refraction, subscribe to one journal which had a small section on optics, read a couple of elementary books on testing vision and he would have absorbed all of the direct optometric education available. Now this does not count background information; there were other readings in physiological optics and related sciences... But practical information was scanty indeed.[3]

The variability in the breadth and depth of the education of optometrists at that time was great. There were some, such as Charles Prentice, with extensive university education in mathematics and physics, and others with only a two-week refraction course who had not finished high school. Even though having training programs is one of the signs of professionalism, those who had served in an apprenticeship of months to years would likely have been better prepared to practice optometry than those who had taken only a two-week or four-week course. As the years went by, the training programs gradually became longer and required more education for entrance into them. Between 1901 and 1914, there were about 42 optometry schools, with curricula typically of three to six months.[2]

OPTOMETRY SCHOOLS AROUND THE BEGINNING OF THE TWENTIETH CENTURY

In an 1899 issue of the *Optical Journal*, there was a Directory of Reputable Optical Colleges.[4] There was no indication of the criteria by which such a list was established. The following schools were listed:

- Atlanta, Georgia: Kellam & Moore's College of Optics.
- Chicago, Illinois: Chicago Ophthalmic College and Hospital, 607 Van Buren St., Dr. H. M. Martin, Pres.
- Chicago, Illinois: Northern Illinois College of Ophthalmology and Otology, Masonic Temple, Drs. J. B. and G. W. McFatrich, Pres. and Sec.
- Chicago, Illinois: McCormick Optical College, 84 Adams St., Dr. Charles McCormick, Pres.
- LaPorte, Indiana: Hutchinson School, J. L. Hutchinson, Supt.
- South Bend, Indiana: South Bend College of Optics, Dr. H. A. Thomson.
- Boston, Massachusetts: Klein School of Optics, 2 Rutland St., August Klein, MD, Pres.
- Boston, Massachusetts: New England Optical Institute, 3 Winter St., C. E. Tucker, Sec.
- Boston, Massachusetts: Dr. Edwin S. Foster, Private, 120 Tremont St.
- Detroit, Michigan: Detroit Optical Institute, Dr. John S. Owen.
- Kansas City, Missouri: Kansas City Optical College, Tenth and Walnut Sts., Dr. J. T. Hamilton.
- New York City: Spencer Optical Institute, 15 Maiden Lane, J. E. Spencer, Pres.
- New York City: American Ophthalmic Institute, 177 Broadway, Dr. R. H. Knowles.
- New York City: L. L. Ferguson, 32 Maiden Lane.
- Syracuse, New York: Syracuse School of Optics, Hitchcock & Morse.
- McMinnville, Oregon: Dr. C. W. Lowe, Private.
- Philadelphia, Pennsylvania: Philadelphia Optical College, 1435 Chestnut St., Dr. C. H. Brown, Pres.
- Toronto, Canada: Optical Institute of Canada, 88 Yonge St., Dr. W. E. Hamill.

Information about many of these schools is limited. The following paragraphs discuss schools for which better documentation exists.

The Northern Illinois College of Ophthalmology and Otology. The Northern Illinois College of Ophthalmology and Otology (NICOO) is one of the predecessor schools of the present-day Illinois College of Optometry. Henry Olin started the Chicago College of Ophthalmology and Otology in 1872. In 1887, James McFatrich joined Olin in his ophthalmology practice and became a member of Olin's faculty. McFatrich took over the school in 1889 when Olin retired. In 1891, McFatrich changed the name of the school to NICOO. George W. McFatrich joined the faculty in 1893.[5] Before 1898, most of their students were doctors of medicine, but after that, the majority of their students were jewelers, dispensing opticians, and refracting opticians.[6]

The Klein School of Optics. The Klein School of Optics was founded in 1894 by August Andreas Klein. Klein came to the United States from Germany when he was 16.[7] He graduated from the Boston University School of Medicine in 1882 and then studied ophthalmology in Germany. The Klein School of Optics had a faculty of seven, including August Klein and three of his children. The one-year curriculum offered instruction in optics, anatomy, pathology, mathematics, physics, dispensing, and refraction.[7] The tuition was $75 for a full course and $30 for a single term. The name was changed to the Massachusetts College of Optometry in 1901 and later became the New England College of Optometry.

The Hutchinson School. In 1886, J. R. Parsons started the Parsons Horological Institute in LaPorte, Indiana, to teach watchmaking.[8,9] In 1888, A. J. Hutchinson went to work for Parsons. Shortly thereafter, Hutchinson resigned, and with J. H. William Meyer, founded the Hutchinson School of Watchmaking and Optics. It is of interest that in 1892, Lydia Moss Bradley purchased the Parsons Institute and moved it to Peoria, Illinois, where it became the Bradley Polytechnic Institute and then later Bradley University. The Bradley Polytechnic Institute offered instruction in optics until about 1926.[10]

Optometric Education 191

An 1896 advertisement for the Hutchinson School said: "Optical Students cannot find a more comprehensive and complete course in Optics than that given at Hutchinson's School for Watchmakers, Engravers and Opticians. Next course commences January 6, 1896. J. H. Wm. Meyer, M.D., Lecturer in Optics...J. L. Hutchinson, Supt., LaPorte, Ind."[4] It may be presumed that the Hutchinson School ceased operation by at least 1912 because the list of optometry schools in the 1912 *Blue Book of Optometrists and Opticians* does not include it.[10]

The South Bend College of Optics. The South Bend College of Optics was founded in 1893.[11] From 1893 to 1901, it offered attendance (live) and correspondence courses. In 1901, it discontinued the attendance courses to concentrate on the correspondence course. In 1912, its president, H. A. Thomson, announced that it would start its attendance courses again.[12] South Bend College of Optics discontinued operation in about 1920.[10] In 1899, it charged $50 for its attendance course and $25 for its correspondence course.[13] In 1903, it announced that its rate had been reduced to $7.50 for the correspondence course and Doctor of Optics diploma.[14]

A 1906 advertisement for the South Bend College of Optics said, "We settle the question of prisms. Our course in optics tells you just when and how to prescribe prisms and when to let them alone." After claiming that their rules for prescribing prisms have "never been known to fail," the advertisement mentions that the course teaches the correction of astigmatism and the use of the ophthalmoscope, retinoscope, and trial set. The school also claimed to be "the most thorough and painstaking optical college in America."[15]

Thomson copyrighted his correspondence course in 1895. It was reprinted in 1975 by Professional Press, with a 30-page historical commentary by Monroe Hirsch.[16] The course consisted of 180 pages in 20 lessons. Each lesson had text and questions to answer, plus a reading assignment from *Hartridge on Refraction*. There were a total of 333 questions.

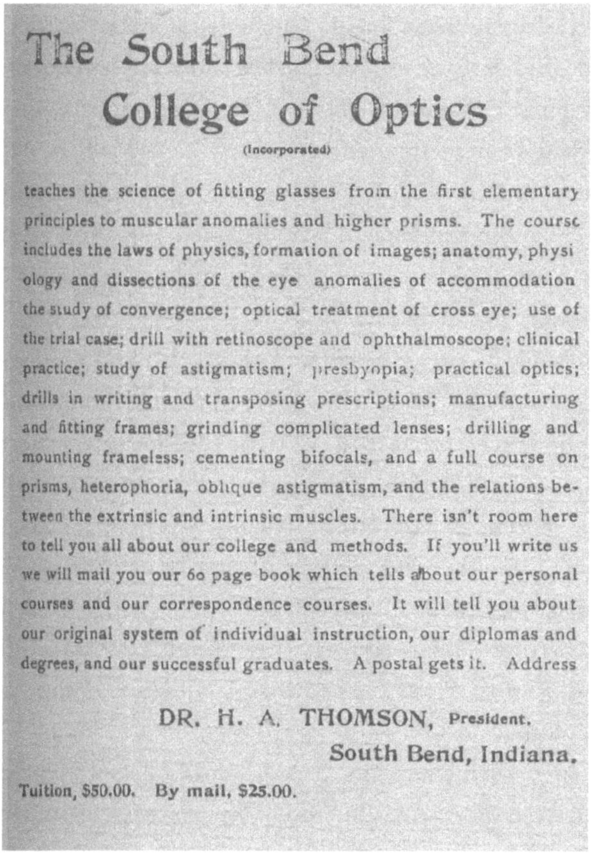

The South Bend College of Optics
(Incorporated)

teaches the science of fitting glasses from the first elementary principles to muscular anomalies and higher prisms. The course includes the laws of physics, formation of images; anatomy, physiology and dissections of the eye anomalies of accommodation the study of convergence; optical treatment of cross eye; use of the trial case; drill with retinoscope and ophthalmoscope; clinical practice; study of astigmatism; presbyopia; practical optics; drills in writing and transposing prescriptions; manufacturing and fitting frames; grinding complicated lenses; drilling and mounting frameless; cementing bifocals, and a full course on prisms, heterophoria, oblique astigmatism, and the relations between the extrinsic and intrinsic muscles. There isn't room here to tell you all about our college and methods. If you'll write us we will mail you our 60 page book which tells about our personal courses and our correspondence courses. It will tell you about our original system of individual instruction, our diplomas and degrees, and our successful graduates. A postal gets it. Address

DR. H. A. THOMSON, President.
South Bend, Indiana.

Tuition, $50.00. By mail, $25.00.

Figure 6.1. An 1899 advertisement for the South Bend College of Optics of South Bend, Indiana. The term optometry was not in common usage at that time, the term optics then often used instead. (Image from *Optical Journal Supplement* 1899;5:53)

Students were instructed not to send in the answers to the questions except for the questions with lessons 18 and 20, which served as the final examination. For all other questions, Thomson sent answers and explanations with the next set of lessons. Students were also advised to purchase a blank notebook and write down the rules that were presented in each lesson, a total of 214 rules in the 20 lessons. The 10-week course sent two lessons to students each week.

A diploma was awarded to those who achieved the requisite score on the final examination. Thomson was not only president of the South Bend College of Optics but also president of the Thomson Optical Company, which sold trial sets and other optical equipment.

Lessons 1-5 covered propagation of light, reflection, refraction by curved surfaces and lenses, spherical aberration, and chromatic aberration. Topics in lessons 6-8 were refraction by the eye, accommodation, and convergence. Lessons 9 and 10 dealt with subjective refraction, the cobalt blue test, estimating refractive error with ophthalmoscopy, and retinoscopy. Hypermetropia, myopia, astigmatism, and anisometropia were the subjects of lessons 11, 12, 13, and 14, respectively. Lessons 15 and 16 were entitled "Practical Work" and looked at general tips in conducting an examination, illuminating and equipping the examination room, order of testing, questions to ask the patient during testing, and prescription of lenses. Retinoscopy was presented in more depth in lesson 17 than the introduction to it in lesson 10.

In lesson 18, the student learned about converting optical crosses to prescriptions, transposing prescriptions, distinguishing types of astigmatism (mixed, simple, compound), lens materials, and ordering lenses and frames. Topics in lesson 19 were heterophoria and prisms. Testing procedures described in this lesson are what we would recognize as the von Graefe and Maddox rod phoria tests. Among the rules that students were told to copy into their notebooks were rules 199 and 200: "In prescribing prisms never give over one-half to two-thirds the full correction.... Patients to whom prisms are given should be requested to return in about two weeks for re-examination of the eyes."[17] In lesson 20, there was further discussion of heterophoria and mention of some common diseases such as cataract, pterygium, glaucoma, nystagmus, and tobacco and alcohol amblyopia as well as the recommendation that: "a hand-book of the different diseases of the eye should be in every optician's library for constant reference and study."[17] Thomson closed lesson 20 with words of encouragement:

Our course of lessons is ended. The course of study upon your part is, I hope, just begun. I have endeavored to guide you on the right path of study and research in this interesting science, until you would have a sufficient understanding of the work to enable you to continue upon your own footing....Hoping that you may attain the highest position in the field which you have chosen, and with many thanks for your kind co-operation in making this course a pleasure and success, I am, Your Friend and Teacher, Dr. H.A. Thomson.[17]

The Philadelphia Optical College. One of the prominent schools in the later nineteenth century and the early twentieth century was the Philadelphia Optical College, which was founded in 1889 by D. V. Brown, W. Reed Williams, and Christian Henry Brown.[18] D. V. Brown at that time was president of the Philadelphia Optical Company and a prominent figure in the optical business. He died in about 1916. There does not appear to have been any family relation between D. V. Brown and C. H. Brown. W. Reed Williams was the treasurer of the Philadelphia Optical Company. C. H. Brown was the initial instructor in the Philadelphia Optical College and seemed to be the major individual in its operation.[19]

It appears that a significant number of persons attended the Philadelphia Optical College. Remarks during a 1917 alumni banquet included the statement that over 2,000 persons had attended.[20] Otto Haussmann, who graduated from the school in 1905 and joined its faculty in 1916, claimed in a memorial tribute to C. H. Brown in the 1930s that "more than 5,000 students enrolled in the Philadelphia Optical College and all of them received Doctor Brown's personal attention."[21]

Those who attended Philadelphia Optical College came from a variety of backgrounds. A news item in the 1908 *Optical Journal* said that some of their students had worked in dentistry, jewelry stores, watchmaking, and engraving.[22] A 1915 news item noted that three of their enrollees were physicians.[23] An 1899 advertisement for the school proclaimed that

"Druggist and Optician will prove a strong combination."[24] Philadelphia Optical College advertised not only in optometric publications, such as *Optical Journal* and *Optometric Weekly*, but also in periodicals for druggists and dentists.[24]

News items in the *Optical Journal* from the Philadelphia Optical College frequently emphasized the successes and leadership positions of graduates. For example, in 1914, graduates were elected to the presidency of the Nebraska State Association of Optometrists, to officer positions in the Florida State Optometric Association, and to the presidency of the Iowa State Board of Optometry, and two graduates gave papers at the Ohio Optical Association meeting.[25,26,27,28] In 1915, a graduate named William V. Nicum was added to the instructional staff of the new optometry school at The Ohio State University, and he recommended the adoption of C. H. Brown's *Optician's Manual* as a textbook there.[29] In 1916, it was reported that graduates Schenmeyer and Jarvis were vice-presidents of the American Optical Association and a graduate named Jenkins was treasurer.[30]

The Indiana University Optometry Library holds a scrapbook of advertisements that the Philadelphia Optical College placed in various periodicals, mostly from 1890 to 1914. The scrapbook is thought to have been compiled by C. H. Brown.[24] A December, 1893 advertisement said, "Our Correspondence Course is all that is needed to make any man a skilled optician, after which our Charter empowers us to award a diploma and confer a degree." In 1900, they advertised six-month, three-month, one-month, special, and post-graduate attendance courses as well as correspondence courses. The one-month, special, and post-graduate courses were for those "already engaged in optical pursuits." In 1903, the degrees awarded by Philadelphia Optical College included Graduate in Optometry, Doctor of Optics, Doctor of Optometry, and Doctor of Refraction.[24] In 1908, the school advertised one-week, two-week, one-month, three-month, or six-month attendance courses, along with correspondence courses. By 1913, the attendance courses ranged from one month to two years in length. A 1914 advertisement said that the attendance courses were "as long or as short as will suffice for individual requirements."[24]

The Philadelphia Optical College did not fare well in the 1920s, when optometry schools were rated by the Education Committee of the International Board of Boards, an organization of optometry boards of examiners. In 1922, a conference on standards in optometric education was held. One of the resolutions of the conference was that "no credits or diplomas for correspondence courses be given..."[31] In 1925, the Philadelphia Optical College was one of the optometry schools that were not rated high enough to even merit an on-site evaluation visit. Despite the poor evaluation, the Philadelphia Optical College continued to operate for a number of years.

The Philadelphia Optical College Correspondence Course. Optometric Historical Society member Charles Letocha provided this author with copies of examination papers from the Philadelphia Optical College correspondence course. The course was taken in August and September of 1914 by Ernest W. Dodd, a relative of one of Dr. Letocha's patients.

Included with the examination paper was a two-page introduction to the course headed "Personal Letter of Advice – Read Carefully." At the top, a blank after "Matriculation No." was stamped with the number 2430. The letter of advice recommended that the student "cultivate habits of study" and "study, study." It was stated that the aim of the course was "to direct your studies and to systemize your knowledge." Students were expected to read and study textbooks, such as C. H. Brown's *Optician's Manual*. One of the two volumes was provided free to students after payment of the enrollment fee. It was noted that all answers on the examination forms would be "critically examined by Dr. Brown." The letter of advice stated that the last lesson was no. 28, "Student's Practice Eye." This was an optional lesson that students received if they purchased a $2 practice eye.

Dodd completed lessons 1 through 27 in August and September of 1914. He received a letter dated October 13, 1914, stating that he was graduating as Doctor of Optics and that a diploma was being sent to him. The examination paper for each lesson consisted of 25 questions with space for answers. Mr.

Dodd's answers were mostly one or two lines, but in some places he squeezed in a three- or four-line answer. The subjects of the 27 lessons are listed in Table 6.1.

Table 6.1. Lessons in the 1914 Philadelphia Optical College correspondence course.

Lesson Number	Lesson Title
1	Anatomy of Eye
2	Mechanism of the Eye
3	Physiology of Vision
4	Dioptrics of the Eye
5	Laws of Light
6	Principles of Optics
7	Institutes of Refraction
8	Lenses
9	Further Study of Lenses
10	Numbering of Lenses
11	Presbyopia – General Principles
12	Presbyopia – Treatment
13	Hypermetropia – General Principles
14	Hypermetropia – Treatment
15	Myopia – General Principles
16	Myopia – Treatment
17	Astigmatism – General Principles
18	Astigmatism – Treatment
19	Anomalies of Ocular Muscles

20	Treatment of Muscular Anomalies
21	The Ophthalmoscope
22	Retinoscopy
23	Method of Examination
24	The Ophthalmometer
25	Theoretic Optics
26	Asthenopia
27	Practical Points

To illustrate the level of difficulty of the questions on the examination papers, here are some of the questions in the lesson on Anomalies of Ocular Muscles:

> 451. Name extra ocular muscles that move the eye.
>
> 452. What is nerve supply of each of the four recti?
>
> 455. What is action of each of the obliques?
>
> 460. Why do accomm., conv., and contraction pupil occur together?
>
> 461. What is punctum prox. of conv. and how determined?
>
> 463. How can the accomm. be lessened or increased?
>
> 464. How can convergence be lessened or increased?
>
> 468. Upon what does diagnosis paralytic strabismus depend?
>
> 471. What is predominant cause of strabismus and how does it act?

> 475. What is the cover test?

It appears that the Philadelphia Optical College continued to operate a correspondence course after C. H. Brown's death late in 1933. It was listed among colleges in the *Blue Book of Optometrists* as late as 1940. The description of the school in the 1936 *Blue Book* gave its location and stated simply, "Established the correspondence system. Offers Personal Extension Course of Home Study which leads to a valid degree in the Science of Optometry."[32]

Remarkably, at least as late as 1954, the Philadelphia Optical College was still offering a correspondence course.[33] Hofstetter[33] expressed concern that it was being sold to "circumstantially gullible" optometrists outside the United States who were not knowledgeable about American educational institutions. He characterized the 1954 correspondence course as "grossly outmoded" based on the examination papers sent to him by an optometrist in Peru, who had completed the course in 1954. The Peruvian optometrist sent Hofstetter examination papers for 12 of the 26 lessons. The subject headings for 11 of those 12 lessons were the same as those in the course taken by Ernest Dodd in 1914.

Hofstetter also referred to the preface for the examination paper for Numbering of Lenses, which stated, "The transition period in the nomenclature of the numbering of lenses is over, and we note the passing of the old inch system, and the adoption of the newer and better Dioptric System. This adds to the difficulty of the subject, because the optometrist must have knowledge of both systems, and a clear understanding of the method of converting one into the other." This exact statement, as well as some of the same examination questions on the inch system, was in the 1914 course. Hofstetter observed that the transition period to the use of diopters "had occurred at least three quarters of a century before 1954." He also noted that "in spite of the abuses attributable to the later owners of the 'chartered' college, it must be said that those who seriously followed through on the lessons and did indeed study Brown's remarkably solid books of the day must have benefited."

The DeMars School of Optometry. Another early optometry school was the DeMars School of Optometry established in 1900 as the DeMars School of Optics.[34] The owner and operator of the school was Louis L. DeMars.[35] He graduated in 1896 from the Northern Illinois College of Ophthalmology and Otology and started a private practice in Minneapolis, Minnesota. In the federal census for 1900 and 1910, he gave his occupation as optician, whereas in 1920 and 1930 he was listed as an optometrist, reflecting the fact that the term *optometrist* was not in common usage in 1900 or 1910. DeMars was one of the charter members of the American Academy of Optometry. One of the aspects of this school that made it notable was that at least two of its graduates became important persons in optometry: Carel C. Koch, who was secretary of the American Academy of Optometry from 1922 to 1925 and from 1944 to 1973, and Ernest H. Kiekenapp, who was secretary of the American Optometric Association from 1922 to 1957.

THE NEW YORK INSTITUTE OF OPTOMETRY AND THE ROCHESTER SCHOOL OF OPTOMETRY'S TWO-YEAR CURRICULA IN 1909

When the optometrists in New York State achieved their licensure law in 1908, they specified that candidates for licensure should have attended at least two years of high school and a two-year optometry course.[36] At that time, no optometry school offered a two-year program, most of them being about three to six months.[37] By 1909, two schools, the New York Institute of Optometry in New York City, and the Rochester School of Optometry in Rochester, New York, were offering two-year programs.

A 1908 advertisement in the *Optical Journal* for the New York Institute of Optometry (NYIO), said that it

> teach[es] Theoretical Optics, including the laws of reflection and refraction, as applied to mirrors, lenses, prisms, and optical instruments. Practical Optics, including the mounting, construction, and adjusting of lenses and prisms. Physiological Optics, covering the dioptric functions of the eye, its anomalies, and their correction by lenses. Theoretical Optometry, covering the principles involved in the methods and instruments used in detecting and measuring the anomalies of the eye. Practical Optometry, covering the demonstration and use of mechanical appliances for measuring the powers of vision. Anatomy, Physiology and Hygiene, including also Ocular Pathology.[38]

The faculty of NYIO, recognized as important optometric leaders and authors of significant optometry books, were Elmer E. Hotaling, E. LeRoy Ryer, Andrew Jay Cross, Robert M. Lockwood, Stephens H. Brooks, and Frederic A. Woll.[39] An advertisement for NYIO in the June 3, 1909, issue of the *Optical Journal* stated that they were offering the "New York State Standard Two-Year (18 months) Course. Complete One-Year (7 to 9 months) Course for Out-of-State Applicants. Post-Graduate Course for Optometrists and Physicians. Special One-Month Courses on Specific Subjects for Advanced Optometrists."[40] NYIO did not offer correspondence courses.[41]

NYIO closed in 1910. Some members of the faculty had resigned because of the difficulty of maintaining their private practices while teaching at the school.[42] Some of its faculty went on to teach in the optometry program at Columbia University, which opened later that same year.

The Rochester School of Optometry was founded in 1902 by physician Arthur H. Bowen.[43] After Bowen's death, B. B. Clark took over as president of the school. The faculty for the two-year curriculum included physicians, optometrists, and a PhD physics professor.

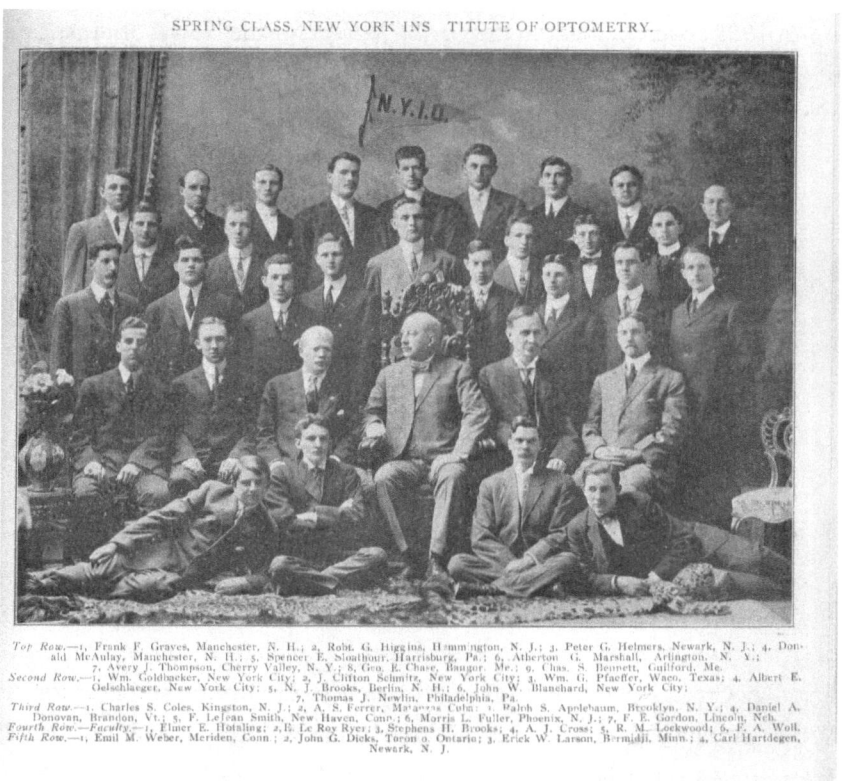

Figure 6.2. A class of students and the faculty of the New York Institute of Optometry in 1909. The faculty, seated in chairs, are, left to right, Elmer E. Hotaling, E. LeRoy Ryer, Stephens H. Brooks, Andrew Jay Cross, Robert M. Lockwood, and Frederic A. Woll. (Image from *The Optical Journal* 1909;23:923)

This expansion of curriculum created controversy. One of the opponents of the longer curriculum was M. B. Ketchum, MD, President of the Los Angeles Optical College and later Dean of the Southern California College of Optometry and Ophthalmology. Ketchum advanced that essential elements of a successful school are individual personal instruction, being equipped with the principal modern instruments used in the profession, and selection of useful textbooks.[44] Ketchum said that the textbooks he found to be most useful were: Henderson's *Lessons* (presumably *Lessons on the Eye* by F. L. Henderson, the third edition of which was published in 1903); *Thorington's Refraction and How to Refract*; both volumes of *The Optician's Manual*, by Brown; *Clinics in Optometry*; Valk's *Squint* (*Strabismus, or Squint, Latent and Fixed* was published by Valk in 1904); Lewis's *Optical Dictionary*; and Haab's *Internal Diseases of the Eye* and *External Diseases of the Eye*.

In 1909, Ketchum[44] suggested that in the first three months of training, the student should be able to demonstrate knowledge of the "anatomy of the eye, ametropia, light, lenses, transposing, neutralizing, etc." Then the student should be "better able to take up the deeper studies, such as amblyopia, asthenopia, the practical use of different instruments and trial case, as well as the study of diseases." He also gave the opinion that state licensure laws should not require specific numbers of hours of instruction in particular areas, but instead curricular design should be the responsibility of the schools.

In contrast, Andrew Jay Cross argued that elevation of the standards of optometric education would benefit the profession and public. One point he made was the importance of understanding theory: "Many old optometrists of long practical experience confess their weakness when it comes to questions of theory. Similar excuses were put forward in medicine and dentistry in their early days, but now it is well known that practitioners whose theories are well grounded have a decided advantage over those who are termed 'empirics'."[45] Cross further emphasized high standards when he said that "efficient schools of optometry must be maintained or else the calling, as a distinct profession, will disappear from off the earth; neither night, correspondence nor mediocre schools of any kind whatsoever will suffice, no matter whether they are run by societies, corporations or individuals."[45]

Harry Martin Bestor, a faculty member at the Rochester School of Optometry, supported the two-year program despite the warnings of some that such requirements were too stringent. Bestor observed that "if optometry is to take a serious and dignified position among professions it seems to me that a two-year course is none too long, and could not be shortened, when you consider the mathematics of the course alone could not be crowded into lesser time."[46] Bestor further suggested that "the weeding out of the charlatan and spectacle peddler by optical laws, and the planting in their places of a dignified and educated class of practitioners, will eventually give to optometry the moral and active support of other professions and the public."[46] Bestor also appealed to readers with the observation that "with general recognition of optometry surely their services will become more valuable and compensation therefore greater."[46]

OPTOMETRY SCHOOL ESTABLISHED AT COLUMBIA UNIVERSITY IN 1910

With the requirements of the New York State licensure law and the closing of the New York Institute of Optometry, a need was recognized for an optometry school at a university.[45,47] Apparently, the efforts of the Rochester School of Optometry would not be sufficient.

In the spring of 1910, it was announced that optometry courses would be started at Columbia University on September 28 of that year.[48] This was a significant step in the history of optometry as this was the first time that an optometry school was to be conducted at a university. Curriculum and instruction were placed in the hands of the Columbia University Department of Physics, and its administration fell under the Extension Teaching Department.[49]

Admissions requirements were the completion of at least two years of high school and being at least 19. Students who had finished high school and who completed the full two years of optometry school were to receive a certificate from the Columbia University Board of Extension Teaching.[48] The tuition was $5 per point, a point being one hour of class or lecture per week, or two hours of laboratory per week, in a semester. This resulted in tuition of $75 for the first term of the first year and $85 for the second term of the first year.[48] The courses in the initial curriculum were as follows:

- First year, first term: Plane Trigonometry, General Physics, Theoretic Optics, Physiologic Optics, Anatomy and Physiology of the Eye.
- First year, second term: General Physics, Theoretic Optics, Practical Optics, Physiologic Optics, Theoretic Optometry.
- Second year, first term: Theoretic Optics, Physiologic Optics, Practical Optics, Theoretic Optometry, Pathologic Conditions of the Eye, Practical Optometry.
- Second year, second term: Theoretic Optics, Physiologic Optics, Practical Optics, Theoretic Optometry, Practical Optometry.[48,50]

Optometrists taught courses in theoretic and practical optometry (Andrew Jay Cross, with some lectures in theoretic optometry by Charles Prentice) and in practical optics (Frederic Woll). Courses in theoretic optics were taught by Assistant in Physics W. W. Stifler. Physiologic optics was taught by Professor of Physics William Hallock.[50] Hallock was head of the Department of Physics at Columbia.[48] Louis R. Welzmiller, MD, was the instructor for the course in pathological conditions of the eye.[50]

Textbooks for theoretic optometry included *Principles of Refraction in the Human Eye*, by Burnett; *System of Ocular Skiametry* by Cross; *Ophthalmic Lenses* by Prentice; and *The Refractive and Motor Mechanism of the Eye* by Souter.[50] Other textbooks used by early classes of Columbia optometry students were *Physics for College Students* by Carhart; *Practical Exercises in Light* by Clay; *Light for Students* by Edser; *The Human Body* by Martin; *Medical Dictionary* by Gould; *Optical Dictionary* by Lewis; *Diseases of the Eye* by May; and *Refraction and Accommodation of the Eye* by Landolt.[51]

There were 21 students taking the course in the fall of 1910; 10

of them, were from New York State, but there were also students from New Jersey, Ohio, Pennsylvania, Indiana, Massachusetts, Michigan, and Missouri.[52]

In 1911, *The Optical Journal and Review of Optometry* announced that A. J. Cross began his lectures in the theoretic optometry class on February 9. Also in attendance was Charles Prentice. Cross started his lecture with a review of some important steps in the history of optics. He included the scientific contributions of Prentice and Prentice's efforts for the legal recognition of optometry. Prentice in turn praised Cross for his work on dynamic retinoscopy and emphasized that it would assume greater significance in the future practice of optometry.[53]

In April of 1911, the president of the optometry student organization at Columbia, Harold W. Eames, wrote a letter to *The Optical Journal and Review of Optometry*.[54]

> Next September Columbia University's Optometry Course will begin its second year. Knowing the interest manifested in the course throughout the country, a word from the students' point of view may be opportune.
>
> The students themselves realize now what opposition was experienced in placing optometry in its proper department, that of physics, rather than in the Department of Medicine, and also what a tremendous opportunity this course presents.
>
> Here, instead of looking up answers to questions in text-books for three or six months, thereby receiving several elaborate diplomas calculated to impress the public eye, the student is given a thorough course in all subjects which relate to the eye and its dioptric functions....
>
> The question is asked, "Why take two years when a three months' course is good enough?" There is just the point. Is it "good enough?"

Glance back over the past few years and note the strides which optometry has made. The fact that 25 States now have optometry laws proves that a higher degree of proficiency is demanded than could be vouchsafed by the three months' course....

In realizing that a university course of instruction is necessary, the public will soon have a higher regard for the optometrist and will naturally give him the preference over oculists in the examination of eyes for glasses....[54]

OPENING OF A SECOND UNIVERSITY-BASED SCHOOL AT OHIO STATE IN 1914

In the 1914 *Blue Book of Optometrists and Opticians*, there is a listing of 27 "optical schools and colleges" in the United States.[55] The brief descriptions of the schools in the *Blue Book* shows significant lack of uniformity. Some gave both attendance and correspondence courses. The length of study varied, with some schools starting a two-year program and some mentioning variable lengths of study, one school giving a range of three months to three years. Various degrees or certificates were offered at different schools, such as Doctor of Optometry, OphD, OptM, OptB, Doctor of Optics, and Full Course certificate.[55]

Of particular importance in optometric education in 1914 was the opening at The Ohio State University of the second university-based optometry school. This was announced in the August 13 issue of *The Optical Journal and Review of Optometry*.[56] In 1908, Charles Sheard, a physics professor at Ohio State, gave a talk to the Ohio State Optical Association. He greatly impressed the optometrists, and they encouraged him to initiate an optometry program at Ohio State.[57,58] University trustees decided at an August 4 meeting to establish the program to begin the next month. Twelve students registered on September 15 and started classes the next day. Charles Sheard served as director of the program, with F. P. Barr of Lancaster, Ohio; C. N. McDonnell of Columbus, Ohio; John C. Eberhardt of Dayton, Ohio; and Clark Sloan of Cleveland, Ohio as lecturers.

The optometry program at Ohio State was known as Applied Optics from 1914 to 1937, and it was operated within the Department of Physics. At first, an optometry certificate was given after the completion of Ohio State's two years of optometry training, which had followed a minimum of two years of high school work. The required courses in the two years at Ohio State were as follows:

- First Year, First Semester: Mathematics, Physics, Anatomy and Physiology, and English (14 credit hours).
- First Year, Second Semester: Theoretical Optics, Practical Optics, Theoretical Optometry (15 credit hours).
- Second Year, First Semester: Theoretical Optics, Physiological Optics, Practical Optics, Theoretical Optometry, Pathological Conditions of the Eye, Practical Optometry (15 credit hours).
- Second Year, Second Semester: Theoretical Optics, Physiological Optics, Physiological Conditions of the Eye, Practical Optometry, Radiant Energy and the Eye, Practice Course (16 credit hours).

The announcement of the program at Ohio State stated that it was "planned to meet the most rigorous of any of the State laws." It further went on to say that "everywhere in Ohio the optometrists are jubilant and agree that now with an optometry department in the State university they must win their campaign for an optometry law."[56] The Ohio State optometry school started in 1914 with a two-year curriculum, but the next year expanded to a four-year curriculum culminating in a Bachelor's degree.

CONFERENCE TO ESTABLISH STANDARDS IN OPTOMETRIC EDUCATION

In January 1922, a meeting called the First Conference to Establish Standards was held in St. Louis, Missouri.[59,60,61] It was funded by the American Optometric Association and attended by representatives of the Executive Council of the AOA, representatives of the International Association of Boards of Examiners in Optometry (sometimes called the International Board of Boards, or IBB), and representatives of the International Federation of Optometry Schools. Attending the conference were the following:

- Oliver Abel, AOA President, St. Louis, Missouri
- George A. Barron, University of Massachusetts, Boston, Massachusetts
- Harry M. Bestor, AOA Executive Council, Rochester, New York
- H. Frank Brown, Missouri College of Optometry, St. Louis, Missouri
- A. P. DeKeyser, DeKeyser Institute of Optometry, Portland, Oregon
- Louis L. DeMars, DeMars School of Optometry, Minneapolis, Minnesota
- Howard C. Doane, IBB Secretary, Boston, Massachusetts
- P. H. Howard, Missouri College of Optometry, St. Louis, Missouri
- Ernest A. Hutchinson, Los Angeles Medical School of Ophthalmology and Optometry, Los Angeles, California
- Theodore Klein, Massachusetts School of Optometry, Boston, Massachusetts
- George W. McFatrich, Northern Illinois College of Ophthalmology and Otology, Chicago, Illinois
- Howard D. Minchin, The Ohio State University, Columbus, Ohio
- W. B. Needles, Needles Institute of Optometry, Kansas City, Missouri
- Joseph I. Pascal, American Institute of Optometry, New York City
- Ernest Petry, Rochester School of Optometry, Rochester, New York

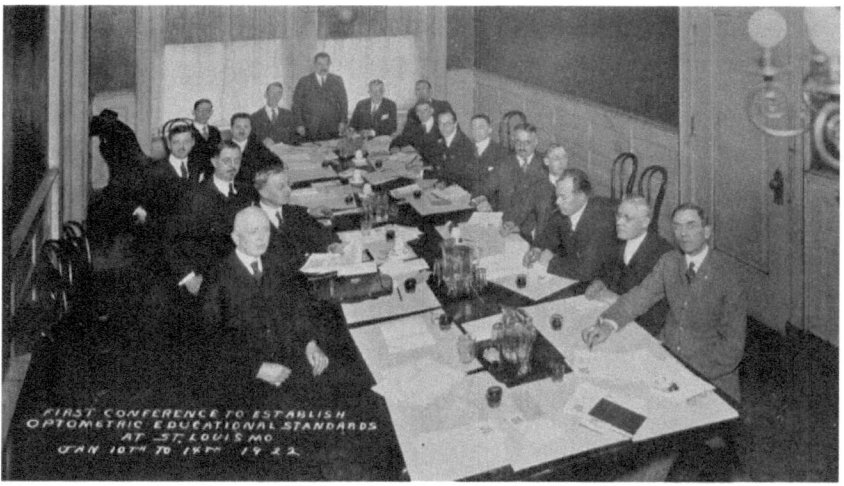

Figure 6.3. First conference to establish standards in optometric education, held in 1922. Clockwise from lower left: George A. Barron, Frederic Woll, Harry M. Bestor, W.B. Needles, Joseph I. Pascal, Ernest Petry, Howard C. Doane (conference secretary), William S. Todd (conference chair), Oliver Abel, Charles Sheard, Howard D. Minchin, Ernest A. Hutchinson, A.P. DeKeyser, Theodore Klein, L.L. DeMars, P.H. Howard, H. Frank Brown, and Claude Wolcott. (Image courtesy of the Archives and Museum of Optometry and The AOA Foundation)

- Charles Sheard, AOA Council on Optometric Education, Southbridge, Massachusetts
- William S. Todd, IBB President, Hartford, Connecticut
- Claude Wolcott, Texas College of Optometry, Dallas, Texas
- Frederic A. Woll, Columbia University, New York City

Several resolutions were passed at this conference. Among them were adoption of uniform standards for evaluation of optometry schools, elimination of apprenticeship provisions in some optometry laws, discontinuation of credits or diplomas for correspondence courses, and adoption of the syllabi for a two-year curriculum prepared by Woll.

As a consequence of the conference, the IBB established a committee to investigate and rate optometry schools.[60] Ernest Eimer chaired the committee, and Woll conducted the evaluations of the schools in 1925 and 1926. There were about 30 schools at that time. Based on preliminary investigations, only 16 of the schools were considered even worthy of onsite inspection. Woll visited those 16 schools, and 11 schools received A, B, or C ratings. To achieve an A rating, the school had to be a nonprofit institution, admit only students with high school education or equivalent, have adequate facilities and staff, have a curriculum of at least two years of 32 weeks or more each, and teach the subjects in Woll's syllabi.[60,61]

Six schools received an A rating: Columbia University, the Los Angeles School of Optometry, The Ohio State University, the Pennsylvania State College of Optometry, the Rochester School of Optometry, and the University of California at Berkeley.[60] The DeKeyser Institute of Optometry and the Massachusetts School of Optometry received B ratings. The Missouri College of Optometry, the Oregon College of Ocular Science, and the Washington School of Optometry were given C ratings. The Northern Illinois College of Ophthalmology and Otology and the Needles Institute of Optometry were not rated, presumably because they were in the process of merging into the Northern Illinois College of Optometry (NICO).[60]

The investigation of optometry schools had a great effect on optometric education. All of the unrated schools, other than NICO, closed. The DeKeyser Institute of Optometry and the Oregon College of Ocular Science merged to form the North Pacific College of Optometry. The Missouri College of Optometry and the Washington School of Optometry, which had gotten C ratings, closed.

The Rochester School of Optometry (RSO), which had achieved an A rating, closed in the late 1920s because the New York optometry law had been changed to make it a requirement that newly qualified optometrists must have an optometry degree from a university. A new optometry school was started at the University of Rochester.[62] At least two faculty members from the RSO, Ernest Petry, Dean at RSO, and Herbert E. Wilder, then served on the optometry faculty at the University of Rochester. The optometry school at the University of Rochester was short-lived, discontinued in 1936.[63]

As a result of these changes, the number of optometry schools in the late 1920s was down to nine: Columbia University, the Los Angeles School of Optometry, the Massachusetts School of Optometry, the Northern Illinois College of Optometry, the North Pacific College of Optometry, The Ohio State University, the Pennsylvania State College of Optometry, University of Rochester, and University of California at Berkeley.

THE FOUNDING OF SIX IMPORTANT OPTOMETRY SCHOOLS

Six important optometry schools that are still operating today were founded between 1919 and 1952. The first of these, the Pennsylvania State College of Optometry, later known as the Pennsylvania College of Optometry, was founded in 1919. The founder and president from 1919 to 1959 was Albert Fitch.[64] In 1923, the Pennsylvania State College of Optometry became the first non-proprietary optometry school to grant a Doctor of Optometry (OD) degree that had been approved by a state legislature.[65]

After years of effort, a committee of the California Optometric Association saw the University of California at Berkeley establish the Curriculum in Optometry in the Department of Physics in 1923.[66,67] Professor of Physics Ralph S. Minor became the director of the program and would later become the school's first dean, a role in which he served until his retirement in 1946. George L. Schneider, who had been a leading member of the California Optometric Association school committee, was made a lecturer in 1923 to give courses in clinical optometry.

The Southern College of Optometry was founded in 1932 in Memphis, Tennessee, as a proprietary school by J. J. Horton, a medical doctor.[68,69] Wilbur Richard Cramer was appointed dean of the college during the 1937-38 school year, and he purchased the school from Horton in

1939. Within a few years, Cramer was able to re-organize the school as a nonprofit institution. Cramer served as president of Southern College of Optometry from 1939 to 1961.

When Newton Wesley and Roy Clunes graduated from the North Pacific College of Optometry in 1939, they started teaching at the school.[70,71,72] In 1941, they purchased the school from its owner, Harry Lee Fording. The entry of the United States into World War II decreased the number of students, and the school suspended operations in 1943. Newton Wesley, who had been in an internment camp for Japanese Americans for a time, relocated to the Midwest, and Roy Clunes joined the U.S. Navy. Wesley and Clunes transferred power of attorney for the school to their good friend Clarence Carkner, who worked with the Oregon Optometric Association to find a university with which the school could be associated. Pacific University entered its first class of optometry students in 1945. An OD degree was to be awarded for a total of five years of pre-optometry and professional optometry study. In the early years of the school, several persons served as dean, including Carol B. Pratt, Wilbur Hulin, Richard Feinberg, and a faculty administrative committee, until James Wahl became dean in 1955. Wahl was dean of the Pacific University College of Optometry until 1963. Faculty members who joined the school in its first years and who subsequently had long careers at the school were Pratt, Detleff Jans, Harold Haynes, Charles Margach, and Anna Berliner. Early part-time faculty members were Clarence Carkner and Hugh Webb. In 1947, three Pacific graduates became the first optometrists to receive OD degrees from a university.[71,73]

Indiana optometrists started talking about the possibility of an optometry school at Indiana University in about 1939 or before.[74,75,76,77] Serious efforts began in 1945 but were met with medical opposition. The impasse was broken by the Indiana optometrists mounting a successful legislative campaign, resulting in a 1951 bill to start an optometry school at Indiana University. Preprofessional classes began in 1951 and professional optometry classes in 1953. The optometry program was started as the Division of Optometry within the College of Arts and Sciences on the Bloomington campus. The initial curriculum consisted of two years of preprofessional study and three years of optometry school, with the graduate receiving a Master of Optometry. Henry Hofstetter was first director of the school, with Merrill Allen and J. Stanley Rafalko as faculty members hired for the school's first year. Eighteen students began optometry studies in the fall of 1953; 12 of the 18 were from Indiana and all of them being men.

A College of Optometry started at the University of Houston in the fall of 1952. At first, their curriculum called for the awarding of the OD degree after five years of college credits: two years of pre-optometry and three years of optometry school.[78,79] In 1956, they announced that after five years, graduates would receive a certificate qualifying them for the practice of optometry, but that an optional fourth year of optometry school, for a total of six years of study, would be required to receive an OD degree. In 1966, they eliminated the certificate program and all students had to complete four years of optometry school, and six years of college credit total to qualify for practice and an OD degree. Charles R. Stewart, who earned his optometry degree and PhD from Ohio State, was dean of the college from 1952 to 1961, followed by Chester H. Pheiffer, who was dean for 17 years.

FORMATION OF THE COUNCIL ON OPTOMETRIC EDUCATION

After a few attempts to establish some form of council on education, the American Optometric Association formed the Council on Optometric Education in 1930, with name changes over the years.[80] In 1934, the Council on Optometric Education and Professional Guidance, with Charles Sheard as chairman, began a three-year study of optometric education.[81] Among their proposals in 1937 were that optometric education should be upgraded in general, and that optometric training should consist of four years of college work with a long range goal of six years total study, two in preprofessional work and four years of optometry school.[82,83] In 1940, the AOA indicated that the Council on Education should serve as an advisor to the International Association of Boards of Examiners in Optometry (or International Board of Boards, IBB) and to optometry schools.[83] Sheard chaired the council from 1934 to 1944, Walter Brown from 1944 to 1945, and H. Ward Ewalt from 1945 to 1951.[84]

In the early 1940s, the AOA Council on Optometric Education (COE) started accrediting optometry schools. The COE discontinued the A, B, and C rating system that had been used by the IBB, using instead the *Manual of Accrediting of Schools and Colleges of Optometry* completed in 1941 by Irvin M. Borish and Eugene Freeman.[85,86,87] Borish and Freeman composed the manual by consulting accreditation manuals from various medical, dental, and other academic accrediting agenices.[88] In 1952, the COE became recognized by the United States Office of Education.[84] The COE has continued as the accrediting body for optometry schools and is now known as the Accreditation Council on Optometric Education.

IBB, NBEO, AND ARBO

Early in the twentieth century, as state licensure laws created state licensing boards, some members of those boards attempted to form national confederations of state boards to share experiences and solutions to common problems. This led to temporary organizations such as the National Board of State Examiners in Optometry, formed in 1909, and the National Organization of State Board Members, formed in 1912.[89]

In 1919, the International Board of Boards (IBB) was formed with William S. Todd serving as the first president.[90,91] Later, it became known as the International Association of Boards of Examiners in Optometry (IAB, although sometimes still referred to as IBB).[92] The IBB or IAB was composed of representatives from optometry boards in various states and provinces in the United States and Canada.[90] When Todd presided over the First Conference on Optometric Standards in 1922, he was president of the IAB. The IAB handled the rating of optometry schools from the 1920s until that function was turned over to the AOA COE in the 1940s.

One of the recommendations of the First Conference on Optometric Standards was that a central examining board be set up to certify eligibility for licensure. It wasn't until 1951 that the IAB worked in conjunction with the Association of Schools and Colleges of Optometry to establish the National Board of Examiners in Optometry (NBEO).[93] Gradually over the years, state licensing boards incorporated the NBEO examinations as part of their licensure requirements.

In 1999, the IAB changed its name to the Association of Regulatory Boards in Optometry (ARBO).[94] In addition to accrediting schools and establishing the NBEO, another contribution of the IBB/IAB/ARBO over the years was playing a role in developing the Treatment and Management of Ocular Disease (TMOD) examination,[92] which was first administered in 1985.

ASSOCIATION OF SCHOOLS AND COLLEGES OF OPTOMETRY

In 1940, representatives of seven optometry schools adopted a resolution to form an association of optometry schools.[95] This led to the formation of the Association of Schools and Colleges of Optometry (ASCO). A loosely organized precursor group, the International Federation of Optometric Schools, had operated for about 20 years until that time.[96] ASCO was founded in 1941, with Albert Fitch of the Pennsylvania State College of

Optometry as president. Fitch was president of ASCO from 1941 to 1945, followed by Clifford Treleaven of Columbia (1945-1949), Ernest Hutchinson of Los Angeles College of Optometry (1949-1951), Kenneth Stoddard of University of California (1951-1953), and Henry Hofstetter of Indiana University (1953-1957).

In addition to overall improvement in optometric education, recurrent themes of meetings in ASCO's first two decades were accreditation, state board examinations, and content of curriculum.[95] In the 1960s and 1970s, ASCO dealt with issues such as construction and facilities, start-ups of new schools, tuition and enrollment levels, impact of expanding scope of optometric practice, and funding sources.

In 1975, ASCO started publishing a quarterly journal entitled *Journal of Optometric Education*. Starting with the Fall 1991 issue (volume 17, number 1), the title was shortened to *Optometric Education*. The last print issue was produced in the fall of 2007 (volume 33, number 1); since then the journal has been available online only.

In the 1980s, ASCO's main effort was in strategic planning. Some of the highest priority elements of the strategic plan were clear definition of the scope of optometric education, curricular enrichment, student aid and recruitment, and faculty recruitment and development.[95]

LENGTH OF CURRICULUM

In the early 1940s, the standard optometry school curriculum was one year of pre-optometry college work and three years of professional optometry school, for a total of four years.[97,98] By the early 1950s, all optometry schools were requiring five years of study, consisting, at most schools, of two years of pre-optometry and three years of optometry school.[99]

In 1951, the American Optometric Association passed a resolution that the OD degree was the appropriate degree for an optometrist.[99] In 1950, six of the ten optometry schools were offering the degree.[99] The primary element needed for the other schools to offer the degree was to increase the curriculum to six years. This would not happen until the 1960s.

CLOSURE OF THE OPTOMETRY SCHOOL AT COLUMBIA UNIVERSITY

In 1954, Columbia University announced that no more optometry students would be admitted, and that its Department of Optometry would close in 1956 after the graduation of its last class.[100,101] The closure was the result of, as one writer put it, "intricate political problems."[102] Enrollments had declined, there was significant opposition from the medical school, and there may have been insufficient support from optometrists.[100,102]

There was also the matter of a law passed by the New York state legislature requiring new candidates for licensure to have a minimum of two years of pre-optometry college credits and four years of optometry school, for a total of six years. In 1926, Columbia had increased to a total of four years, and in 1949, to two years of pre-optometry and three years of optometry school, for a total of five years.[103] The increase mandated by the state legislature would have meant another year of optometry and would have made the granting of the O.D. degree a possibility. The burden of additional staff and facilities for a fourth year, and the degree question stiffened existing opposition to the program.

The closing was a great loss to optometry, primarily because of the pride of having an optometry school at a prestigious university, but also because of the perception that nationwide optometry school enrollments were too low.[104] Through efforts of several optometrists, the clinical and research components of the school were transferred, in April of 1956, to a new entity that they called the Optometric Center of New York. One of the optometrists in that effort, Isidore Finkelstein, who was on the Columbia optometry faculty from 1926 to 1956, became its first director.[101,105] After

Finkelstein's resignation in 1957, Alden N. Haffner became the executive director of the center. In 1971, a new optometry school started at the State University of New York (SUNY), in New York City with Haffner as the dean, and in 1975, the programs of the Optometric Center of New York were merged into the SUNY College of Optometry.[105]

GRADUATE PROGRAMS OFFERED BY OPTOMETRY SCHOOLS

One of the problems facing optometric education in the mid-twentieth century was having sufficient numbers of optometrists qualified for university faculty positions, by virtue of having Master's or PhDs. To address that need, some optometry schools made arrangements with the graduate schools at their universities to institute graduate programs leading to MS and PhD degrees in physiological optics. The term *physiological optics* was taken from the title of the famous book by Hermann von Helmholtz, which was a comprehensive review of the science of vision.[106]

Ohio State was the first optometry school to start such a program, with Glenn Fry as its director. In 1938, Howard Haines and Herbert Mote became the first to receive MS degrees there. The first PhD was awarded in 1942 to Henry Hofstetter.[106] The University of California at Berkeley was the next school to start a graduate program in physiological optics, and it gave its first MS and PhD degrees in 1949 and 1950, respectively. In the 1950s, Pacific University started offering an MS program, with degrees given in either physiological optics or clinical optometry. The physiological optics program at Indiana University awarded its first MS degree in 1956 and its first PhD degree in 1962. By the early 1980s, there were also graduate programs at the University of Houston, the State University of New York, and the University of Alabama Birmingham. Data on the numbers of graduates through 1990 and the origins of each of the programs at that time are given in Table 6.2 from a 1993 publication.[106]

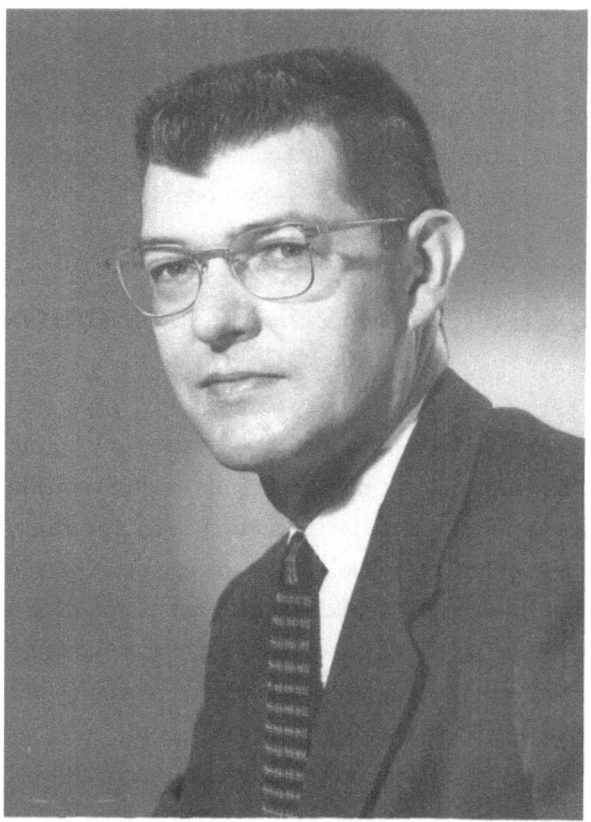

Figure 6.4. Henry W. Hofstetter (1914-2002), first recipient of a Ph.D. degree in physiological optics from a graduate program associated with an optometry school. (Image courtesy of Indiana University School of Optometry)

Table 6.2. Data through 1990 for MS and PhD programs associated with optometry schools.

School	No. of MS degrees	First MS degree granted	No. of PhD degrees	First PhD degree granted	First program director
Ohio State	109	1938	33	1942	Glenn Fry
Berkeley	40	1949	51	1950	Kenneth Stoddard
Indiana	70	1956	46	1962	Henry Hofstetter

Pacific	54*	1954	0	-	Ronald Everson**
Houston	40	1972	23	1976	Donald Pitts
SUNY	16	1973	3	1984	Alan Lewis
Waterloo	30	1974	7	1980	No one person
Montreal	14	1975	0	-	Michel Millodot
Alabama	23	1981	11	1981	Ellen Takahashi

*Numbers are approximate because university records did not distinguish between degrees in clinical optometry or physiological optics from those in psychology or education.
**Before 1964, graduate programs were administered by the Pacific University Graduate School dean. Incomplete records suggest that about three MS degrees in clinical optometry or physiological optics were granted before 1964, when Everson became director of the Graduate Program in Physiological Optics.

In the early years of these graduate programs, the vast majority of the PhD students were optometrists; through 1970, only three of the 42 who earned PhDs were not. After 1970, more and more nonoptometrists entered these graduate programs. Another early trend was that a large majority of graduates took faculty positions at optometry schools. Later, increasing numbers were employed in industry, nonoptometric academic institutions, and other situations. Beginning in the late twentieth century, these graduate programs started identifying themselves as programs in vision science rather than physiological optics. Because physiological optics/vision science is such a broad discipline, its graduate programs have produced faculty who have taught in all areas of optometry school curricula, and research personnel for a variety of settings.[107]

OPTOMETRY SCHOOLS AND LENGTH OF CURRICULUM IN THE 1960S

From the mid-1950s when the optometry school at Columbia University closed to the fall of 1969 when the school at the University of Alabama Birmingham opened, there were 10 optometry schools in the United States: the Illinois College of Optometry, Indiana University, the Los Angeles College of Optometry, the Massachusetts College of Optometry, The Ohio State University, Pacific University, the Pennsylvania College of Optometry, the Southern College of Optometry, the University of California at Berkeley, and the University of Houston.

In the early 1960s, nine of the 10 schools required a minimum of two years of college pre-optometry study followed by three years of optometry school.[108] The exception was the Pennsylvania State College of Optometry, which, starting in 1955, required a total of six years, two years of pre-optometry and four years of optometry school, with the OD degree awarded at the end of the fourth year.[108,109] At the University of Houston and the Massachusetts College of Optometry, professional qualifying degrees were earned after three years of optometry school, but students could take an optional fourth year to earn an OD.[108] Although the minimum requirement for optometry school entrance was two years of college study, many students had more than that. For example, at the Pennsylvania College of Optometry from 1961 to 1968, entering students averaged 3.3 years of previous college credit.[110]

By 1965, six optometry schools were requiring six years of study, two years pre-optometry and four years of optometry school.[111] By 1967, all 10 schools had initiated six-year programs.[109] Six years of study allowed optometry schools at public universities to award the OD degree because their governing boards required six years of study, minimum, for the granting of a doctoral degree. The last school to adopt the OD was the University of California School of Optometry at Berkeley.[112] They awarded their first OD degrees in 1970. Reasons given for the expansion to four years at University of California, for example, were advancements in physiological optics and optometry, along with increased interest in visual performance, as well as the opinion of alumni that there should be expanded coverage of ocular disease, pharmacology, contact lenses, pediatric and geriatric optometry, and practice management.[112]

A CALL FOR ADDITIONAL SCHOOLS

It was widely accepted in the 1960s that there was a shortage of health care professionals, including optometrists. One study estimated that 750 new optometry graduates were needed annually in the United States to make up for retirements and population increases.[113] The actual number of graduates nationwide was between 300 and 400 each year from 1956 to 1965,[114] yet the number of registered optometrists in the United States dropped from 22,136 in 1956 to 20,610 in 1966.[115]

Writing in 1967, Baldwin[116] agreed with the United States Public Health Service that there was a need for more optometrists. A commonly accepted standard was that there should be one optometrist per about 7,000 population. He argued that there should probably be more optometrists than that, due to "the expansion of valid methods for improving human visual performance." When speaking of the number of optometrists, he said, "The gap between the supply and the need is in grave danger of becoming wider."[116] At that time, optometrist-to-population ratios varied from one optometrist to about 5,000 people in Illinois and Oregon to one optometrist for approximately 18,000 population in some states in the southeastern U.S. Baldwin noted that increasing the number of optometrists could be achieved by increasing enrollments at individual schools or by increasing the number of schools.

Enrollment ceilings were established by the COE for each school, based on factors such as admission standards, rate of attrition, faculty, curriculum, achievement standards, physical facilities, clinical program, financial status, research activity, demand for graduates, current enrollment, and particularly, the COE's last evaluation of the school.[117] Baldwin was in favor of those ceilings, and he agreed with the assessment of the COE that the number of schools should be increased. Baldwin argued against increased tuition income being a financial incentive to schools to increase their enrollments because he calculated that tuition could not be expected to provide more than about half of the expense of educating one student, regardless of the number of students. He suggested that the number of schools be at least doubled and that new schools be established at universities. Addressing concerns about an adequate number of qualified faculty for a greater number of schools, he did not expect that to be troublesome because the number of those completing PhD degrees in physiological optics and related areas was increasing. He also argued that practicing optometrists could be recruited by the schools to faculty positions if salaries were made competitive.[116]

Baldwin's call for a doubling of the number of schools was not achieved until 2009. In the 1960s there were, however, increases in enrollments at each of the 10 schools. The increases in enrollments from 1960-61 to 1964-65 ranged from 14% at the Los Angeles College of Optometry to 103% at the Pennsylvania College of Optometry.[112] The number of optometry school graduates in the United States increased from fewer than 400 per year from 1956 to 1965 to between 400 and 500 each year from 1966 to 1970.[114]

OTHER ASPECTS OF OPTOMETRIC EDUCATION IN THE 1960S

Federal legislation in 1963 and 1965 provided funds to health profession schools for construction grants, educational improvement grants, student loans, and scholarships.[118,119] The aim of this funding was to increase the numbers of graduates as well as to improve the quality of professional education. All 10 optometry schools took advantage of this funding.[109]

One potential measure of the level of education offered could be the degrees earned by faculty. In 1962, 77% of optometry faculty held a doctorate degree: an OD in 49% of faculty, a PhD in 19% of faculty, and another doctorate in 8%.[113] In the 1960s, there were six programs designed for optometrists to complete graduate degrees.[120] The University of California at Berkeley, Indiana University, and the Ohio State University offered MS and PhD programs in physiological optics. An MS degree in perceptual psychology, physiological optics, or clinical optometry could be pursued at Pacific University. Optometrists who had completed five years of pre-optometry and optometry college credit could also attend programs at the University of Houston or the Massachusetts College of Optometry to complete an OD.[120] From 1961 to 1970, Indiana University awarded 39 MS and 12 PhD degrees in physiological optics, the University of California at Berkeley granted 10 MS and eight PhD degrees in physiological optics, Ohio State awarded seven MS and three PhD degrees, and Pacific granted 11 MS degrees.[106]

In 1969, the number of optometry schools in the United States increased to 11 with the opening of a school at the University of Alabama Birmingham. They started with a class of eight students in the fall of 1969 to become the first university connected optometry school in the southeastern United States.[121] It was also the first optometry school designed to be incorporated into a university-based academic health sciences complex.

In the 1960s, the number of optometry school applicants was increasing over the levels in the late 1950s, and the grade point averages of entering students were higher than in previous decades.[122] For 1962, the ratios of applications to entering students at the 10 optometry schools ranged from 1.27 to 1 to 3.53 to 1.[113] Levine and Baldwin[122] recommended that in addition to grade point average, information from interviews, letters of recommendation, a personal data form, and tests such as the Graduate Record Exam and an occupational interest test, and a personality profile could be useful in selecting students from the applicant pool. They further recommended that optometry should construct a national selection test for optometry applicants, with the assistance of a testing organization. Within a few years, the Optometry College Admission Test (OCAT, now OAT) was developed.[123,124]

THE HAVIGHURST REPORT

In the early 1970s, the American Optometric Association made a $90,000 grant to the National Commission on Accrediting to make a study of optometric education. Twelve persons, including two past presidents of the AOA (H. Ward Ewalt and Charles E. Seger) and two heads of optometry schools (A. N. Haffner and Alfred A. Rosenbloom), and various authorities in educational development and accrediting and health care education, were appointed to the Commission on the Study of Optometric Education. Robert J. Havighurst, Professor of Education and Human Development at the University of Chicago, was named study director.

Between June 1971 and December 1972, Havighurst met with members of the Commission, students and faculty at all optometry schools in the United States and one in Canada, presidents or deans of optometry schools, and staff and officers of the AOA. The results of the study were summarized in a 128-page soft-cover book.[125]

Among the recommendations coming from the study were the following: (1) Practitioners should be required to take continuing education courses to maintain licensure. (2) All schools should have some faculty with both OD and PhD degrees. (3) Optometry faculty salary scales should approximate those of other health science schools, such as dentistry. (4) Optometry faculty should have time available for research and service activities; the amount of time should approximate one-third of a full-time faculty member's time. (5) There should be more opportunities for graduate training and research. (6) The optometry school curriculum should give greater emphasis to ocular disease and pharmacology, public and community health, social and behavioral sciences related to vision, and optometry practice specialty areas. (7) Standards for vision science libraries should be developed. (8) Optometry schools should cooperate with organizations that provide continuing education. (9) Several new optometry schools associated with universities or health science centers should be established. (10) The optometric profession should continue to study itself so that it can make a wise plan for the future. Within the following decades these recommendations were largely met.

FOUR NEW SCHOOLS BETWEEN 1971 AND 1980

In April 1971, New York Governor Nelson Rockefeller signed bills authorizing the establishment of the State University of New York (SUNY) College of Optometry. Classes started in September 1971. The founding president was Alden N. Haffner, who was the executive director of the Optometric Center of New York, a nonprofit institution. Haffner served as the SUNY College of Optometry president from 1971 to 1979, and again from 1987 to 2005, with time in between as the vice chancellor for research, graduate studies, and professional programs for the SUNY system. At first, the College of Optometry occupied space where the Optometric Center of New York had operated a clinic, but soon the college rented additional space, and then in 1976, consolidated both facilities in one 130,000-square-foot location where it remained for the next quarter century.[126] The inaugural class starting in September 1971 consisted of 23 students.[127]

The College of Optometry at Ferris State College (now the Ferris State University Michigan College of Optometry) entered 21 students in September of 1975. This was the culmination of efforts of the Michigan Optometric Association, although it had originally envisioned the school at one of Michigan's larger universities. Ferris State President Robert Ewigleben was successful in arguing that the optometry school would be a natural fit with Ferris State's Opticianry and Optometric Technician programs.[128] The College of Optometry's first dean was Jack W. Bennett, who served in that role until 1988 when he became dean at the Indiana University School of Optometry. The faculty members during the school's first two years were Robert L. Carter, Michael Keating, and Vincent King.[128]

The next optometry school to open was at Northeastern Oklahoma State University in Tahlequah where 24 students started classes in the fall of 1979. One of the attributes of that location that made an optometry school feasible was that Tahlequah was the capital of the Cherokee Nation and the site of an Indian Health Service, U.S. Public Health Service hospital, where an optometry clinic could be incorporated.[129,130] The first dean of the college was Chester H. Pheiffer, who had previously been dean at the University of Houston College of Optometry. The faculty in the first year of the program were Hank G. Van Veen, Lesley L. Walls, and M. Gary Wickham. David A. Goss joined the faculty in August of 1980 and Harry O. House in January of 1981.

The College of Optometry at the University of Missouri St. Louis started classes in the fall of 1980 and had 32 students graduate in May 1984.[131] Efforts to establish the school began in 1967 when the Missouri Optometric Association appointed Jerry Franzel chairman of a task force for that purpose.[132,133] The founding dean was Jerry L. Christensen. Faculty who started at UMSL in the first few years of the optometry school, and subsequently taught there for 25 or more years, include G. A. Franzel, Ralph Garzia, William Long, and Carol Peck.[134]

ADDITIONS TO CURRICULUM RELATED TO PATHOLOGY AND PHARMACOLOGY IN THE 1970S

The 1970s saw increases in coursework in ocular and systemic disease, and pharmacology at all optometry schools, corresponding to the expansion in scope of practice occurring in many states.[135] For example, required courses in pathology and pharmacology in the optometry curriculum at Indiana University listed in the 1969-70 Bulletin were four semester hours in general and ocular pathology, eight semester hours of applied ocular pathology, and one semester hour of ocular pharmacology. In contrast, required disease-related coursework in the 1979-80

Bulletin included four semester hours of medical and ocular microbiology, four semester hours of general pathology, three semester hours of ocular physiology and biochemistry, six semester hours of ocular disease, six semester hours of general and ocular pharmacology, and three semester hours of physical diagnosis.

Optometry school curricula in the 1970s also showed expanded coverage of biological basic sciences. For example, among the changes at the University of California at Berkeley were expansion of the ocular anatomy course and incorporation of additional courses in neuroanatomy and ocular embryology.[136] Implementation of ocular disease management in the teaching clinics was a challenge but was aided at many schools by external rotations.

ACCELERATED OPTOMETRY PROGRAM FOR PHDS

In 1972, the Massachusetts College of Optometry (later named the New England College of Optometry/NEWENCO), established a program in which students with earned PhDs in the sciences could obtain an OD in an accelerated two-year program. Similar two-year programs were already in existence in some medical and dental schools. The initial planners for the accelerated OD program at NEWENCO were William R. Baldwin and John H. Carter, and its first director was Norman E. Wallis. The program made extensive use of seminars and independent study. By 1976, the program had graduated 22 ODs.[137] One of the motivating factors in establishing the program was a shortage of optometric educators, and many of the graduates did take faculty positions at optometry schools. For example, in the summers of 1981 and 1982, when the Northeastern State University College of Optometry in Oklahoma was expanding its faculty in the third and fourth years of its existence, three of the 10 faculty hired were graduates of the accelerated OD program at NEWENCO: Lynn Cyert, George Fulk, and Roger West.

In 1983, Pease reported on 10 years of experience with the accelerated OD program.[138] From 1972 to 1981, 85 students were enrolled in the program, and 74 (69 men and five women) had graduated. The most common original fields of the students were physics, psychology, biochemistry, and biology. Their mean age was 37, with a range of 27 to 54. Curricular content was "essentially the same" as in the four-year curriculum, and the number of clock hours in clinical rotations was the same. The primary areas of employment of the 66 graduates in the first eight years of the program were optometry practice (37) and teaching/research (20), with 18 of the latter having full-time positions at optometry schools.[138]

By 1994, the entrance requirement of a PhD in science had been modified to a doctorate-level degree in medicine or science.[139] Through 1995, there were 140 graduates of the NEWENCO accelerated OD program.[140] Out of 101 who responded to a survey, 37% were self-employed and 35% were employed in education and/or research. Among the respondents were faculty members at 12 optometry schools and two medical schools. Two-thirds were members of the American Optometric Association and one-third were members of the American Academy of Optometry. Their performance on basic science and clinical science sections of the National Board Examination in Optometry far exceeded national averages.

CHANGES IN NUMBERS OF OPTOMETRY SCHOOL APPLICANTS IN THE 1970S

From 1969-70 to 1974-75, the number of persons submitting applications to optometry schools increased from 1,400 to 3,622, the total number of applications increased from 1,744 to 8,328, and thus the number of applications per applicant also showed an increase (from 1.2 to 2.3).[141] Explanations for the increased number of applicants could include increase in numbers of female applicants to optometry school, increasing recognition of optometry, high regard for health care workers by the public at this time, and possible deferment from military service during the Vietnam War.

The number of applicants who matriculated at an optometry school increased from 783 in 1969-70 to 1,000 in 1974-75. Thus, the percentage of applicants who were admitted to an optometry school decreased from 55.9% in 1969-70 to 27.6% in 1974-75.[141]

The numbers of applicants to medical and dental school also showed increases from 1969-70 to 1974-75. At the time, there were 10 times as many medical schools as optometry schools and five times as many dental schools as optometry schools. So in terms of numbers of persons, the increases were greater for medicine and dentistry, but on a percentage basis the increases for optometry were greater. From 1969-70 to 1974-75, the number of persons applying to dental schools increased by 45%, to medical schools by 73%, and to optometry schools by 159%.[141]

The number of applicants per acceptance at optometry schools increased in the years between 1969-70 to 1974-75 from 1.8 to 3.6, at medical schools from 2.3 to 2.9, and at dental schools from 2.4 to 2.6. Thus, the applicant-to-acceptance ratio was lower for optometry than for dentistry and medicine in 1969-70 but higher in 1974-75.[141]

The number of optometry school applications increased again from 8,328 in 1974-75 to 9,164 in 1975-76, but after the startling increases in numbers of optometry school applications from 1969-70 to 1975-76, the numbers of applications decreased each year in the rest of the 1970s.[142] The number of applications decreased to 6,185 in 1979-80.[142]

THE FIRST YEAR-LONG RESIDENCIES

The first year-long residency in optometry was in vision therapy at the State University of New York College of Optometry. It started in 1974 with four residents: Stanley Appelbaum, Harvey Estren, Kenneth Koslowe, and Robert Sanet.[143,144] A residency started at the Veterans

Administration hospital in Kansas City in 1975 became the first residency accredited by the COE.[145] The first resident in that program was Thomas Stelmack.[145] By 1979, there were 18 residency programs offered by 10 optometry schools.[146] Areas of emphasis of those residencies included general optometry, ocular disease, low vision, vision therapy, pediatric optometry, and contact lenses.[146]

SUMMIT ON OPTOMETRIC EDUCATION (1992-1994)

In 1992, Richard L. Hopping observed that "at no previous time in the history of the optometric profession has there been a greater need for the full cooperation of the entire profession in order to move the educational establishment and thus the profession forward to an even higher level."[147] In 1992 through 1994, a series of eight conferences were held to evaluate the status of optometric education and to study what should be done to prepare for the future. Over 200 participants represented the American Academy of Optometry, the American Foundation for Vision Awareness, the American Optometric Association, the American Optometric Foundation, the American Optometric Student Association, the Association of Schools and Colleges of Optometry, the College of Optometrists in Vision Development, IAB, the National Board of Examiners in Optometry, the National Optometric Association, the Optometric Extension Program, and faculties of each of the optometry schools. Representatives of the corporate sponsors—Alcon, Allergan, CIBA, and Vistakon—also attended. The eight conferences were (1) the Georgetown Conference, examining a broad range of topics, March 19-22, 1992; (2) the Scope of Optometric Practice Conference, July 9-12, 1992; (3) the Curriculum Conference, July 30-August 1, 1992; (4) the Conference on Optometric Students, January 10-12, 1993; (5) the Conference on Optometric Research, April 1-4, 1993; (6) the Conference on Graduate Education, Residencies, and Fellowships, August 26-29, 1993; (7)

the Conference on Financing Optometric Education, November 18-21, 1993; and (8) the Action Plan Conference, October 8-11, 1994.

Richard L. Hopping served as chairman of the Summit on Optometric Education Conferences. Hopping; L. Edward Elliot, president of the American Optometric Association in 1991-92; and Larry DeCook, president of the AOA in 1994-95, were the only persons to attend all eight conferences.[148]

Among the concepts discussed at the conference on scope of practice were what constitutes entry-level competence and the need for optometry to practice primary, secondary, and tertiary levels of care. Factors identified as affecting scope of practice included matters such as public welfare, professional judgment, education, training, and new technologies.

The 1978 Association of Schools and Colleges of Optometry's curriculum model had significant impact in the 1980s, but by the 1990s its limitations were beginning to be recognized. Its emphasis on knowledge limited its ability to keep up with expansion of scope of practice. Developing an understanding of concepts, learning problem-solving skills, and gaining an appreciation for lifelong learning came to be considered more important than the knowledge of facts. The expansion of learning in the biological sciences also required additional facilities and equipment.

It was agreed that research was essential for the future survival and growth of optometry. To make efficient use of resources, the importance of collaboration between optometric institutions and other professions studying vision was emphasized. The idea of a training program for optometric clinician-scientists was also discussed.

It was observed that graduate programs and residencies could serve as a vehicle for expansion of the scope of optometric practice and for certification in optometric subspecialties. The need for recruitment of graduate students, for informing graduate students about uniquely optometric areas of study, for a strategic plan for residencies, and for the development of fellowships in optometry were among areas identified as requiring attention.

Coming out of the conferences, perhaps the greatest sense of urgency could be felt in the section on financing optometric education.[148] In conference documents, it was stated that the resource gap was "really big, not just big." Identified areas of need included meeting increased operating costs, resources needed for expansion of scope, maintenance and expansion of faculty and infrastructure, expansion of research, replacement of reduced government scholarship funding, provision of adequate student loans and financial aid, and resources for new technology.

DISCUSSION ON THE NUMBER OF OPTOMETRY SCHOOLS

One matter discussed at the Summit on Optometric Education, which has received a great deal of attention in the following years, was whether additional optometry schools should be started. At that time, there were 16 optometry schools in the United States. Hopping[147] pointed out the great increase in optometry graduates in the eight years following the end of World War II due to the very large classes admitted at some schools (see Appendix 2). He stated, "Had the profession not graduated the number of optometrists that it did at that time…we would not be the major provider in the eye/vision care field today and we would not have captured our distribution system and the primary care position that the profession enjoys today."[147] Hopping noted that there were many factors affecting manpower needs in the health professions and that longitudinal manpower studies should be conducted on a regular basis. He also suggested that appropriate ratios of faculty, space, library volumes, and patient encounters per student should be evaluated.

Jack Bennett[149] pointed out that in 1976, the AOA recommended a total of 22 schools, but in 1984, it changed the recommendation to four new schools for a total of 19. Bennett listed the the following reasons in favor of additional schools: (1) There is a need for additional optometrists, particularly in light of expanding scope of care, aging of the population, and unmet needs in areas such as low vision and rehabilitation. (2) An optometry school is a political resource for legislative and regulatory matters. (3) Schools are resources for needed research. (4) Schools have a positive impact on the professional image perceived by the public, funding agencies, governmental entities, and other professions. (5) Schools have an important role in continuing education. Bennett also gave as a significant argument against the addition of new schools that it would dilute financial and faculty resources and the applicant pool. He concluded that additional schools were warranted but only under appropriate conditions in areas of need.

Earle Hunter[150] was of the opinion that additional schools were not needed because existing schools could increase or decrease the number of students admitted to adjust to perceived changes in manpower needs. Lorraine Voorhees[151] observed that schools can improve the professional image of optometry by being a center for research and specialty patient care, but she felt that overall, there were more arguments for not having more schools: (1) Manpower projections do not suggest a need for additional graduates. (2) The applicant pool is not large enough to ensure high academic standards for all admitted students. (3) Financial support is a limiting factor. (4) There may not be adequate financial aid for students. (5) There may not be enough qualified individuals for additional faculty positions.

INCREASING CURRICULAR EMPHASIS ON OCULAR DISEASE AND PHARMACOLOGY

The expansion of curricular elements devoted to disease and pharmacology continued through the closing decades of the twentieth century. For example, comparing the 1979-80 and 1999-2001 Bulletins for the Indiana University School of Optometry, there was an increase of three semester credit hours in courses on general and ocular pathology and on ocular disease. Looking at the 1981-82 and 2000-2002 Bulletins for the Northeastern State University College of Optometry in Oklahoma, the increase was seven semester credit hours. Over those time spans, there was a decrease of one credit hour in courses on geometrical and physical optics at both schools.

A 1983 comparison of lecture hours on pharmacology given to medical students and to optometry students at Indiana University in Bloomington indicated that the total number of hours was the same, but there was more emphasis on ocular pharmacology in the optometry curriculum and more breadth of coverage in the medical school curriculum.[152] Similar results were found in a 1985 study comparing 41 optometry, medical, and dental schools in 14 states.[153]

The vast majority of respondents to a survey of optometrists graduating from Indiana University School of Optometry before 1995 supported the trend of increasing curricular emphasis on ocular disease, but they also strongly felt that optometrists should continue to be very good at all aspects of eye and vision care, including refraction, basic binocular vision problems, and contact lenses, as well as ocular disease.[154] In support of the latter response was the fact that an average of 93% of the respondents' income was derived from traditional optometric services, compared to an average of 7% from treatment of ocular diseases.

The increasing prominence of disease-related material in optometry school curricula has continued into the twenty-first century. For instance, Northeastern State University had two more courses in ocular and systemic disease and medical treatment topics in 2020 than it had in its 2000-2002 catalog. Pacific University had more than twice as many courses in basic biological sciences, disease, and pharmacology in 2020 than it had in its 1973-74 bulletin.

INCREASING NUMBER OF OPTOMETRIC RESIDENCY PROGRAMS

The number of accredited optometry residency programs increased in the 1980s and 1990s, going to more than 20 programs in 1983, more than 40 in 1986, and more than 60 in 1995. In 1996, that jumped up to 82 accredited residency programs.[155] Haffner observed that factors explaining the increase in residency programs included expansion in scope of optometric practice and "need for advanced clinical skills generally and for concentrated specialized skills."[155] A total of 139 positions in 82 residency programs in 1996 made it possible for about 10% of optometry school graduates to pursue residency education. In 2019, there were more than 450 residency positions in 250 residency programs, making residency positions available for about 25% of optometry graduates.[156] The majority of residency programs in 2013 through 2019 were in ocular disease and primary eye care.[156]

EIGHT NEW OPTOMETRY SCHOOLS BETWEEN 1981 AND 2017

We have already seen that in 1967, when there were 10 optometry schools and a perceived shortage of optometrists, Baldwin recommended doubling the number of optometry schools and in 1976, the American Optometric Association recommended an increase to 22 schools.[116,149] The number of schools reached those levels early in the twenty-first century, despite later concerns there would be too many students enrolled.[150,151,157,158,159,160]

The School of Optometry at the Inter American University of Puerto Rico opened in 1981, with Henry Hofstetter as acting dean for a semester and Arthur Afanador following him as dean.[161] The College of Optometry at Nova Southeastern University in Fort Lauderdale, Florida, entered its first class in 1989. At that time, the name of the university was the Southeastern University of the Health Sciences, and in 1994, it merged with Nova University to form Nova Southeastern University.[162] Stewart Abel was the first dean.

Three schools started operation in 2009. The Midwestern University Arizona College of Optometry opened in Glendale, Arizona, with Hector C. Santiago as founding dean after he had served as dean of the school in Puerto Rico for several years.[163] The Rosenberg School of Optometry at the University of the Incarnate Word, a private Catholic university in San Antonio, Texas, had H. S. Ghazi-Birry as its first dean.[164] The third school to open in 2009 was the Western University of Health Sciences College of Optometry in Pomona, California. Elizabeth Hoppe was the founding dean.[165]

The Massachusetts College of Pharmacy and Health Sciences School of Optometry, Worcester, Massachusetts, enrolled its first class in 2012. Lesley L. Walls, who had previously been dean at the Northeastern State University College of Optometry and Pacific University, and president of the Southern California College of Optometry was the school's first dean.[166] The University of Pikeville Kentucky College of Optometry opened in 2016 with Andrew Buzzelli as founding dean, and Michael Bacigalupi taking over as dean in 2018.[167,168] The Midwestern University Chicago College of Optometry in Downers Grove, Illinois, started operation in 2017. Sunny Sanders was the founding dean, with Melissa Suckow being appointed the next dean in 2018.[169,170] Data on the numbers of optometry schools and optometry school graduates by year can be found in Appendix 2.

RECRUITING RACIALLY AND ETHNICALLY DIVERSE STUDENTS

In 1969-70, only 6% of students enrolled in optometry schools in the United States were members of a racial minority group.[171] In 1971, the

American Optometric Association and the National Optometric Association jointly operated a federally sponsored minority student recruitment project.[172] This was followed by the NOA's Project to Increase Minority Optometric Manpower, which existed from 1972 to 1980, supported by the federal Health Careers Opportunity Program. Also in the 1970s and 1980s, several optometry schools operated summer programs and other initiatives to recruit students from racial minority groups.[173,174]

The percentage of students from these groups increased to 12% in 1982-83, 21% in 1988-89, and 33% in 1996-97. However, most minority groups remained under-represented, as the preponderance of the increase was due to large increases in numbers of Asian students (see Appendix 2 for data).

In 2006, ASCO launched its Developing a Diverse Applicant Pool in Optometric Education Mini-Grant Program to fund programs and projects at optometry schools.[175] The number of Asian students continued to increase, showing a doubling from 1996-97 to 2016-17, but other minority groups remained under-represented.[170,176] A 2017 ASCO report suggested that the previous decade showed "both success and opportunity for increasing diversity," and called for actions such as developing pipeline programs and doing a better job of marketing the profession.[175]

INCREASING STUDENT INDEBTEDNESS

In 2005, one optometric educator correctly predicted that rising student indebtedness resulting from large increases in tuition would become a significant challenge to optometry schools.[177] In 1979-80, the average expenditure for tuition, fees, supplies, and costs other than room and board was $3,273 for in-state residents, and $5,428 for non-residents,[178] about $11,000 and $17,000, respectively, in 2020 dollars. Tuition and fees were about three times as much in 2018-19, based on data from ASCO.[179] Average student indebtedness was $99,000 in 2001-02 and $181,000 in 2018-19,[179,180] an increase of about 28% in 2020 dollars.

Improvements and curricular expansion in optometric education have been an essential part of the advancement of optometry. Academic optometry has often led the elevation of optometric care. Among the continuing challenges optometry schools face are funding, incorporation of new teaching and clinical technologies, and teaching the expanding scope and knowledge base in a four-year curriculum.

Chapter 6: Notes

1. Gregg JR. *The Story of Optometry*. New York, NY: Ronald Press, 1965:218-221.
2. Sheard C. Optometric education and professional advancement. *Optom Weekly* 1942;33:1085-1089.
3. Gregg JR. New era in optometric education. *J Am Optom Assoc.* 1964;35:291-294.
4. *Optical J Supplement.* 1899;5:31.
5. Miller AR, Brown JM. *Optometry in America: A History of the Illinois College of Optometry 1872-1997.* Chicago, IL: Illinois College of Optometry, 1996:19-24,129.
6. Miller & Brown, 23.
7. Moline SW. *Century of Vision: The New England College of Optometry, An Anecdotal History of the First Hundred Years.* Boston, MA: New England College of Optometry, 1994:3-7.
8. Reed DR. The Indiana optometry heritage: The first optometrist in LaPorte. *Indiana J Optom.* 1999;2:19-20.
9. Brown A. Bradley University and its watchmaking past. www.peoriamagazines.com/print/7998.
10. Goss DA. A historical list of optometry schools in the United States. *Hindsight* 2012;43:82-89.
11. *Blue Book of Optometrists and Opticians.* Chicago, IL: The Optometrist and Optician, 1912:16.
12. Thomson HA. New attendance course announced by the South Bend College of Optics. *Optical J Rev Optom.* 1912;29:1421.
13. *Optical J Supplement.* 1899;5:53.
14. *Optical J.* 1903;12:144.
15. *Optical J.* 1906;17:378.
16. *Dr. Thomson's 1895 Correspondence Course in Optics with Historical Commentary by Monroe J. Hirsch.* Chicago, IL: Professional Press, 1975.
17. *Dr. Thomson's*, 171-180.
18. Three new members added to the faculty of the Philadelphia Optical College. *Optical J Rev Optom.* 1916;37:1505.

19   Goss DA. Christian Henry Brown (1857-1933) and the Philadelphia Optical College. *Hindsight* 2010;41:114-121.
20   Philadelphia alumni give notable banquet: Speeches by Dilworth, Moore, Hagerty, Haussmann and others. *Optical J Rev Optom.* 1917;39:1419-1421.
21   Haussmann OG. A tribute to the late Dr. C. H. Brown, pioneer educator in optometry. *Optical J Rev Optom.* 1934;71(2):30.
22   Philadelphia Optical College notes. *Optical J.* 1908;21:261.
23   Philadelphia Optical College personals. *Optical J Rev Optom.* 1915;35:852.
24   Brown CH. [Scrapbook containing clippings of advertisements and brochures for optometric courses and servies, 1890-1931]. Microfilm, Indiana University Optometry Library.
25   Philadelphia Optical College personals. *Optical J Rev Optom.* 1914;33:1058.
26   Philadelphia Optical College personals. *Optical J Rev Optom.* 1914;34:117.
27   Philadelphia Optical College notes. *Optical J Rev Optom.* 1914;34:584.
28   Philadelphia Optical College personals. *Optical J Rev Optom.* 1914;34:943.
29   Philadelphia Optical College notes. *Optical J Rev Optom.* 1915;35:1362.
30   School notes: Philadelphia Optical College. *Optical J Rev Optom.* 1916;38:548.
31   Christensen JL. The first conference to establish optometric standards. *Optom Vis Sci.* 1996;73:428-434.
32   *Blue Book of Optometrists*, 13th ed. Chicago, IL: Professional Press, 1936:32.
33   Hofstetter HW. An early correspondence course. *Newsletter Optom Hist Soc.* 1984;15:33-36.
34   Goss DA. Louis L. DeMars and the DeMars School of Optometry. *Hindsight* 2014;45:65-66.
35   L.L. DeMars. *J Am Optom Assoc.* 1945;16:212.
36   Petry E. Optometric educational standards. *Optical J Rev Optom.* 1920;46:1585-1587.
37   Hofstetter HW. *Optometry: Professional, Economic, and Legal Aspects.* St. Louis, MO, 1948:297.
38   *Optical J* 1908;23:39.
39   *Optical J* 1908;23:46.
40   *Optical J* 1909;23:895.
41   *Optical J* 1909;23:347.
42   Closing of the New York Institute of Optometry. *Optical J.* 1909;24:828.
43   Goss DA. Glimpses of American optometric education 100 years ago as revealed in the pages of *The Optical Journal* of 1909. *Hindsight* 2009;40:117-128.
44   Ketchum MB. The best methods for an optometrical school. *Optical J.* 1909;25:61-62.
45   Cross AJ. Higher education in optometry: A plea for appreciation and co-operation. *Optical J.* 1909;25:82-85.
46   Bestor HM. Two-year course not too long. *Optical J.* 1909;25:108-109.
47   Ryer EL. Some of the effects of the N.Y. optometry law. *Optical J.* 1910;25:256-260.

48 Prentice CF. Optometry in Columbia University, New York. *Optical J.* 1910;25:857-861.
49 Southall JPC. Courses in optics and optometry in Columbia University. *J Optical Soc Am.* 1921;5:184-192.
50 Columbia University issues prospectus of optometry course. *Optical J Rev Optom.* 1911;28:327-328.
51 Books used in Columbia optometry course. *Optical J Rev Optom.* 1913;31:46.
52 Class of optometry students at Columbia University organize an association and elect officers. *Optical J Rev Optom.* 1910;26:1229.
53 Lectures in theoretic optometry begun at Columbia University by Prof. A. Jay Cross. *Optical J Rev Optom.* 1911;27:478.
54 Eames HW. Columbia students on work of first year in the optometry course. *Optical J Rev Optom.* 1911;27:929.
55 *Blue Book of Optometrists and Opticians*, 2nd ed. Chicago, IL: The Optometrist and Optician, 1914:23-26.
56 Ohio recognizes optometry. *Optical J Rev Optom.* 1914; 34:565-566.
57 History of the College of Optometry at The Ohio State University. http://optometry.osu.edu/aboutTheCollege/history.cfm.
58 Hebbard FW. *The Ohio State University College of Optometry.* Undated unpublished typescript, Ohio State University Library.
59 Todd WS, ed. *Report of First Conference to Establish Optometric Standards.* Hartford, CT: American Optometric Association Department of Education, 1922.
60 Hofstetter, 297-299.
61 Woll FA, ed. *First Revision of Optometrical Syllabuses and Standards*, rev. ed. International Association of Boards of Examiners in Optometry, 1935.
62 Enoch JM. A jewel in the crown: The program in optometry at the University of Rochester in New York. Part I. The founding of the program. *Hindsight* 2005;36:20-28.
63 Enoch JM. A jewel in the crown: the program in optometry at the University of Rochester in New York; Part II. The termination of the program. *Hindsight* 2005;36:35-37.
64 Wolfberg MD. Contributions to optometry by Albert Fitch. *Hindsight* 2009;40:136-138.
65 Lewis TL. Celebrating 75 years at the Pennsylvania College of Optometry. *J Am Optom Assoc.* 1996;67:188-192.
66 Morgan MW. University of California: School of Optometry. *J Am Optom Assoc.* 1968;39:643-646.
67 Fiorillo J. *Berkeley Optometry: A History.* Berkeley, CA: University of California School of Optometry, 2010.
68 Tully JL. *The History of the Southern College of Optometry 1932-1992.* Dissertation for the Doctor of Education degree, University of Memphis, 1999.
69 Maples WC. 75 years of progress. *J Behav Optom.* 2007;18:114,133.

70　Baker WJ, ed. The twenty-fifth anniversary of the College of Optometry at Pacific University. *Oregon Optometrist* 1970;37:4-25.
71　Wesley NK. *Contacts: One Hundred Years Plus.* New York, NY: Vantage Press, 1988:23-27.
72　Fletcher SK. The College of Optometry at Pacific University celebrates its 50th year. *J Am Optom Assoc.* 1995;66:599-601.
73　Miranda G, Read R. *Splendid Audacity: The Story of Pacific University.* Seattle, WA: Documentary Book Publishers, 2000:87-91.
74　Borish IM. Indiana University: Division of Optometry. *J Am Optom Assoc.* 1968;39:270-276.
75　Moshos F. Establishment of the optometry program at Indiana University. *J Optom Ed.* 1976;2(3):22-25.
76　Interview with Dr. Henry Hofstetter. *Indiana J Optom.* 1998;1:20-22.
77　Goss DA. History of the Indiana University Division of Optometry. *Indiana J Optom.* 2003;6:28-74.
78　Pheiffer CH. University of Houston: College of Optometry. *J Am Optom Assoc.* 1968;39:926-932.
79　Stewart CR. *The Founding Years: University of Houston College of Optometry 1952-1961.* Georgetown, TX: Armadillo Publishing, 2003.
80　Gregg JR. *American Optometric Association: A History.* St. Louis, MO: American Optometric Association, 1972:125.
81　Gregg, 144.
82　Gregg, 152.
83　Gregg, 167-168.
84　Koetting RA. *The American Optometric Association's First Century.* St. Louis, MO: American Optometric Association, 1997:60.
85　Hofstetter, 299.
86　Abrahamsen N. History of the Council. *J Am Optom Assoc.* 1967;38:275-278.
87　Gregg, 206-207, 219-220.
88　Baldwin WR. *Borish.* Springfield, MA: Bassette, 2006:72-74.
89　Gregg, 45, 54.
90　Hofstetter, 62-63.
91　Freitag ML, Gordon DR. International Association of Boards of Examiners in Optometry: 75 years of optometric history. *Optom Ed.* 1994;19:73-74.
92　Koetting, 62.
93　Hofstetter HW. The National Board of Examiners in Optometry. *J Am Optom Assoc.* 1951;23:224-226.
94　*ARBO History.* www.arbo.org.
95　Christensen J. A history of ASCO. *Optom Ed.* 1991;17:10-19.
96　Gregg, 377.
97　Sheard C. Optometric education and professional advancement. *Optom Weekly* 1942;33:1085-1089.

98 American Optometric Association Council on Education and Professional Guidance. Facts regarding optometric education and professional advancement. *J Am Optom Assoc.* 1943;14(6);160-169.

99 Koch CC. Six-year professional courses for optometry. *Am J Optom Arch Am Acad Optom.* 1951;28:438-440.

100 Koch CC. Columbia to close undergraduate optometry course. *Am J Optom Arch Am Acad Optom.* 1954;31:252-253.

101 Enoch JM. Isidore Finkelstein, O.D., Ph.D. (January 6, 1905 – March 13, 1965), optometric scientist and scholar, inspirational teacher, and stalwart of the profession: A tribute! *Hindsight* 2002;33:9-14.

102 Gregg JR. *The Story of Optometry.* New York, NY: Ronald Press, 1965:223.

103 Columbia University to inaugurate five-year course: Outline of curriculum. *Optical J Rev Optom.* 1949;86(5):54.

104 Greenspon W, et al. Report of the Council on Education and Professional Guidance. *J Am Optom Assoc.* 1955;27:95-98,100.

105 Haffner AN. Guest editorial: Opportunity in adversity. *J Am Optom Assoc.* 1996;67:307-312.

106 Goss DA. A history of M.S. and Ph.D. programs offered by schools and colleges of optometry in North America. *Optom Vis Sci.* 1993;70:616-621.

107 Bailey JE, Brookman KE. A study of graduate education in physiological optics in the United States: 1938-1989. *Optom Vis Sci.* 1993;70:511-516.

108 Baldwin WR. Modern optometric education. *J Am Optom Assoc.* 1962;33:667-672.

109 Hazlett RD, Hofstetter HW. Optometric education in the United States. *J Am Optom Assoc.* 1967;38:927-935.

110 Fischer AF. Pennsylvania College of Optometry. *J Am Optom Assoc.* 1968;39:1109-1113.

111 Baldwin WR. Optometric education: Portent for the profession. *J Am Optom Assoc.* 1965;36:332-334.

112 Morgan MW, Peters HB. Optometry at the University of California. *J Am Optom Assoc.* 1965;36:1059-1067.

113 Morgret F. Optometric education in the United States. *J Am Optom Assoc.* 1963;34:785-795.

114 Goss DA. Numbers of optometry graduates since 1925. *Hindsight* 2014;45:81-84.

115 Havighurst RJ. *Optometry: Education for the Profession.* Washington, DC: National Commission on Accrediting, 1973:39.

116 Baldwin WR. Do we need more schools of optometry? *J Am Optom Assoc.* 1967;38:293-296.

117 American Optometric Association Council on Education. Enrollment ceilings. *J Am Optom Assoc.* 1967;38:288-292.

118 Seger CE. The council on optometric education. *J Am Optom Assoc.* 1967;38:271-272.
119 Morgan MW. Federal support of undergraduate optometric education. *J Am Optom Assoc.* 1967;38:284-287.
120 Armed Forces Liaison Committee of the Association of Schools and Colleges of Optometry. Graduate programs for optometrists. *J Am Optom Assoc.* 1961;32:808-809.
121 Naff D. Profile: University of Alabama in Birmingham. *J Optom Ed.* 1976;1:142-144.
122 Levine NR, Baldwin WR. Achievement and aptitude tests in selection of optometry students. *Am J Optom Arch Am Acad Optom.* 1968;45:840-850.
123 Wallace WL, Levine NR. Optometry college admission test. *Am J Optom Physiol Opt.* 1974;51:872-886.
124 Levine NR. Coping with the admission's avalanche: The role of ASCO's OCAT committee. *J Optom Ed.* 1975;1:34-41.
125 Havighurst.
126 State University of New York College of Optometry. *History and Mission.* www.suny.opt.edu/about/history_and_mission
127 1st SUNY College of Optometry president dies. *Eyecare Business,* June 23, 2016. www.eyecarebusiness.com/news/2016/1st-suny-college-of-optometry-president-dies
128 Saladin JJ, Carter RL. *Vision Realized: A History of the MCO.* Big Rapids, MI: Ferris State University, 2012.
129 Frankovic JG. Northeastern Oklahoma State University College of Optometry: Its conception and establishment, 1973-1979. Seminar paper presented in Hist 5433, Northeastern State University, in partial fulfillment of the requirements for the M.A. degree, 2008.
130 Eger MJ. Optometry's new college in Oklahoma. *J Am Optom Assoc.* 1983;54:467-470.
131 UMSL University Bulletin 2020-21. College of Optometry. General information. www.bulletin.umsl.edu/collegeofoptometry
132 Brechler F. Formation of the School of Optometry at the University of Missouri-St. Louis. *Optom Vis Sci.* 1994;71:584-589.
133 UMSL College of Optometry. *Founding History.* http://optometry.umsl.edu/About Us/history.html
134 UMSL College of Optometry EyeWire newsletters, 2005-2008. www.umsl.edu/~optometry/Alumni and Friends/EyeWire Archives.html
135 Optometry curriculum model: A report of the Curriculum Committee of the ASCO Council on Academic Affairs. *J Optom Ed.* 1978;4(1):11-22.
136 Godske S, Carter J. University of California, Berkeley, School of Optometry. *J Optom Ed.* 1978;4(2):4-6.
137 Butterfield P. The second time around: A look at MCO's accelerated program for Ph.D.'s. *J Optom Ed.* 1976;2:17-20.

138 Pease PL. The accelerated O.D. program: The two-year program after ten years. *J Optom Ed.* 1983;8:15-19.
139 Heath DA, Caruso J, Chauncey DM. Developing innovative programs for unique student populations. *J Am Optom Assoc.* 1994;65:865-871.
140 Chauncey DM. The accelerated doctor of optometry program: Outcomes assessment. *Optom Ed.* 1998;23:108-113.
141 Levine NR, Levine L. A study of applicants to colleges of optometry in the U.S. *J Am Optom Assoc.* 1976;47:616-623.
142 Boucher JA. Optometric education. *J Am Optom Assoc.* 1980;51:359-363.
143 Suchoff I. The first year-long optometric residency education program. *Hindsight* 2010;41:122-125.
144 Estren H. Recollections of participation in the first year-long optometric residency program. *Hindsight* 2010;41:126-128.
145 Amos JF. A brief history of optometric residency education. *J Am Optom Assoc.* 1987;58:374-376.
146 Bleything WB. The optometric residency: Its bloom. *J Optom Ed.* 1979;5:16-21.
147 Hopping RL. What should be the proper size and number of optometric schools? *J Am Optom Assoc.* 1992;63:808-811.
148 Gregg JR, ed. *The Georgetown Summit: A Critical Assessment of Optometric Education.* St. Louis, MO: American Optometric Association, 1995.
149 Bennett JW. The pros and cons of developing additional schools and colleges of optometry. Typescript of paper presented at the Summit on Optometric Education, 1993.
150 Hunter EL. The pros and cons of developing additional schools and colleges of optometry. *J Am Optom Assoc.* 1992;63:865-866.
151 Voorhees LI. Topic: Discuss the pros and cons of developing additional schools and colleges of optometry. Typescript of paper presented at the Summit on Optometric Education, 1993.
152 Hegeman S. Comparison of pharmacology courses for optometry and medical students, Indiana University, Bloomington. *J Optom Ed.* 1983;9:22-23.
153 Waigandt M, Waigandt A. An analysis of pharmacology training in schools of optometry, medicine and dentistry. *J Optom Ed.* 1985;10:20-25.
154 Grosvenor T, Goss DA. A survey of Indiana University School of Optometry alumni. *Optom Ed.* 1998;23:114-120.
155 Haffner AN. Optometric residency education: Past, present, and future. *Optom Ed.* 1997;22:82-86.
156 National Matching Service Inc. ORMatch Statistics 2021. www.natmatch.com/ormatch/statistics.html
157 Cheezum T. How many schools are too many? *Optom Times.* 2013;5(6):8.
158 Elder KH, et al. Optometric profession debates increase in number of schools. *Primary Care Optom News.* November 2011. www.healio.com/optometry/primary-care-optometry/...

159 Mullen CF. Challenges and opportunities in optometry and optometric education. Sept. 14, 2017. www.charlesmullen.com/optoemtric-education-challenges-opportunities/#enrollment
160 Kekevian B. How the diploma deluge is reshaping optometry. *Rev Optom.* Feb. 15, 2018. www.reviewofoptometry.com/article/how-the-diploma-deluge-is-reshaping-optometry
161 Hofstetter HW. School of Optometry at Inter American University. *J Optom Ed.* 1981;7(1):20-21.
162 Nova Southeastern University. *About NSU: History.* 2020. www.nova.edu/about/history.html
163 Santiago named first dean of Arizona College of Optometry. *AOA News* 2008;47(2):6.
164 ASCO welcomes new school. *AOA News* 2009;47(14):31.
165 Preliminary approval for Western University College of Optometry. *AOA News* 2008;46(14):7.
166 Berman M. Letter from the Dean. Massachusetts College of Pharmacy and Health Sciences. www.mcphs.edu/academics/school-of-optometry/letter-dean
167 University of Pikeville names dean. *Optom Times.* April 8, 2014. www.optometrytimes.modernmedicine.com/print/381494
168 University of Pikeville names dean of Kentucky College of Optometry. Association of Presbyterian Colleges and Universities. May 10, 2018. www.presbyteriancolleges.org/in_the_news/view/952/university_of_pikeville_names_dean_of_kentucky_college_of_optometry
169 Midwestern University opens new Chicago College of Optometry. *Primary Care Optom News.* May 16, 2016. www.healio.com/news/optometry/20160516/midwestern-university-opens-new-chicago-college-of-optometry
170 Midwestern University names Suckow as Dean of Chicago College of Optometry. *Vision Monday.* Jan. 17, 2018. www.visionmonday.com/latest-news/article/midwestern-university-names-suckow-as-dean-of-chicago-college-of-optometry
171 Association of School and Colleges of Optometry. Annual Surveys of Optometric Educational Institutions. Data in email to the author from Joanne Zuckerman, Manager, Data Services and Special Projects, ASCO, August 26, 2021.
172 Email to the author from Edwin C. Marshall, Emeritus Professor of Optometry, Indiana University, September 1, 2021.
173 Sherman J. Minority recruitment for a minority profession. *J Am Optom Assoc* 1973;44:68-70.
174 Marshall EC. An experiment in health careers recruitment: A summer program at Indiana University. *J Am Optom Assoc* 1975;46:1284-1292.
175 Chu GY, Kalaczinski L, Russo D, Leasher J, Elder K, Fink B. Diversity in our colleges and schools of optometry. *Optom Ed* 2017;43(1). www.journal.opted.org/article.diversity-in-our-colleges-and-schools-of-optometry

176 Association of Schools and Colleges of Optometry. Past Student Data Reports. www.optometriceducation.org/data-reports/annual-student-data-report
177 Lewis AL. In: Think tank: optometric education. *Optom Ed* 2005;31:10-11.
178 Association of Schools and Colleges of Optometry. Annual survey of optometric educational institutions. *J Optom Ed* 1980;6:23-28.
179 Association of Schools and Colleges of Optometry. Student Data Report 2018-2019. www.optometriceducation.org/data-reports/annual-student-data-report
180 Association of Schools and Colleges of Optometry. Student Data Report 2019-2020. www.optometriceducation.org/data-reports/annual-student-data-report

Chapter 7
Optometry Publications

As optometry transitioned from trade to profession, publications in both periodical and book form proliferated, and they have been important in the dissemination and expansion of the knowledge base of optometry.

OPTOMETRY PERIODICALS

There have been numerous optometric periodicals. They have served various educational, organizational, communication, and research roles. The first periodicals devoted exclusively to optometry appear to have been *Johnston's Eye Echo*, published by J. Milton Johnston, from 1886 to 1891, and *The Optician*, published by Frederick Boger from 1891 to 1894. In 1895, Boger started *The Optical Journal*, which became *Optical Journal and Review of Optometry* and then later *Review of Optometry*, the title it retains today. Hofstetter[1] wondered why an optometry magazine didn't start until 600 years after the invention of eyeglasses, and centuries after formation of spectacle makers guilds in Europe. He speculated:

> Until the latter part of the 19th century, the security of the optometrist's comfortable livelihood had been virtually unchallenged. At that point, though, came the invasion of the ophthalmic field by the medical professional, which for 600 years had re-

mained quite aloof except for an occasional spoofing of eyeglasses. Perhaps not until then were optometrists anxious for the collegial communication a journal can afford.

In the materials from the correspondence course used by the South Bend School of Optics in the late 1890s and early 1900s, the following statements appear:

> In reply to a number of inquiries from the class as to the best periodical devoted to opticians I would say that *The Optical Journal* published by Mr. F. Boger...is the only journal in the United States published in the interest of optics and opticians exclusively. It is a wide-awake, up-to-date monthly and none of the class can afford to be without it. It contains news of the optical societies and optical legislation, as well as a great many technical and practical articles from a large staff of paid contributors.[2]

Another significant early optometry periodical was *Optometric Weekly*. It was started with the title *Practical Optometrist and Optician* by Chicago optometrist Lionel Topaz. After various changes in title, it became *Optometric Weekly* in 1928. In 1978, it became a monthly titled *Optometric Monthly*, which continued until 1985.

Speaking of the *Optical Journal and Review of Optometry* and *Optometric Weekly*, Gregg had this to say: "The early vigor of the optometric publications was an important factor in the development of optometry...They deserve much credit...educational materials the optometrist received, news of professional affairs, and editorial suggestions were the priceless assets he derived from the optometric journals of the day.[3]

Journals that were of a scholarly nature and that published research papers are the journals published by the American Optometric Association and the American Academy of Optometry. The AOA started publish-

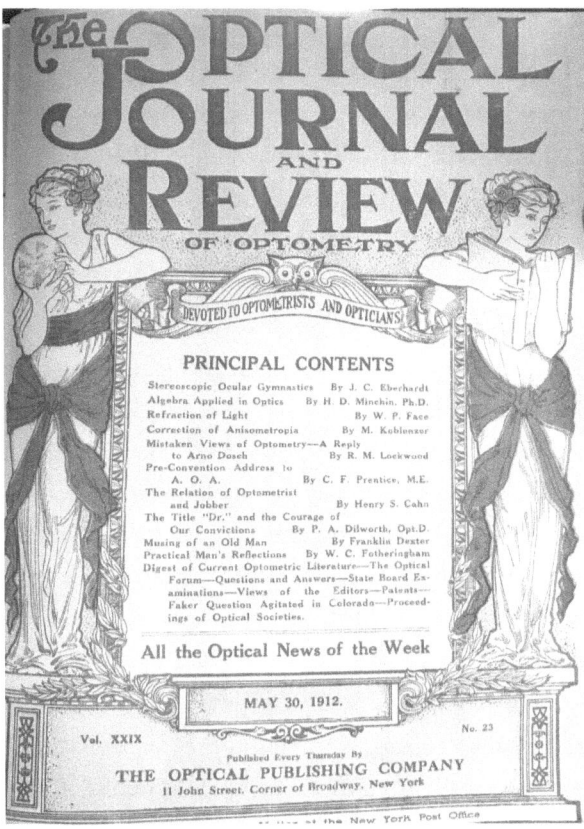

Figure 7.1. A cover from *The Optical Journal and Review of Optometry* in 1912. It was a widely read periodical among optometrists and was published weekly at that time. It continues to the present as *Review of Optometry*. (Image from a photograph taken by the author)

ing the *AOA Messenger* in 1926.[4] Its title changed to the *Organizer* in 1929 and then the *Journal of the American Optometric Association* in 1930. Starting in 1978, after a journal review board was organized, papers submitted for publication were refereed. In 2000, the title of the AOA's journal was changed to simply *Optometry*. Unfortunately, financial concerns forced the discontinuation of the journal in 2012.[5]

The journal published by the American Academy of Optometry

has the title *Optometry and Vision Science* today. Its beginnings can be traced to the *Northwest Journal of Optometry*, started in 1924, as a joint publication of the Minnesota, North Dakota, and South Dakota state optometric associations.[6,7] In 1925, it changed title to *American Journal of Optometry*, also representing state associations of Iowa, Nebraska, and Oklahoma, and in 1928, it started an association with the American Academy of Optometry.[8] The journal had title changes to *American Journal of Optometry and Archives of the American Academy of Optometry* in 1941, *American Journal of Optometry and Physiological Optics* in 1974, and *Optometry and Vision Science* in 1989.

Through the twentieth century, optometry became more heavily involved in research, and optometry research journals gained in prominence. The Academy's journal became the leading optometry research journal. Other prominent optometry research journals include *Ophthalmic and Physiological Optics* started in 1896, which is published in the United Kingdom and can be traced back to the *British Dioptric and Ophthalmometric Review*; *Clinical and Experimental Optometry* started in 1919, which is published in Australia and had its origins as the *Commonwealth Optometrist*; and *Journal of Optometry* started in 2008, which is published in Spain.[9,10]

In a 1996 paper, Jurkus and Dujsik[11] reported that there were 105 English language periodicals relating to the eye care field at that time. In 1993, they had conducted a survey of faculty at 16 optometry schools in the United States, and they listed 77 periodicals available in one optometry school library. Respondents were asked to indicate one of the following four answers, as their reading habit for each of the periodicals: *don't read, skim/glance, read part regularly (read specific articles but not entire journal)*, or *always read (read most of the journal, every issue)*. A total of 263 completed surveys were returned out of 586 distributed. More than half of the respondents marked 10 journals as being at least skimmed regularly. Fifty-eight different publications were marked as *read* or *always read*, indicating quite varied reading habits. Refereed journals that had the highest percentages of

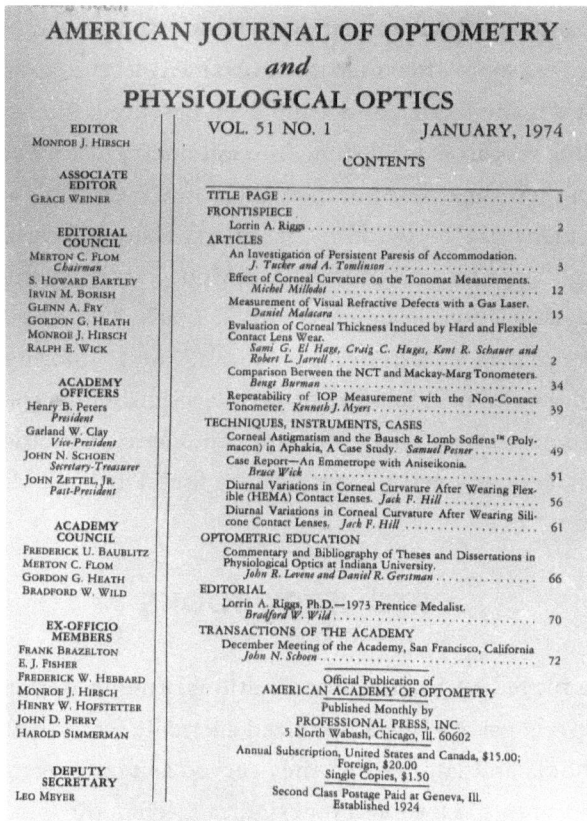

Figure 7.2. The title of the journal published monthly by the American Academy of Optometry changed from *American Journal of Optometry and Archives of the American Academy of Optometry* to *American Journal of Optometry and Physiological Optics* in January, 1974 with this issue. In 1989 the title of the journal changed to *Optometry and Vision Science*. (Image from a photograph taken by the author)

respondents marking *read* or *always read* were the *Journal of the American Optometric Association* (72%), *Journal of Optometric Education* (42%), *Optometry and Vision Science* (40%), *Archives of Ophthalmology* (40%), and *American Journal of Ophthalmology* (34%). Non-refereed periodicals that were *read* or *always read* by the most respondents were *AOA News* (65%), *Review of Optometry* (52%), *Optometric Management* (40%), and *Contact Lens Spectrum*

(35%). The authors observed that periodicals received as a membership benefit were read more often than those obtained by subscription.

There are many lesser known and even obscure periodicals that can be outstanding resources for delving into optometry history and studying the events of their time. Some of these often rare periodicals are available online, but many can be found in optometry school libraries or at the Archives and Museum of Optometry (AMO), located at the American Optometric Association headquarters in St. Louis. The AMO holds collections of more than 50 historical periodicals.[12] More information on the periodicals discussed here, plus other periodicals including specialty periodicals on contact lenses, vision therapy, optometric education, practice management, and optometry history, can be found in Appendix 3.

OPTOMETRY BOOKS

Books have played an important educational role in optometry, both before comprehensive and standardized curricula were available at optometry schools and later, when they served as textbooks in rigorous academic programs. Optometry periodicals from the opening years of the twentieth century, like *Optical Journal*, were filled with advertisements for books on topics such as retinoscopy, optometric testing procedures, and elementary geometrical optics. Offering advice in 1921 to his fellow optometrists on how to advance their practices and their profession, Eugene Wiseman wrote that "the cost of any book is small and it is almost certain that you can easily obtain from any one of them an idea that can be worth many times the investment."[13] In writing about the principles on which optometry practice should be conducted, E. LeRoy Ryer and Elmer Hotaling suggested that "not to know many books and not to know them well is to miss keen joy, deny ourselves encouragement and inspiration, and reduce immeasurably the chances of success."[14]

The proliferation of optometry books beginning in the late nineteenth century and early twentieth century was important in the dissemination of optometric knowledge and helped to spark a scholarly tradition in optometry. As optometry advanced, the sophistication, depth of knowledge presented, and breadth of topics examined in optometry books expanded and progressed. The following paragraphs consider a sampling of the most pivotal or most prominent optometry books since the late nineteenth century. Additional detail on the history of optometry books can be found in Appendix 4.

William Bohne can be said to be the first American author of a textbook written for optometrists (or opticians as they were known at that time).[15,16] The first edition of Bohne's *Handbook for Opticians* was published in 1888, with second and third editions appearing in 1892 and 1895. Recognizing that his book was "something new," Bohne wrote in the preface to the first edition that "my book may be the pioneer to open the road for other writers."[17]

The beginning of the twentieth century saw a surge in interest in retinoscopy. George A. Rogers' books, *Skiascopy: A Treatise on the Shadow Test in Its Practical Application to the Work of Refraction* (1899) and *The Shadow Test in Ocular Diagnosis* (1905) provided instruction in retinoscopy.[18] Books by Andrew Jay Cross, *A System of Ocular Skiametry* (1903) and *Dynamic Skiametry in Theory and Practice* (1911), were important in the development and popularization of dynamic retinoscopy.[19]

Robert M. Lockwood wrote several practical and popular little books between 1903 and 1907, including *The Principles of Optometry* (1903) and *Skiascopy without the Use of Drugs* (1906).[18] Christian Henry Brown's *Optician's Manual* was first published in 1897. It went through several editions, with a split into two volumes in 1902 and a change in title to *Optometrist's Manual* in 1921. Brown's book covered a broad range of topics in practical optics and optometry.[20]

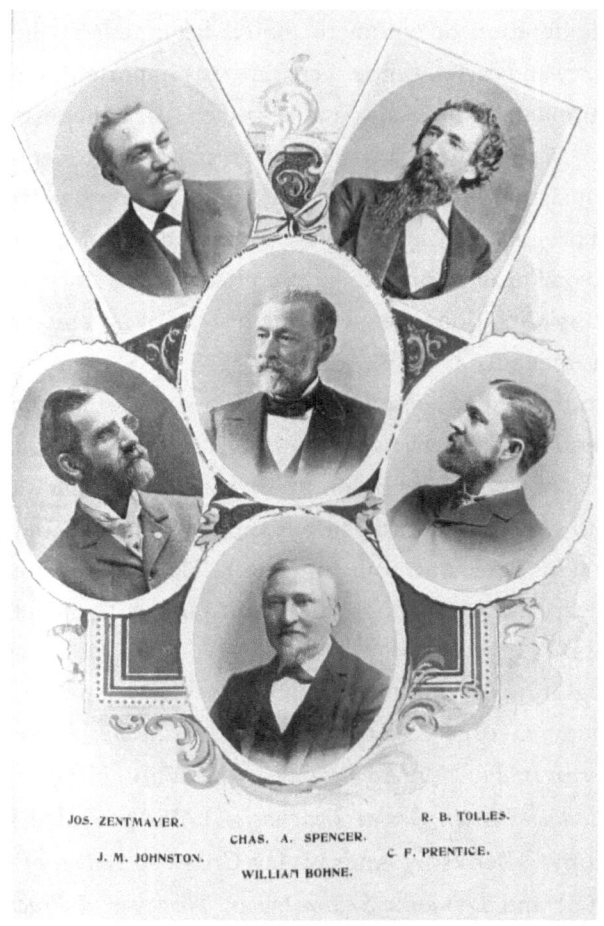

Figure 7.3. Frontispiece from William Bohne's book, *Handbook for Opticians*, showing leading individuals in nineteenth century optics and optometry. Joseph Zentmayer (1826-1888), top left, Charles Spencer (1813-1881), center, and Robert Tolles (1823-1883), top right, were innovative makers of lenses, microscopes, telescopes, and optical instruments. J.M. Johnston (1844-1930), center left, was publisher of the first periodical devoted exclusively to optometry. Some of Charles Prentice's (1854-1946), center right, contributions to optometry were discussed in chapter 2. William Bohne (1827-1906) is pictured bottom center. (Image from Bohne W. *Handbook for Opticians*, 3rd ed. New Orleans, LA: Griswold, 1895).

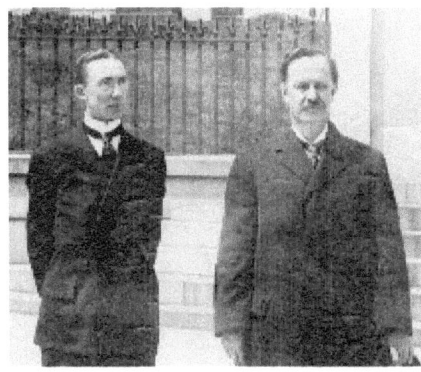

Figure 7.4. E. LeRoy Ryer (1880-1972), left, and Robert M. Lockwood (1857-1920). Both were frequent contributors to optometric periodicals and authors of important optometry books. (Image courtesy of the Archives and Museum of Optometry and The AOA Foundation).

English optometrist Lionel Laurance first published *Visual Optics and Sight Testing* in 1921, with the book progressing to a fourth edition in 1936. Its coverage included ocular anatomy, ocular optics, ophthalmic optics, vision science, and testing procedures.[21] Illustrative of its wide acceptance is the statement by Irvin Borish: "Although many concepts, and even instrumentation, varied between England and the United States, this volume remained the basic text in the field until it was replaced by *Clinical Refraction* in 1949."[22]

Charles Sheard was the author of several significant publications for optometry, some of which were collected in a volume commemorating his work.[23] Perhaps his most important book was *Dynamic Ocular Tests* (1917). In it he spelled out a routine of 18 tests in an optometric examination. Later Sheard expanded his sequence to 20 tests.[24] Sheard's list of tests appears to have led to the numbered list of tests in the 21-point examination popularized by the Optometric Extension Program.[25,26]

Many optics books have been written for optometry students. The most notable and most complete of the early ones was *Mirrors, Prisms, and Lenses: A Textbook of Geometrical Optics* (first edition, 1918) by James P.C. Southall, long-time director of the optometry school at Columbia University.[27] The third edition added a nearly 100-page chapter on physical and physiological optics.

In *Building Optometry* (1921), Eugene Wiseman forcefully argued in favor of professionalism.[28] He stressed practicing in an upstairs office rather than a street-level store, giving good service, building a strong knowledge base, having proper equipment, charging fees for services, avoiding the use of advertisements, and participating in optometric organizations. Wiseman's book included several photographs of professional optometry offices, one of which is shown in Figure 5.6.

An optometrist who has largely been forgotten is Ray Morse Peckham.[29] His 1926 book *The Modern Treatment of Ocular Imbalances* can be viewed as the first book on optometric vision therapy. It explained the use of an instrument with prism slides to measure phorias and fusional vergence ranges, and how it could be used for anti-suppression training and improvement of accommodation and vergence function. He also discussed the treatment of hyperphoria and amblyopia. In the foreword to the 1928 second edition, E. LeRoy Ryer praised Peckham for "his brilliant exposition of the true underlying principles" of binocular imbalances, in noting that their root cause was usually functional rather than anatomical.[30]

In 1941, Ryer and E lmer E. Hotaling published *Optometric Procedure: Basic and Supplementary*, in which they expressed principles for conducting an optometry practice.[31] They advocated thorough knowledge, mastery of instruments, an efficient floor plan, knowledge of optometry history, adequate equipment, an orderly and complete examination, a well-used library, ethical and professional practice, and an optometrically trained assistant.

Optometry: Professional, Economic, and Legal Aspects was published in 1948 by Henry Hofstetter.[32] It was important in providing a one-source summary of a great deal of information and data on those aspects of optometry, including historical background of optometry, legal status, licensure and board examinations, governmental relations, ethics, types of practice, earnings and fees, office accounting, international optometry, optometric education, and distribution of optometrists. Another important book published in 1948 was *How to Succeed in Optometry* by practice management consultant Ralph Barstow.[33] In it he expounded on the nature of successful professional practice and how it can be achieved.

Many would agree that the most famous book in optometry is *Clinical Refraction* by Irvin M. Borish. The first edition was published in 1949 and the second in 1954. The best known version of the book was the 1970 third edition, which expanded to more than twice as many pages as the second edition with the contributions of 19 collaborators.[34] A completely new book, *Borish's Clinical Refraction*, under the editorship of William J. Benjamin and with contributions from 46 authors, including Borish, was published in 1998. A second edition was published in 2006.

A book that deepened optometric interest in the relationships of vision problems, near work, and school performance was *Notes on a Dynamic Theory of Vision* (1954) by educational consultant Darell Boyd Harmon.[35] An important book in presenting the OEP testing sequence and analysis was *Visual Analysis*, first published in 1952 by Leo Manas.[36] A more detailed second edition appeared in 1958, and the better known and significantly expanded third edition was published in 1965.

Monroe J. Hirsch and Ralph E. Wick produced three significant books in the 1960s. They edited *Vision of the Aging Patient* (1960) and *Vision of Children* (1963) with broad coverage of geriatric and pediatric optometry, and they wrote *The Optometric Profession* (1968), examining some of the history of optometry and analyzing the structure of the profession at the time of their writing.[37]

Although contact lens textbooks started appearing in the 1940s,[38] the best known and most widely used for many years was *Contact Lens Practice* by Robert Mandell. It was first published in 1965, and it continued to a fourth edition, published in 1988, with twice as many

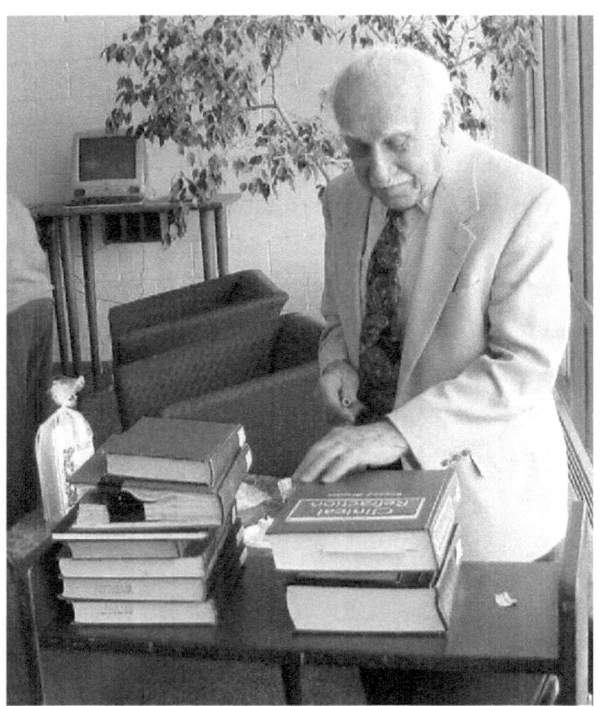

Figure 7.5. Irvin M. Borish (1913-2012) with a collection of books he authored and contributed to. At the top of the stack on which his left hand is resting is the first edition of Borish's *Clinical Refraction*, edited by William J. Benjamin (1998), and at the bottom of that stack is Borish's most famous book, the third edition of *Clinical Refraction* (1970). (Image courtesy of Indiana University School of Optometry)

pages as the first edition. A reviewer called it "the definitive contact lens textbook."[39]

In the 1970s and 1980s, there was an increase in the number of well-written books in some of the specialty areas of optometry. An example is *Binocular Anomalies* by John R. Griffin. The first edition was published in 1976, and it proceeded to a fifth edition in 2010. One review called *Binocular Anomalies* "a standard text in the field of binocular vision."[40]

Through much of the twentieth century, optometrists learned ocular disease from books written by ophthalmologists for ophthalmologists. As optometric scope of practice expanded, more books on ocular disease and pharmacology were written by optometrists and optometry school faculty members. An example of one of the best books in that area is *Clinical Ocular Pharmacology* edited by Jimmy D. Bartlett and Siret D. Jaanus. The first edition was published in 1984 and a fifth edition in 2008.

An optometry author known for the clarity and readability of writing in several textbooks was Theodore Grosvenor.[41,42] His best known book was *Primary Care Optometry* (first edition, 1982; fifth edition, 2007).

Two excellent books, which between them provide wide coverage of testing, diagnosis, and management for vision care, are *Diagnosis and Management in Vision Care* (1987) edited by John F. Amos and *Clinical Procedures in Optometry* (1991) edited by J. Boyd Eskridge, John F. Amos, and Jimmy D. Bartlett.[43] Borish wrote a foreword for each of them, expressing the view that their organization and authoritativeness made them important for the profession. Borish wrote that *Diagnosis and Management in Vision Care* represented "a significant contribution and a major impact on the potential clinical processes of the profession."[44] In the foreword to *Clinical Procedures in Optometry*, he wrote that the goal of the editors to assemble a complete text of clinical procedures to promote consistency of testing procedures across the profession was a very important objective for the future of optometry.[22]

Other commentators would likely identify many additional books worthy of being considered among the most prominent optometry books. In fact, in a survey seeking opinions on what would be the most important twentieth-century optometry books, input from 21 respondents resulted in a list of 106 books.[45,46] Reflecting upon the observation of Borish that "the literature fashioned within and by a profession is obviously intended to guide the evolution of that profession"[44] leads to the recognition that optometry periodicals and books will continue to be an important element for the future of the profession.

Chapter 7: Notes

1. Hofstetter HW. Why did it take so long? *Rev Optom.* 1991;128(1):39.
2. *Dr. Thompson's 1895 Correspondence Course with Historical Commentary by Monroe J. Hirsch.* Chicago, IL: Professional Press, 1975:147-148.
3. Gregg JR. *The Story of Optometry.* New York, NY: Ronald Press, 1965:185-186.
4. Christensen JL. History of the Journal of the American Optometric Association. *J Am Optom Assoc.* 1985;56:852-858.
5. Carlson D. A message to readers. *J Am Optom Assoc.* 2012;83(1):np.
6. Hirsch MJ, Weiner G. History of the *American Journal of Optometry. Am J Optom Arch Am Acad Optom.* 1968;45:43-57.
7. Gregg JR. *History of the American Academy of Optometry 1922-1986.* Washington, DC: American Academy of Optometry, 1987:156-163.
8. Flom MC. How did our Academy journal start and become preeminent? *Optom Vis Sci.* 2005;82:1011-1013.
9. Goss DA. Literature and information in vision care and vision science. *Optom.* 2008;79:670-686.
10. Elliott DB, Handley N. A historical review of optometry research and its publications: Are optometry journals finally catching up? *Ophthal Physiol Opt.* 2015;35:245-251.
11. Jurkus J, Dujsik G. Reading habits of optometric educators. *Optom Ed.* 1996;21:90-93.
12. Hébert K. Rare ophthalmic periodicals: The historiography of the profession at risk. *Hindsight* 2018;49:57-61.
13. Wiseman EG. *Building Optometry.* Philadelphia, PA: Keystone, 1921:189.
14. Ryer EL, Hotaling EE. *Optometric Procedure: Basic and Supplementary.* Southbridge, MA: American Optical, 1941:28.
15. Goss DA. William Bohne (1827-1906), author of *Handbook for Opticians*, first textbook by an American optometrist. *Hindsight* 2011;42:14-16.
16. Aitken MJ. The incunabula of American optometry. *Hindsight* 2012;43:19-24.
17. Bohne W. Extract from Preface of first edition. *Handbook for Opticians*, 3rd ed. New Orleans, LA: Griswold, 1895:5-6.
18. Goss DA. Robert M. Lockwood and George A. Rogers, early twentieth-century optometry authors. *Optom Vis Sci.* 2010;87:190-194.
19. Goss DA. Biographical sketches. *Hindsight* 2016;47:32-41.
20. Goss DA. Christian Henry Brown (1857-1933) and the Philadelphia Optical College. *Hindsight* 2010;41:114-121.
21. Goss DA. Biographical notes on Lionel Laurance. *Hindsight* 2012;43:107-109.
22. Borish IM. Foreword. In: Eskridge JB, Amos JF, Bartlett JD, eds. *Clinical Procedures in Optometry.* Philadelphia, PA: Lippincott, 1991:ix.
23. Sheard C. *The Sheard Volume: Selected Writings in Visual and Ophthalmic Optics.*

Philadelphia, PA: Chilton, 1957.
24 Sheard C. Considerations regarding the analysis and interpretation of data on ocular accommodation and convergence. *Am J Optom.* 1934;11:412-422, 448-460, 1935;12:52-61.
25 Borish IM. 21 points. *Newsletter Optom Hist Soc.* 1987;18:23-24.
26 Hendrickson H. 21 points and more. *Newsletter Optom Hist Soc.* 1987;18:55-56.
27 Goss DA. Biographical notes on James P. C. Southall. *Hindsight* 2013;44:9-12.
28 Goss DA. Eugene Wiseman (1885-1967), optometric practitioner, organizer, innovator, and writer. *Hindsight* 2010:41:71-78.
29 Goss DA. Ray Morse Peckham (1876-1944) and his optometric writings. *Hindsight* 2010;41:9-14.
30 Ryer EL. Foreword. In: Peckham RM. *The Modern Treatment of Binocular Imbalances with Genothalmic Kratometer,* 2nd ed. Geneva, NY: Shur-on Standard Optical Company, 1928:v-viii.
31 Goss DA. E. LeRoy Ryer (1880-1972) and Elmer E. Hotaling (1887-1950), optometric leaders and authors, and partners in optometry practice. *Hindsight* 2011;42:52-59.
32 Koch CC. "Optometry" by Hofstetter. *Am J Optom Arch Am Acad Optom.* 1948;25:507-508.
33 Goss DA. Ralph Barstow (1884-1968), optometric practice management advisor and author of *How to Succeed in Optometry. Hindsight* 2011;42:94-96.
34 Benjamin WJ. Preface. In: Benjamin WJ, ed. *Borish's Clinical Refraction.* Philadelphia, PA: W. B. Saunders, 1998:xiii-xv.
35 Goss DA. Darell Boyd Harmon (1898-1975). *Hindsight* 2018;49:81-83.
36 Goss DA. Biographical notes on five authors associated with the Northern Illinois College of Optometry. *Hindsight* 2011;42:106-111.
37 Goss DA. Biographical notes on Monroe Hirsch and Ralph Wick: Optometric leaders and co-authors of three significant books. *Hindsight* 2014;45:25-28.
38 Goss DA. Authors of the first contact lens textbooks: Beacher, Feinbloom, and Obrig. *Hindsight* 2015;46:27-31.
39 Efron N. Book review: *Contact Lens Practice. Clin Exp Optom.* 1989;72:67.
40 Daum KM. Book review: *Binocular Anomalies: Diagnosis and Vision Therapy. Optom Vis Sci.* 1996;73:438.
41 Strong JG. Theodore P. Grosvenor: Foundation head of the optometry course at University of Auckland. *Clin Exp Optom.* 2003;86:346-349.
42 Grosvenor T. Clinical optometry textbooks. *Hindsight* 2007;38:40-46.
43 Goss DA. Jess Boyd Eskridge, optometric educator and author. *Hindsight* 2012;43:103-106.
44 Borish IM. Foreword. In: Amos JF, ed. *Diagnosis and Management in Vision Care.* Boston, MA: Butterworths, 1987:xi-xii.
45 Goss DA, Penisten DK. Most important 20th-century optometry books. *Hindsight* 2004;35:36-40.

46 Goss DA. Two more important 20th-century optometry books. *Hindsight* 2004;35:43.

Appendix 1
A Historical List of Optometry Schools in the United States

One estimate suggests that there were about 60 optometry schools operating for various periods of time, between 1872 and 1901 in the U.S., about 42 between 1901 and 1914, about 36 from 1914 to 1922, and about 30 from 1922 to 1926.[1] As a result of the efforts to improve standards in optometric education in the 1920s, the number of schools decreased and then remained fairly constant around 9 to 12 from 1927 to the early 1970s, before gradually increasing to 17 by 1989 and then to more than 20 in the twenty-first century. This appendix represents an attempt at an historical list of optometry schools in the United States.

EXTINCT SCHOOLS

The following is a list of extinct schools of optometry. It was compiled from the lists of schools in the *Blue Book of Optometrists;* from a list of extinct schools in a 1977 issue of the *Newsletter of the Optometric Historical Society* that had been compiled from the files of the International Library, Archives, and Museum of Optometry;[2] and from mentions of schools in other publications.[3,4,5,6]

Some of the different listings may represent name changes in continuing schools. Previous names of existing schools are also included. This list does not indicate how active the schools were. It is likely that all major schools no longer in existence are included in this list, but it also seems likely that some minor short-lived schools may not be listed.

The years in parentheses are the years in which the schools were listed in the *Blue Book of Optometrists*. The *Blue Book of Optometrists* was first published in 1912 and then published every other year thereafter through most of its existence. Because the listings began in 1912 and were printed only every other year and the criteria for inclusion in the *Blue Book* are unclear, the years of inclusion likely do not accurately represent the starting and ending years of operation of many of the schools. Where the correct starting and ending years are known, they are noted in brackets.

- American Institute of Optometry, New York, NY (1916-1924)
- American Medical College Optometry Department, St. Louis, MO
- American Optical College, Detroit, MI (1912-1914)
- Appleton College of Optometry, Seattle, WA (1922)
- Atlantic University School of Optometry, Virginia Beach, VA (1932)
- Aydelotte-McCormick College of Ophthalmology, Dixon, IL (1934)
- Bates' School of Optometry, New York, NY
- Bradley Horological Institute, Peoria, IL (1914-1916) [started 1886]
- Bradley Polytechnic Institute, Peoria, IL (1918-1926)
- California College of Optics, San Francisco, CA (1918)
- California College of Optometry, San Francisco, CA (1920-1924) [started 1904]
- Chicago College of Optometry, Chicago, IL (1948-1954) [formerly Monroe College of Optometry, merged with Northern Illinois College of Optometry in 1955]
- Chicago Ophthalmic College, Chicago, IL
- Chicago Ophthalmic College and Hospital, Chicago, IL
- Chicago School of Refraction (1916), Chicago, IL
- Columbia Optical College, St. Paul, MN (1914, 1920-1926)
- Columbia University, New York, NY (1912-1954) [1910-1956]
- DeKeyser Institute of Optometry, Portland, OR (1916-1926) [founded

A Historical List of Optometry Schools in the United States 267

in 1910, merged with the Oregon College of Ocular Sciences in the 1920s to form the North Pacific College of Optometry]
- Delaware Ophthalmic College
- DeMars School of Optics, Minneapolis, MN (1912-1922) [started 1900]
- Denver Optical College, Denver, CO (1912)
- Detroit Optical Institute, Detroit, MI
- Donders School of Optometry, Los Angeles, CA (1918)
- J.C. Eberhardt's Optometry Courses, New York, NY
- Ferguson's School of Optometry, New York, NY
- Foster School of Optics, Boston, MA
- Franklin Institute, Passaic, NJ (1914-1918)
- Harden Optical College, Denver, CO (1912, 1918)
- Harden Optical College, Cleveland, OH (1920-1926)
- Indiana State College of Optics, South Bend, IN
- Interstate Institute of Optometry, Litchfield, IL (1912-1914)
- Iowa College of Optometry, Des Moines, IA
- Jacksonian Optical College, Jackson, MI
- Johnston Optical Institute, Chicago, IL
- Johnston Optical Institute and College of Ophthalmology, Chicago, IL
- Kansas City Optical College, Kansas City, MO
- Kansas City School of Optometry
- Kansas School of Optics, Saco, ME (1912-1918)
- Kansas School of Optics, Atascadero, CA (1920)
- Kansas School of Optics, Topeka, KS [started about 1901]
- Kellam and Moore's College of Optics, Atlanta, GA
- Kentucky State College of Optometry, Mt. Sterling, KY (1940) [1935-1945]
- King School of Optics, New York, NY
- Klein School of Optics, Boston, MA [started 1894, became Massachusetts School of Optometry in 1901]
- Knowles' School of Optometry, New York, NY

- Leader Optical College, Topeka, KS
- Lincoln Optical College, Lincoln, NE
- Los Angeles College of Optometry, Los Angeles, CA (1950-1972) [name change to Southern California College of Optometry in 1972]
- Los Angeles Medical School of Ophthalmology and Optometry, Los Angeles, CA (1912-1920) [name change to Los Angeles School of Optometry in 1922]
- Los Angeles Optical College, Los Angeles, CA [merged with Southern California Eye College in 1909]
- Los Angeles School of Optometry, Los Angeles, CA (1922-1930, 1934-1948) [name change to Los Angeles College of Optometry in 1949]
- Lowe's School of Optometry, McMinnville, OR
- James Maguire, St. Paul, MN (1912)
- Manhattan School of Optics of the City of New York, NY
- Maryland Optical College, Baltimore, MD
- Massachusetts College of Optometry, Boston, MA (1952-1972) [1950-1976, when it became New England College of Optometry]
- Massachusetts School of Optometry, Boston, MA (1912-1950) [1901-1950, when it became Massachusetts College of Optometry]
- McCormick Medical College, Chicago, IL (1914-1918, 1924-1926)
- McCormick Neurological College, Chicago, IL
- McCormick Optical College, Chicago, IL
- Monroe College of Optometry, Chicago, IL (1940-1946) [started in 1936 as Midwestern College of Optometry, name change to Monroe College of Optometry in 1937, name change to Chicago College of Optometry in late 1940s]
- Milwaukee College of Optometry, Milwaukee, WI (1920)
- Missouri College of Optometry, St. Louis, MO (1914-1926)
- Nebraska College of Optics, Lincoln, NE (1920)
- Needles Institute of Optometry, Kansas City, MO (1912-1926) [1907-1926]

- New England Optical Institute, Boston, MA
- New Orleans Optical College, New Orleans, LA (1914-1926)
- New York Institute of Optometry, New York, NY [1908-1910]
- The New York Preparatory School, New York, NY
- New York School of Optometry, New York, NY
- New York University, New York, NY
- Northern Illinois College of Ophthalmology and Otology, Chicago, IL (1912-1926) [name changed to NICOO in 1891, merged with Needles Institute of Optometry in 1926]
- Northern Illinois College of Optometry, Chicago, IL (1928-1954) [formed through a merger in 1926, merged with Chicago College of Optometry in 1955 to form Illinois College of Optometry]
- North Pacific College of Optometry, Portland, OR (1928-1942) [started in the 1920s, suspended operations during World War II]
- Northwest College of Optometry, Seattle, WA (1924)
- Omaha Optical Institute, Omaha, NE (1914-1922)
- Oregon College of Ocular Sciences, Portland, Oregon (1922-1924) [founded in 1919, merged with DeKeyser Institute of Optometry in the 1920s to form the North Pacific College of Optometry]
- Pennsylvania College of Optics and Ophthalmology, Philadelphia, PAa (1914-1920)
- Pennsylvania College of Optometrists, Philadelphia, PA (1918-1920)
- Pennsylvania College of Optometry, Pittsburgh, PA
- Pennsylvania State College of Optometry, Philadelphia, PA (1920-1964) [started in 1919, name changed to Pennsylvania College of Optometry]
- Philadelphia Institute of Optometry, Philadelphia, PA (1914-1916)
- Philadelphia Optical College, Philadelphia, PA (1912-1940) [started in 1889]
- Post Graduate Eye Institute, Chicago, IL (1932)
- Physicians and Surgeons Optical College, Denver, CO (1912-1920)
- Reynolds Optical College, Portland, OR (1912)

- Rochester School of Optometry, Rochester, NY (1912-1926) [1902-1926]
- Rowley Ophthalmological College, St. Louis, MO
- Seattle College of Optometry, Seattle, WA
- School of Optometry of Monroe University, Chicago, IL (1938)
- South Bend College of Optics, South Bend, IN (1912-1920)
- Southern California Eye College (1914)
- Southern California College of Optics
- Southern California College of Optometry and Ophthalmology, Los Angeles, CA (1912)
- Southwestern College of Optometry, Kansas City, MO
- Southwestern Optical College, Kansas City, MO (1912-1922)
- Spencer Optical Institute, New York, NY (1912-1914)
- St. Louis College of Optometry, St. Louis, MO
- St. Louis College of Physicians and Surgeons, St. Louis, MO
- Stone School of Optics, St. Paul, MN (1912-1922)
- Syracuse School of Optics, Syracuse, NY
- Texas College of Optometry, Dallas, TX (1922-1924)
- Trowbridge School of Optometry, Chicago, IL
- University of Illinois, Champaign, IL (1924)
- University of Massachusetts, Boston, MA (1922)
- University of Rochester, Rochester, NY, (1926-1932) [first students admitted,1926; closure of program, 1936]
- University of Southern California, Los Angeles, CA (1932)
- Washington School of Optometry, Spokane, WA (1914-1928)
- Western Ophthalmology Institute, San Francisco, CA (1914-1918)

SOME CHANGES IN NAME AND LOCATION OF EXTINCT SCHOOLS

The Kansas School of Optics appears in the list of extinct schools above in Topeka, Kansas while the Kansas School of Optics was listed in the *Blue*

Book in Maine and California. This was a correspondence school operated by James Littlefield, and the different locations represent the moves that he made during his lifetime.[7]

There was an entry in the 1912 *Blue Book* for a James Maguire school in St. Paul, Minnesota. In the 1914 through 1926 *Blue Books*, the Columbia Optical College is described as being in St. Paul with James Maguire as the president, so these are presumably the same school.

The teaching of optometry in the late nineteenth and early twentieth century was sometimes done in conjunction with the teaching of horology (watch and clock-making). It has been suggested that the first school of horology was the Parsons Horological Institute, opened in 1886, in LaPorte, Indiana, by J. R. Parsons.[8] Its department of optics was the start for some optometrists.[9] In 1892, Lydia Moss Bradley purchased the school and moved it to Peoria, Illinois. It may have been known as Parsons Polytechnic Institute for a time because a history of the Indiana Association of Optometrists states that one of its charter members, I. M. Rowe, took a course in 1894 at Parsons Polytechnic Institute, in Peoria.[10] In 1897, it was dedicated as Bradley Polytechnic Institute with the inclusion of a horology department. In 1946, Bradley Polytechnic Institute was renamed Bradley University.[11]

One of the schools listed in the *Blue Book* was the Kentucky State College of Optometry. It was founded in 1935 by William Dayton Walden (1911-1988) with the name Walden College of Optometry and Technology.[12] The school was rechartered with the name Kentucky State College of Optometry in 1937. It closed in 1945.

ALTERNATIVE NAMES FOR SCHOOLS

It is possible that some schools may have, at times, been referred to by the name of the proprietor rather than the actual name of the school as with James Maguire mentioned above. For example, I have read of two optometrists who were said to have taken a six-month night course at Benson's College of Optometry in San Francisco.[13] Optometrist Ernest A. Benson (1872-1960) was president of the California College of Optometry, which opened in 1904 in San Francisco.[14] So it appears that the California College of Optometry and Benson's College of Optometry may well have been the same school.

NUMBERS OF GRADUATES BY SCHOOL IN THE 1940S

A 1944 survey conducted under the auspices of the American Optometric Association reported the school from which 12,534 practicing optometrists graduated.[15] The survey did not include between 1,800 and 2,000 optometrists who were in military service at the time of the survey. The data are given in Table A1.1.

Table A1.1. Number of graduates among 12,534 practicing optometrists in 1944

Name of School	Number of Graduates
Columbia University	524
Chicago Ophthalmic College*	93
DeMars School of Optometry*	93
Klein School of Optics**	51
Los Angeles School of Optometry	710
Massachusetts School of Optometry	458
McCormick Medical College*	166
Monroe College	61
Needles Institute*	860
Northern Illinois College of Optometry	2,898

Ohio State University	227
Pennsylvania College of Optics*	64
Pennsylvania State College of Optometry	678
Philadelphia Optical College*	476
Rochester School of Optometry*	302
Southern College of Optometry	175
Southern California College of Optics*	39
Southwestern Optical College*	104
University of California	290
University of Rochester*	42
Other	4,223

* Not still in operation in 1944 at the time of the survey.
** Changed its name to the Massachusetts School of Optometry in 1901.

PRESENT-DAY OPTOMETRY SCHOOLS

From the late 1940s to the early 1970s, the number of optometry schools remained fairly stable at 10 to 12. Although four schools opened during those years, those were offset by one closure (the optometry school at Columbia University in 1956) and one merger (the Chicago College of Optometry merged with the Northern Illinois College of Optometry to form the Illinois College of Optometry in 1955). Three schools opened in the 1970, and three in the 1980s. No more optometry schools opened until 2009 when three more started.

As of 2019, the Association of Schools and Colleges of Optometry (ASCO) listed 23 member schools and colleges.[16] The current names of those schools, as given at the ASCO website and the years of their original founding are as follows:

- Illinois College of Optometry (Chicago, IL), with one of its predecessor schools, the Chicago College of Ophthalmology and Otology founded in 1872
- New England College of Optometry (Boston, MA), 1894
- Southern California College of Optometry at Marshall B. Ketchum University (Fullerton, CA), 1904
- The Ohio State University College of Optometry (Columbus, OH), 1914
- Pennsylvania College of Optometry at Salus University (Philadelphia, PA), 1919
- University of California at Berkeley School of Optometry (Berkeley, CA), 1923
- Southern College of Optometry (Memphis, TN), 1932
- Pacific University College of Optometry (Forest Grove, OR), 1945 (a continuation of the North Pacific College of Optometry, founded in the 1920s)
- Indiana University School of Optometry (Bloomington, IN), 1951 (preprofessional classes started in 1951; first professional courses in 1953)
- University of Houston College of Optometry (Houston, TX), 1952
- University of Alabama at Birmingham School of Optometry (Birmingham, AL) 1969
- State University of New York State College of Optometry (New York, NY), 1971
- Michigan College of Optometry at Ferris State University (Big Rapids, MI), 1975
- Northeastern State University Oklahoma College of Optometry (Tahlequah, OK), 1979
- University of Missouri at St. Louis College of Optometry (St. Louis, MO), 1980
- Inter American University of Puerto Rico School of Optometry (Bayamon, Puerto Rico), 1981

- Nova Southeastern University College of Optometry (Ft. Lauderdale, FL), 1989
- M idwestern University Arizona College of Optometry (Glendale, AZ), 2009
- University of the Incarnate Word Rosenberg School of Optometry (San Antonio, TX), 2009
- Western University of Health Sciences College of Optometry (Pomona, CA), 2009
- Massachusetts College of Pharmacy and Health Sciences School of Optometry (Worcester, MA), 2012
- University of Pikeville Kentucky College of Optometry (Pikeville, KY), 2016
- Midwestern University Chicago College of Optometry (Downers Grove, IL), 2017

SOME NAME CHANGES OF EXISTING SCHOOLS

Illinois College of Optometry (ICO) traces its origin to the Chicago College of Ophthalmology and Otology started in 1872. With a change in ownership in 1891 from Henry Olin to James McFatrich, the name of the school changed to the Northern Illinois College of Ophthalmology and Otology (NICOO). Another of the predecessor schools of ICO was the Needles Institute of Optometry, started in 1907 in Kansas City. William Needles purchased NICOO in 1922, and in 1926 he merged NICOO and the Needles Institute of Optometry to form the Northern Illinois College of Optometry. In 1936, physician Reuben Seid started another of ICO's predecessor schools, the Midwestern College of Optometry, which had name changes to Monroe College of Optometry in 1937 and to the Chicago College of Optometry in the late 1940s. The Northern Illinois College of Optometry and the Chicago College of Optometry merged in 1955 to form ICO.[17]

The New England College of Optometry had its start as Klein School of Optics in 1894 and was started by physician August Andreas Klein. In 1901, the name of the school was changed to the Massachusetts School of Optometry. In 1950, its name was changed to the Massachusetts College of Optometry and, in 1976, to the New England College of Optometry.[18]

The origin of the Southern California College of Optometry, as described by James Gregg,[19] was in the Los Angeles School of Ophthalmology and Optometry, founded by Marshall B. Ketchum in 1904. Another school, the Southern California Eye College, was started in 1908 by oculists T. J. Ruddy and M. M. Ring. In 1909, the name of Ketchum's school was changed to the Los Angeles Optical College and Post Graduate School for Opticians. The Southern California Eye College merged with the Los Angeles Optical College to form the Southern California College of Optometry and Ophthalmology in 1909. In 1911, the name of the school changed to the Los Angeles Medical School of Ophthalmology and Optometry. In 1922, the name of the school became the Los Angeles School of Optometry. In 1930, the school operated as part of the University of Southern California (USC) in the Department of Physics-Optics. In 1933, the school separated from USC and again assumed the name Los Angeles School of Optometry. Later name changes were to the Los Angeles College of Optometry in 1949 and to the Southern California College of Optometry (SCCO) in 1972.[19] In 2013, SCCO added a physician assistant and pharmacy program and became known as Marshall B. Ketchum University.

The North Pacific College of Optometry had its origins in the 1920s. It operated in Portland, Oregon, until its suspension during World War II. The charter and assets of the school were transferred to Pacific University in Forest Grove, Oregon, and the College of Optometry started there in 1945.[20,21] One reference says that the DeKeyser Institute of Optometry was founded in 1910 and the Oregon College of Ocular Sciences was founded in 1919 with the North Pacific College of Optometry being formed in 1921 from their merger.[20] Pacific University's magazine also gives 1921 as the year of the merger.[22] However, the year of the merger was more likely 1926 or 1927 because that would be more consistent with the listings of schools in the *Blue Book of Optometrists* and because both the DeKeyser Institute of Optometry and the Oregon College of Ocular Sciences were among the schools evaluated by the International Boards of Boards in 1925 and 1926.[23] Pacific University, in 2002, created the College of Education (formerly School of Education), which now includes the School of Communication Sciences & Disorders, and in 2006, Pacific created the College of Health Professions, bringing together existing and new programs including physical therapy, occupational therapy, clinical psychology, dental hygiene, pharmacy, physician assistant studies, healthcare administration, and audiology. Programs in both the Colleges of Education and Health Professions collaborate interprofessionally with the College of Optometry.

The Pennsylvania College of Optometry began as the Pennsylvania State College of Optometry in 1919. In 2008, the Pennsylvania College of Optometry established Salus University. The following programs are offered by Salus University: the Pennsylvania College of Optometry, the College of Health Sciences, Education and Rehabilitation, and the Osborne College of Audiology.[24]

Appendix 1: Notes

1. Hofstetter HW. *Optometry: Professional, Economic, and Legal Aspects*. St. Louis MO: Mosby, 1948:297.
2. Hofstetter HW. 66 or more optometry schools. *Newsletter Optom Hist Soc.* 1977;8:18-20.
3. Gregg JR. *The Story of Optometry.* New York, NY: Ronald Press, 1965:219.
4. Cox ME. *Optometry, the Profession: Its Antecedents, Birth, and Development.* Philadelphia, PA: Chilton, 1957:45.
5. Hofstetter HW. Jacksonian Optical College. *Newsletter Optom Hist Soc.* 1991;22:39-40.
6. Hofstetter HW. Delaware Ophthalmic College. Notes on early schools. More notes on extinct schools. Another extinct college. *Newsletter Optom Hist Soc.* 1977;8:50-52.

7   Goss DA. James E. Littlefield, author of *Optometry: The Littlefield System of Eye and Nerve Measurements. Hindsight* 2010;41:92-99.
8   Brown A. Bradley University and its watchmaking past. Peoria Magazines, 2012. www.peoriamagazines.com/print/7998
9   Goss DA. Century-old optometry practices. *Hindsight* 1998;29:23.
10 Anonymous. Origins of an association. *Newsletter Optom Hist Soc.* 1983;14:37-44.
11 Bradley University. *History.* www.bradley.edu/about/history
12 Hofstetter HW. An academic rise and demise. *Newsletter Optom Hist Soc.* 1986;17:3-5.
13 Fiorillo J. *Berkeley Optometry: A History.* Berkeley, CA: University of California, 2010:11,337.
14 Fiorillo, 80-81.
15 Hofstetter HW. *Optometry: Professional, Economic, and Legal Aspects.* St. Louis, MO: Mosby, 1948:296.
16 Association of Schools and Colleges of Optometry. ASCO Member Schools and Colleges. www.optometriceducation.org/about-asco/asco-member-schools-and-colleges
17 Miller AR, Brown JM. *Optometry in America: A History of the Illinois College of Optometry 1872-1997.* Chicago, IL: Illinois College of Optometry, 1996.
18 Moline SW. *Century of Vision: The New England College of Optometry, An Anecdotal History of the First Hundred Years.* Boston, MA: New England College of Optometry, 1994.
19 Gregg JR. *Origin and Development of the Southern California College of Optometry, 1904-1984.* Fullerton, CA: Southern California College of Optometry, 1984.
20 Bleything W. Pacific University College of Optometry. *Oregon Encyclopedia.* Portland, OR: Portland State University, 2009. www.oregonencyclopedia.org/entry/view/pacific_university_college_of_optometry/
21 Miranda G, Read R. *Splendid Audacity: The Story of Pacific University.* Seattle, WA: Documentary Book Publishers, 2000.
22 Optometry through the decades. *Pacific Magazine* 2020;53(1):11.
23 Christensen JL. The first conference to establish optometric standards. *Optom Vis Sci.* 1996;73:428-434.
24 Salus University. Academics.www.salus.edu/

Appendix 2
The Changing Optometry Student Body: Data on Optometry Students and Graduates

This appendix presents data on optometry students and graduates in order to illustrate some historical trends and changes over several decades.

NUMBERS OF OPTOMETRY SCHOOL GRADUATES

Concern about the production of too many new optometry graduates is not a recent phenomenon. In 1946, Edmund Richardson, president of the American Optometric Association, suggested that the large numbers of graduates coming out of optometry schools after World War II should be directed toward areas of need for their services, so that they didn't enter commercial practice.[1] Some of the issues brought up by those who opposed increasing numbers of graduates included concerns about the oversupply of optometrists, the quality level of an enlarged applicant pool, and adequate numbers of qualified faculty.[2,3,4] Balanced against that were factors such as increasing population, changing age and demand demographics, and the expanding scope of optometric practice (see Chapter 6). One comment of interest is that the large increase in numbers of optometrists following World War II "enabled the optometric profession to become and remain the dominant eye/vision care provider in this nation."[5] For many years, the optimum ratio of optometrists to population given by the AOA was one optometrist for every 7,000 persons.[6]

Manpower studies have tried to assess needs for new graduates. For example, a manpower study commissioned by the AOA and the Association of School and Colleges of Optometry, completed in 2014, suggested that there would be a more than adequate supply of optometrists through 2025.[7]

Table A2.1. Numbers of Optometry Schools and Graduates Compared to U.S. Population

Year	Approximate Number of U.S. Optometry Schools	Number of Graduates	U.S. Population (Millions)
1925	30	154	115.8
1926	30	205	117.4
1927	9	195	119.0
1928	9	203	120.5
1929	9	180	121.8
1930	9	192	123.1
1931	9	215	124.0
1932	9	246	124.8
1933	9	338	125.6
1934	9	264	126.4
1935	9	310	127.3
1936	9	203	128.1
1937	9	375	128.8
1938	10	532	129.8
1939	10	666	130.9
1940	10	608	132.1

1941	10	373	133.4
1942	9	418	134.9
1943	9	336	136.7
1944	9	326	138.4
1945	10	157	139.9
1946	10	217	141.4
1947	10	528	144.1
1948	10	1452	146.6
1949	10	1934	149.2
1950	10	1572	152.3
1951	11	961	154.9
1952	12	636	157.6
1953	12	684	160.2
1954	12	674	163.0
1955	12	473	165.9
1956	11	333	168.9
1957	10	355	172.0
1958	10	349	174.9
1959	10	323	177.8
1960	10	375	180.7
1961	10	319	183.7
1962	10	334	186.5
1963	10	350	189.2
1964	10	384	191.9
1965	10	377	194.3

1966	10	413	196.6
1967	10	481	198.7
1968	10	477	200.7
1969	11	441	202.7
1970	12	445	205.1
1971	12	528	207.7
1972	12	683	209.9
1973	12	691	211.9
1974	12	684	213.9
1975	13	806	216.0
1976	13	905	218.0
1977	13	920	220.2
1978	13	980	222.6
1979	14	1051	225.1
1980	15	1083	227.2
1981	16	1092	229.5
1982	16	1112	231.7
1983	16	1147	233.8
1984	16	1188	235.8
1985	16	1113	237.9
1986	16	1058	240.1
1987	16	1106	242.3
1988	16	1034	244.5
1989	17	1145	246.8
1990	17	1115	249.6

1991	17	1137	253.0
1992	17	1150	256.5
1993	17	1167	259.9
1994	17	1125	263.1
1995	17	1219	266.3
1996	17	1210	269.4
1997	17	Not available	272.7
1998	17	1237	275.9
1999	17	1340	279.0
2000	17	1343	282.2
2001	17	1329	285.0
2002	17	1324	287.6
2003	17	1324	290.1
2004	17	1307	292.8
2005	17	1282	295.5
2006	17	1242	298.4
2007	17	1321	301.2
2008	17	1342	304.1
2009	20	1357	306.8
2010	20	1356	309.4
2011	20	1332	311.6
2012	21	1404	313.9
2013	21	1567	316.2
2014	21	1569	318.3
2015	21	1557	320.6

2016	22	1666	322.9
2017	23	1658	325.0
2018	23	1667	326.7
2019	23	1722	328.2

Sources of data on numbers of graduates:
1925-1941: Sheard[8]; 1942-1979: Boucher[9]; 1980-2019: Association of Schools and Colleges of Optometry. Note: 1925 represents the data for school year 1924-25, 1926 the data for 1925-26, 1927 for 1926-27, etc., from Sheard and Boucher.)
Source of U.S. population estimates: www.census.gov and www.multpl.com/united-states-population/table

The large decrease in number of optometry schools after 1925-26 was due to accreditation standards, which were introduced in the 1920s, resulting in the closing of many schools.[10,11] The decrease in the number of graduates in the early and mid-1940s was due to World War II. The very large numbers of graduates in 1948 through 1950 resulted from increased enrollments at some schools to accommodate the many World War II veterans who attended school on the GI Bill.

LEVELS OF COLLEGE TRAINING BEFORE ENTERING OPTOMETRY SCHOOL

Levels of college training for optometry school matriculants are shown in Table A2.2. At the beginning of the twentieth century, there were generally no academic requirements for admission to optometry school.[12] In 1944, only 19% of practicing optometrists had attended college before entering optometry school.[12] Optometry school entrance requirements were gradually added, and by the early 1940s, they were increasing to a minimum of one year of college credit. This has incrementally increased to the present standard of four years of pre-optometry college work although some students with exceptional academic records can gain admittance after three years of college.

The Changing Optometry Student Body

Each year from 1999 to 2019, at least 90% of optometry students had a Bachelor's degree or higher entering optometry school. Of course, there have always been a number of students who exceed the minimum requirements for admittance. In each of the years from 1999 to 2019, 1% to 3% of entering students had a Master's or doctorate degree.

Table A2.2. Percent of United States optometry students with college training and college degrees before entering optometry school.

Year	Percent with college training	Percent having Bachelor's degree or higher	Source
1924	3	<1	Estimated from Hofstetter[12] Figs. 18-19
1925	14	1	Estimated from Hofstetter[12] Figs. 18-19
1926	15	<1	Estimated from Hofstetter[12] Figs. 18-19
1927	13	1	Estimated from Hofstetter[12] Figs. 18-19
1928	10	<1	Estimated from Hofstetter[12] Figs. 18-19
1929	13	2	Estimated from Hofstetter[12] Figs. 18-19
1930	12	1	Estimated from Hofstetter[12] Figs. 18-19
1931	15	2	Estimated from Hofstetter[12] Figs. 18-19
1932	15	3	Estimated from Hofstetter[12] Figs. 18-19
1933	20	3	Estimated from Hofstetter[12] Figs. 18-19
1934	19	3	Estimated from Hofstetter[12] Figs. 18-19
1935	10	2	Estimated from Hofstetter[12] Figs. 18-19
1936	15	2	Estimated from Hofstetter[12] Figs. 18-19
1937	18	2	Estimated from Hofstetter[12] Figs. 18-19
1938	22	4	Estimated from Hofstetter[12] Figs. 18-19
1939	24	4	Estimated from Hofstetter[12] Figs. 18-19
1940	35	6	Estimated from Hofstetter[12] Figs. 18-19
1941	39	7	Estimated from Hofstetter[12] Figs. 18-19
1970	100	41	Seger[13]
1973	100	49	Seger[14]
1977	100	64	J Optometric Education[15]
1978	100	64	J Optometric Education[16]

1979	100	65	J Optometric Education[17]
1980	100	66	J Optometric Education[18]
1981	100	63	J Optometric Education[19]
1982	100	62	J Optometric Education[20]
1983	100	61	J Optometric Education[21]
1984	100	64	J Optometric Education[22]
1987	100	62	Data provided by ASCO[23]
1989	100	76	ASCO Survey[24]
1990	100	67	ASCO Survey[25]
1991	100	71	ASCO Survey[26]
1999	100	92	Data provided by ASCO[23]
2000	100	90	Data provided by ASCO[23]
2001	100	90	Data provided by ASCO[23]
2002	100	90	Data provided by ASCO[23]
2003	100	91	Data provided by ASCO[23]
2004	100	91	Data provided by ASCO[23]
2005	100	92	Data provided by ASCO[23]
2006	100	92	Data provided by ASCO[23]
2007	100	93	Data provided by ASCO[23]
2008	100	94	ASCO website[27]
2009	100	93	ASCO website[27]
2010	100	94	ASCO website[27]
2011	100	96	ASCO website[27]
2012	100	97	ASCO website[27]
2013	100	96	ASCO website[27]
2014	100	96	ASCO website[27]
2015	100	96	ASCO website[27]
2016	100	95	ASCO website[27]
2017	100	96	ASCO website[27]
2018	100	96	ASCO website[27]
2019	100	96	ASCO website[27]

ASCO = Association of Schools and Colleges of Optometry

PRE-OPTOMETRY GRADE POINT AVERAGES

Not only have the years of pre-optometry training increased, but the available data (see Table A2.3) indicate an increase in pre-optometry grade point averages since the 1960s. Some of this increase can be attributed to grade inflation, which has been estimated at an average increase in GPA of about 0.1 per decade from the 1960s to the 2010s.[28]

Table A2.3. Mean pre-optometry grade point averages (GPA).

Year	Overall mean GPA	Range of mean GPAs for ASCO member schools	Source
1965	2.46		Seger[14]
1966	2.50		Seger[14]
1967	2.56		Seger[14]
1968	2.62		Seger[14]
1969	2.59		Seger[14]
1970	2.67		Seger[14]
1971	2.80		Seger[14]
1972	2.91		Seger[14]
1973	3.00		Seger[14]
1975	3.27		Boucher[9]
1976	3.25		Boucher[9]
1977	3.29	2.89 – 3.53	J Optometric Education[15]
1978	3.30	2.91 – 3.53	J Optometric Education[16]
1979	3.31	2.90 – 3.58	J Optometric Education[17]
1980	3.28	2.87 – 3.48	J Optometric Education[18]

1981	3.19	2.80 – 3.40	J Optometric Education[19]
1982		2.86 – 3.38	J Optometric Education[20]
1983		2.91 – 3.40	J Optometric Education[21]
1984		2.70 – 3.40	J Optometric Education[22]
2009		3.03 – 3.57	ASCO website[27]
2010		3.33 – 3.87	ASCO website[27]
2011		3.28 – 3.92	ASCO website[27]
2012		3.03 – 3.73	ASCO website[27]
2013		3.02 – 3.65	ASCO website[27]
2014		3.08 – 3.61	ASCO website[27]
2015		2.94 – 3.66	ASCO website[27]
2016		2.94 – 3.62	ASCO website[27]
2017		3.20 – 3.70	ASCO website[27]
2018		2.90 – 3.72	ASCO website[27]
2019		3.04 – 3.75	ASCO website[27]

Note: For some years, the available data were the overall mean GPAs for all entering optometry students, and for some years the data available were mean GPAs for entering students at each of the ASCO member schools. In the latter case, the table gives the range from the school with the lowest mean entering GPA to the school with the highest mean entering GPA.

PERCENTAGES OF WOMEN AMONG APPLICANTS AND ENTERING STUDENTS

A survey conducted by the American Optometric Association in 1944 found that about 3% of practicing optometrists were women.[29] The pattern of so few women in optometry persisted until the 1970s. The percentage of women optometry school applicants increased from 5% in 1971 to 19% in 1977.[30] The proportion of women among optometry students throughout the last quarter of the twentieth century increased until they reached a majority. These trends are shown in Table A2.4.

Table A2.4. Percentages of women among optometry school applicants and among entering optometry students.

Year	Percentage among applicants	Percentage among entering students	Source
1971	5		Levine[30]
1972	7		Levine[30]
1973	9		Levine[30]
1974	13		Levine[30]
1975	14		Levine[30]
1976	18		Levine[30]
1977	19	20	Levine[30]; J Optometric Education[15]
1978		20	J Optometric Education[16]
1979		23	J Optometric Education[17]
1980		25	J Optometric Education[18]
1981		27	J Optometric Education[19]
1982		29	J Optometric Education[20]
1983		34	J Optometric Education[21]
1984		35	J Optometric Education[22]
1989		50	ASCO Survey[24]
1990		51	ASCO Survey[25]
1991		53	ASCO Survey[26]
1992		55	Trends in Optometric Education[31]
2008		65	ASCO website[27]
2009		62	ASCO website[27]
2010		64	ASCO website[27]
2011		66	ASCO website[27]

2012		63	ASCO website[27]
2013		65	ASCO website[27]
2014		68	ASCO website[27]
2015		69	ASCO website[27]
2016		70	ASCO website[27]
2017		65	ASCO website[27]
2018		68	ASCO website[27]
2019		70	ASCO website[27]

RACIAL DIVERSITY OF OPTOMETRY STUDENTS

Table A2.5. Numbers of students from racial minority groups enrolled in optometry schools in the United States.

School Year	African American	Hispanic or Latino	American Indian or Alaska Native	Asian	Foreign National	Native Hawaiian or other Pacific Islander	Other or Unknown	Two or More Races	Percent of Student Body	Total Enrollment, All Students
1969-70	15	23	2	72	18				6	
1970-71	15	27	2	97	25				5.9	
1971-72	22	37	1	107	33					
1972-73	37	40	4	131	43					
1973-74	52	39	5	141	42					
1974-75	73	45	5	153	40					
1975-76	83	55	8	166	37				8.9	
1976-77	89	46	12	157	30				8.1	
1977-78	79	55	7	153	49				8.1	
1978-79	62	66	11	166	53				8	
1979-80	56	67	13	208	51				8.8	
1980-81	57	80	12	243	40				9,5	
1982-83	71	107	19	296	59				12	
1983-84	88	123	18	293	62				12.9	
1984-85	96	116	20	269	62				12.7	
1985-86	111	126	20	313	78				14.6	
1986-87	116	136	13	352	86					
1987-88	117	139	22	410	84				15.7	

Year										
1988-89	130	280	26	462	84				20.9	
1992-93	144	314	18	698	211	9			28	4998
1994-95	139	318	20	818	232	3			29.5	5201
1995-96	120	330	19	930	219	7			31.7	5150
1996-97	122	312	19	1019	241	11			33.2	5210
1999-2000	120	275	29	1307	265	15	1			5464
2000-01	126	268	27	1357	247	16	19			5428
2001-02	141	282	31	1357	300	2	38			5414
2002-03	163	294	31	1254	322	11	62			5362
2003-04	171	302	35	1244	285	10	77			5354
2004-05	177	273	30	1212	338	1	101			5369
2005-06	189	273	29	1252		14	221			5377
2006-07	175	271	26	1306		20	327			5488
2007-08	172	255	19	1380		17	364			5556
2008-09	169	249	20	1465		9	370			5595
2009-10	165	258	24	1601		8	437			5832
2010-11	164	274	25	1708		4	464			6060
2011-12	189	274	24	1834		13	417			6289
2012-13	195	292	35	1925		20	416			6555
2013-14	204	302	37	1926		30	448			6676
2014-15	209	350	41	1976		30	401			6797
2015-16	183	383	40	1931		15	460	151		6900
2016-17	195	436	41	2088		13	438	149		7024
2017-18	192	455	34	2187		13	380	147		7124
2018-19	194	474	39	2177		21	438	141		7175
2019-20	229	521	41	2177		15	518	177		7244

Sources of data: 1969-70 to 2005-06, Association of Schools and Colleges of Optometry. Annual Surveys of Optometric Educational Institutions. Data in email to the author from Joanne Zuckerman, Manager, Data Services andSpecial Projects, ASCO, August 26, 2021. 2006-07 to 2019-20, Association of Schools and Colleges of Optometry. Past Student Data Reports. www.optometriceducation.org/data-reports/annual-student-data-report

Note: Empty cells indicate data which were not available in the source documents. Numbers include students in all four years of optometry school, so individuals were counted in multiple years.

Appendix 2: Notes

1. Richardson EF. Our increased student body: Asset or catastrophe? *Optical J Rev Optom.* 1946;83(22):46,49,51.
2. Hunter EL. The pros and cons of developing additional schools and colleges of optometry. *J Am Optom Assoc.* 1992;63:865-866.
3. Haffner AN. Urgent challenges to optometric education. *J Am Optom Assoc.* 1995;66:666-667.
4. Byrne J. Optometric profession debates increase in number of schools. *Primary Care Optom News* Nov., 2011. www.healio.com/news/optometry/20120225/optometric-profession-debates-increase-in-number-of-schools
5. Hopping RL. What should be the proper size and number of optometric schools? *J Am Optom Assoc.* 1992;63:808-811.
6. Pennell MY, DeLong MB. Optometric education and manpower. *J Am Optom Assoc.* 1970;41:941-956.
7. The Lewin Group. Eye Care Workforce Study: Supply and Demand Projections, Final Report, Prepared for American Optometric Association and the Association of Schools and Colleges of Optometry, April 25, 2014.
8. Sheard C. Optometric education and professional advancement. *Optom Weekly* 1942;33:1085-1089.
9. Boucher JA. Optometric education. *J Am Optom Assoc.* 1980;51:359-363.
10. Hofstetter HW. 75 years: A good beginning in optometric education. *Optical J Rev Optom.* 1966;103:72-74.
11. Goss DA. A historical list of optometry schools in the United States. *Hindsight* 2012;43:82-89.
12. Hofstetter HW. *Optometry: Professional, Economic, and Legal Aspects.* St. Louis, MO: Mosby, 1948:297-307.
13. Seger CE. A year of educational activity. *J Am Optom Assoc.* 1971;42:331-336.
14. Seger CE. Report to AOA House of Delegates: Optometric education 1974. *J Am Optom Assoc.* 1974;45:918-925.
15. Optometric Educational Institutions 1977-78. *J Optom Ed.* 1978;4(2):27-30.
16. American Optometric Association Council on Optometric Education. Annual Survey of Optometric Educational Institutions 1978-79. *J Optom Ed.* 1980;5(4):27-31.
17. American Optometric Association Council on Optometric Education. Annual Survey of Optometric Educational Institutions 1979-80. *J Optom Ed.* 1980;6(2):23-28.
18. American Optometric Association Council on Optometric Education. Annual Survey of Optometric Educational Institutions 1980-81. *J Optom Ed.* 1982;7(3):22-27.
19. American Optometric Association Council on Optometric Education. Annual Survey of Optometric Educational Institutions 1981-82. *J Optom Ed.* 1982;8(2):24-29.
20. American Optometric Association Council on Optometric Education. Annual Survey

of Optometric Educational Institutions 1982-83. *J Optom Ed.* 1984;9(3):24-29.
21   American Optometric Association Council on Optometric Education. Annual Survey of Optometric Educational Institutions 1983-84. *J Optom Ed.* 1985;10(3):26-30.
22   American Optometric Association Council on Optometric Education. Annual Survey of Optometric Educational Institutions 1984-85. *J Optom Ed.* 1986;11(3):26-30.
23   Association of Schools and Colleges of Optometry. Data. Email from Joanne Zuckerman, Manager, Data Services and Special Projects, ASCO, April 7, 2015.
24   Association of Schools and Colleges of Optometry. *Annual Survey of Optometric Educational Institutions: Survey Results July, 1989-June, 1990.* On file, Indiana University Optometry Library, Bloomington, IN.
25   Association of Schools and Colleges of Optometry. *Annual Survey of Optometric Educational Institutions: Survey Results July, 1990-June, 1991.* On file, Indiana University Optometry Library, Bloomington, IN.
26   Association of Schools and Colleges of Optometry. *Annual Survey of Optometric Educational Institutions: Survey Results July, 1991-June, 1992.* On file, Indiana University Optometry Library, Bloomington, IN.
27   Association of Schools and Colleges of Optometry. www.opted.org/past-student-data-reports/
28   Rojstaczer S, Healy C. Grading in American colleges and universities. *Teachers College Record*, 2010. www.tcrecord.org/Content.asp?ContentId=15928
29   Hofstetter HW. *Optometry: Professional, Economic, and Legal Aspects.* St. Louis, MO: Mosby, 1948:313-314.
30   Levine NR. Characteristics of applicants to schools and colleges of optometry 1971-72 to 1977-78: Changes, lack of changes, trends. *J Optom Ed.* 1978;4(2):8-14.
31   Association of Schools and Colleges of Optometry. Trends in optometric education 1989-90 to 1992-93. On file, Indiana University Optometry Library, Bloomington, IN.

Appendix 3
A History of Selected Optometric Periodicals

The first optometry periodicals appeared in the late 19th century, and numerous optometry periodicals have come and gone. Their geographical reach has varied, and the information presented has varied, including educational material, organization news, industry developments, and research results.

In 1948, Hofstetter[1] listed 49 optometric periodicals then being published in the United States. The list included national journals, regional and state journals, optometry school publications, and periodicals produced by organizations. Hofstetter[2] also compiled a worldwide list of 409 serial publications related to vision science that had been published before 1948. In 1990, Carlson[3] compiled a list of 206 English language optometry and ophthalmology journals, most of which were no longer in existence. This appendix is not a comprehensive review of optometric periodicals, but rather a brief history of some of the most significant American optometric periodicals.

PERIODICALS FOR JEWELERS WITH OPTICAL CONTENT

Jewelers' Circular was a periodical started in about 1870. In 1886, it started an "Optical Department" with a series of articles by C. A. Bucklin.[4] In 1900, *Jewelers' Circular* purchased *Jewelers' Weekly*, and it became the

Jewelers' Circular-Weekly. In 1901, the optical feature was expanded with regular weekly contributions by George A. Rogers,[4] and E. LeRoy Ryer published frequent optometry articles in *Jewelers' Circular-Weekly* from 1903 to 1905.[5] The optical department of this periodical split off to form a new serial publication, *Optical Review*, in 1907.

The Keystone, the magazine of the Keystone Watch Case Company, was started in about 1881 and continued to 1934 when it was purchased by *Jewelers' Circular-Weekly*.[4] *The Keystone* had various subtitles at different times, but at one point it was *A Monthly Journal Devoted to the Interests of the Watch, Jewelry, and Optical Trades*.[6] In 1909, *Keystone Magazine of Optometry* split off from *The Keystone. Keystone Magazine of Optometry* continued as *Optical Age* from 1921 to 1924.

JOHNSTON'S EYE-ECHO

The first periodical in the United States, and possibly the world, devoted exclusively to optometry was *Johnston's Eye-Echo*.[7,8] It was published by J. Milton Johnston (1844-1930), who was born in western New York. He served in the Civil War and then attended Adrian College in Michigan, and Northwestern University in Illinois. In 1880, after nine years as a Methodist minister, he joined his brothers in the Johnston Optical Company founded by his brother George in Detroit, Michigan. He soon recognized the need for an optical periodical. The first issue of *Johnston's Eye-Echo* was the January-February 1886 issue.

Johnston's Eye-Echo was published in six issues per year, each containing about four pages, from 1886 to 1891.[8,9] In each issue, Johnston included lessons that he called "Eye Studies." Each following issue contained questions on the previous lesson, and then in the issue after that, the answers to the questions were given. During 1891, Johnston changed the title to *Eye Light*. From 1893 to about 1895, Johnston published another periodical titled *Our Vision*.

In 1892, Johnston published a 228-page book, *Eye Studies: A Series of Lessons on Vision and Visual Tests*, which was revised and enlarged from a compilation of lessons he had written for the *Eye-Echo* and *Eye Light*.[10] In 1895, Johnston started an optometry school, which included correspondence courses. In 1905, he moved to Portage, Wisconsin, where he practiced optometry.[8]

OPTICAL JOURNAL AND REVIEW OF OPTOMETRY

Today's *Review of Optometry* is the optometry periodical that has had the longest publishing history although it has had several name changes. It started as a monthly and then later was a weekly, then a biweekly, and once again a monthly. It was started in 1895 as *Optical Journal* by Frederick Boger (1866-1936).

Boger got his start in the publishing business as a teenager, working as an employee of the publisher of *Jewelers' Circular*.[11] In 1891, Boger started a monthly periodical that he called *The Optician*. The lead article in the first issue was "A metric system of numbering and measuring prisms" by Charles F. Prentice.[12] *The Optician* was not financially successful, and in 1894, Boger ceased its publication.[13]

In March of 1895, Boger launched *The Optical Journal*. The first issue contained an article on optical glass by William Bohne. It also included Boger's call for the formation of a national association of opticians.[14] He continued to work toward the formation of that organization, and from 1898 to 1900, even though he was not an optician or optometrist, he served as the first secretary of the American Association of Opticians, which later became the American Optometric Association. In 1910, he was made the first honorary member of the American Association of Opticians.[15]

The Optical Journal published educational articles, opinion pieces, extensive news, and many advertisements, and it achieved the prosperity that Boger's previous publication had not. It also absorbed several other periodicals. The Focus was started in 1901 by George A. Rogers; it became a publication of the Northern Illinois College of Ophthalmology and Otology when Rogers began teaching there the next year, and soon after that Boger purchased it. In 1906, Boger purchased Optical Instrument Monthly, which had started publication in 1905, and in 1910, he acquired Optical Review, which had begun in 1907.[11] With the acquisition of Optical Review in 1910, the title of the periodical was changed to Optical Journal and Review of Optometry.

Frederick A. McGill, who had been editor of Optical Review, became editor of Optical Journal and Review of Optometry. The journal was published by the Optical Publishing Company with V. S. Mulford, who, with his father, had been publisher of Jewelers' Circular Weekly and Optical Review, as president, and Frederick Boger as vice-president and treasurer.[15] Boger retired in 1913. In 1927, the journal became part of United Publishers Corporation and in the 1930s, part of the Chilton Company.

When Frederick McGill died in 1936, his associate for 18 years, Maurice E. Cox, became the editor of Optical Journal and Review of Optometry.[15] Cox continued as editor until 1965 and as publisher until 1968. Cox was named a vice president of the Chilton Company in the late 1950s.[16] Cox wrote a series of articles on the history of optometry in Optical Journal and Review of Optometry, from October 1945 to January 1947, which were issued in a 48-page booklet in 1947 titled Optometry, the Profession: Its Antecedents, Birth, and Development. A revised 72-page edition of the book was published in 1957. Its contents clearly show his familiarity with events in optometry history and his admiration for the optometrists who led its development. Cox received an honorary Doctor of Ocular Science degree from the Northern Illinois College of Optometry, clear recognition of his dedication to optometry.[17] In 1984, Cox also received a Recognition

Certificate from the Optometric Historical Society for significant contributions to awareness of optometry history.[18]

In 1977, the title of the periodical changed to *Review of Optometry*, a title it retains at the present time. For a number of years, the Chilton Company had *Chilton's Review of Optometry* on the cover, so sometimes it is indexed in library catalogs as *Chilton's Review of Optometry*.

OPTOMETRIC WEEKLY

In 1910, while practicing optometry in Chicago, Lionel Topaz started publishing a periodical titled *Practical Optometrist and Optician*. In 1912, the title was changed to *Optometrist and Optician*, and then in 1919, to *Optometric Weekly and the Optometrist and Optician*. For five decades, from 1928 to 1978, it was published as *Optometric Weekly*. In February 1978, it became a monthly and the title was changed to *Optometric Monthly*, which was published until May 1985 at which point it was merged with *International Contact Lens Clinic* to form *International Eyecare*, which was published from June 1985 to December 1986. Like *Optical Journal and Review of Optometry*, *Optometric Weekly* published clinical review articles, opinion pieces, news items, and related material rather than peer-reviewed research. It was a widely read publication.

Topaz founded Professional Press, which published not only *Optometric Weekly* but also *Eye, Ear, Nose, and Throat Monthly*, *Optical Index*, the *Blue Book of Optometrists*, the *Red Book of Ophthalmologists*, and many optometry books. His son, Martin Topaz, and grandson, Peter Topaz, followed him into management of Professional Press.

According to an obituary,[19] Lionel Topaz was born in Finland, but most sources[20,21,22] and several federal censuses say that he was born in Russia. He immigrated to England in 1897 and then settled in the United States in 1903. He graduated from optometry school at the Northern

Illinois College of Ophthalmology and Otology in Chicago in 1905.[20] Lionel Topaz was active in the American Optometric Association.

In 1943, Lionel Topaz's children, Mae, Oscar, and Martin, made a gift to The Ohio State University to establish the Lionel Topaz Memorial Library of Visual Science there. Ohio State was chosen for the gift because of the high esteem Topaz had for Charles Sheard, the first director of Ohio State's optometry school.[20,21]

One obituary notice for Lionel Topaz stated that "his purposeful writings contributed towards the upbuilding of the exclusive ethical practice of professional optometry, now generally accepted as the normal standard of refractive practice."[22] Many other optometrists expressed their high regard for him in tributes in *Optometric Weekly*.[23] In speaking about optometric periodicals in the early decades of the twentieth century, Gregg[24] observed that: "the independent journals, such as *The Weekly*, spoke effectively and well for the profession...Topaz in his editorials spoke strongly for professionalism, education, and research."

OPTOMETRIC WORLD

Western Optical World was published from 1917 to 1944. In 1944, its title was changed to *Optical World*, and then in 1947, to *Optometric World*. It ceased publication in 1975. Its content included educational articles, news communications, historical pieces, and related material.

An optometrist readily recognized as being associated with *Optometric World* and who also served in other important capacities in optometry, was Arthur E. Hoare. He contributed many articles and was associate editor from 1962 to his death in 1971. Hoare was born in Australia and attended Battersea Polytechnic School in London and Otago University in Dunedin, New Zealand.[25] A few months before his ordination as a Presbyterian missionary, he was drafted into the British Army.[26] Serving for four years during World War I, he was wounded twice and nearly had to have a foot amputated.[26,27] His military experiences led him to "the philosophy that he could better reconcile doctrine with the idea of tangible service to people than with spiritual leadership."[27]

Influenced by his brother, a California MD who was taking courses at the Los Angeles Medical School of Ophthalmology and Optometry run by M. B. Ketchum, Hoare enrolled there and completed optometry school in 1922.[26,27] He subsequently taught at the school in the 1920s and again in the 1940s,[28] and he practiced in Los Angeles.

Hoare was very active in the American Optometric Association, serving as trustee from 1926 to 1929, director of the Department of Education, and as the first chairman of the Council on Optometric Education.[26] He was a member of the Board of Trustees of the Los Angeles School of Optometry from 1928 to 1948, serving as an officer many of those years.[28] He was an editor of the *California Optometrist*, the magazine of the California Optometric Association.[28] He was recognized by the American Academy of Optometry with an Honorary Life Fellowship, and he received an honorary DOS degree from the Los Angeles College of Optometry in 1962.

Hoare was a charter member of the Optometric Historical Society and a member of its first Executive Board from 1970 until his death in 1971. Hofstetter noted that Hoare "felt so keenly…that optometry's history is magnificent."[27] Hoare was described as a "gifted writer, brilliant orator and true friend who…marked the course of the future of optometry."[26]

AMERICAN JOURNAL OF PHYSIOLOGICAL OPTICS

The *American Journal of Physiological Optics* was a quarterly journal published from 1920 to 1926 by the American Optical Company and edited by Charles Sheard. It published research papers and review articles by leading vision scientists, optometrists, and ophthalmologists.

JOURNALS PUBLISHED BY THE AMERICAN ACADEMY OF OPTOMETRY AND THE AMERICAN OPTOMETRIC ASSOCIATION

One of the signs of the maturity of a profession is the publication of scholarly journals. For many years, the leading scholarly optometric journals in the United States were those published by the American Academy of Optometry (AAO), which continues today, and the American Optometric Association (AOA), which was dissolved in 2012.

AMERICAN JOURNAL OF OPTOMETRY / OPTOMETRY AND VISION SCIENCE

The journal known today as *Optometry and Vision Science* had its origin in January 1924 as the *Northwest Journal of Optometry*, a publication of the Minnesota, North Dakota, and South Dakota state optometric associations.[29] In August, 1925, the journal was renamed the *American Journal of Optometry*, then also representing the Nebraska, Iowa, and Oklahoma state optometric associations.[30] By 1928, it was the official journal of 11 state optometric associations. Starting in May 1928, the journal became a news outlet of the American Academy of Optometry. In 1934, the journal no longer represented individual state associations, and it was associated only with the American Academy of Optometry.

The Academy also separately published volumes of the papers presented at its fourth through eighteenth annual meetings, starting in 1927.[31] The thirteenth such volume, *Transactions of the 18th Annual Meeting of the American Academy of Optometry*, was published in 1939. In 1940, an AAO committee decided to merge its publications. The first issue of the merged publication, the *American Journal of Optometry and Archives of the American Academy of Optometry*, appeared in January

1941 (volume 18, number 1). The journal became a leading journal for clinical optometry and vision science, and it had several thousand subscribers.[30]

The founder of the journal, its editor from 1924 to 1968, and the owner of the company that published it from 1924 to 1973, was Carel C. Koch. Koch attended Washington University in St. Louis and then the DeMars School of Optometry in Minneapolis. His optometric education was interrupted by service in the United States Army, but he returned to the DeMars School and graduated in 1919. The unusual instructional organization of the DeMars School made such an interruption manageable. Two years of study were required for completion. The complete course of lectures was only six months, but each student was required to attend the complete set of lectures four times.[32] Advanced students also did clinical work. Koch completed optometry school in 1919 and set up practice in Minneapolis. Koch and Jack I. Kurtz, who shared practice space with him, were among the first optometrists in Minnesota to practice in professional offices.[33]

Koch was a charter member of the American Academy of Optometry and was secretary of the AAO from 1922 to 1925 and again from 1944 to 1973. He was chairman of the AAO in 1929 and later on its Committee on Interprofessional Relations and Long Range Planning Committee. He also served on several boards and commissions of civic and community organizations in Minneapolis. Among various awards and recognitions he received were honorary degrees from the Chicago College of Optometry and the Pennsylvania College of Optometry.[33,34] Writing in 1968, Hirsch and Weiner said, "The *Journal* and its editor have been vital forces influencing the transition [of optometry] from a trade to a profession."[33] An obituary notice said that Koch was "a great man whose intelligence, charm, love and dedication to his profession permeated everything he did...He inspired us to a life of scientific professional service through optometry, of dedication to the visual welfare of mankind, and of contribution to our fellow practitioners."[34]

In 1968, Monroe J. Hirsch, who had been associate editor since 1953, became the editor, and he served as editor through 1976. Merton Flom was an interim editor in 1977 and 1978. In 1974, the title of the journal was changed to the *American Journal of Optometry and Physiological Optics*.[35] The company publishing the journal was Professional Press in 1974 and 1975, and then, starting in 1976, Williams & Wilkins.

William M. Lyle was editor of the journal from 1979 to 1996. Newcomb and Eger stated that he "had served with distinction as the Journal's fourth Editor" and "he had substantially improved the quality of the Journal in many ways..."[36] The most visible changes in the journal during Lyle's tenure occurred in 1989, when the title of the journal changed to *Optometry and Vison Science*, and there was an increase in the page size and a change in color of the cover to the sea-foam green used in the academic regalia for optometry.

William Lyle was born in Canada and graduated from the College of Optometry of Ontario in Toronto in 1938. After practicing in Kirkland Lake, Ontario, and Winnipeg, he entered the Canadian military in 1940. He left the military with the rank of Captain in 1946, after serving in Europe during World War II.[37] He then returned to practice in Winnipeg, and while there, served as president of the Canadian Association of Optometrists and took additional courses in biochemistry, microbiology, genetics, and statistics at the University of Manitoba. In 1960, Lyle enrolled in the physiological optics graduate program at Indiana University. He completed an MS degree in 1962 and his PhD in 1965. That same year, Lyle joined the faculty of the College of Optometry of Ontario. Then in 1967, he became one of the first five faculty members in the University of Waterloo School of Optometry, where he taught for many years.

A tribute to William Lyle for his service as the *Optometry and Vision Science* editor noted:

Typically, upon accepting the responsibility or the editorship, Bill Lyle took a series of courses about editing from the American Medical Writers Association and a 6-month leave of absence from his teaching duties so he could put all his time and energy into the task....Throughout his career, as his history reveals, Bill has never hesitated to sacrifice his time, effort, and even his realm, toward consistently elevating his capacity to meet his accepted obligations – toward his own education, toward the profession's status, toward meeting his own sense of responsibilities....To anyone who reviews the publications of the academy as they have matured throughout the years, the development of the Journal during his editorial tenure is obvious – in physical format, in the type of articles published, in its increasing degree of scientific involvement, in circulation, and in the growing coalition of respected investigators.[38]

Editors following William Lyle have included Mark Bullimore, Anthony Adams, and Michael Twa. Throughout its history, the *American Journal of Optometry/ Optometry and Vision Science* has been an outlet for some of American optometry's best writing and research, and it has matured into a leading international journal of clinical optometry and vision science. A cumulative index for volumes 1 through 44 (issues published in 1924 to 1967), compiled by Grace Weiner, was published in 1968, and a second cumulative index for volumes 45 to 60 (1968 to 1983), prepared by Alison Howard and Grace Weiner, was published in 1985. A diskette with an index for volumes 45 to 70 (1968 to 1993), prepared by T. David Williams, was produced in 1994.

JOURNAL OF THE AMERICAN OPTOMETRIC ASSOCIATION / OPTOMETRY

The origins of the *Journal of the American Optometric Association* can be traced to the bulletin titled *The AOA Messenger*, which was first published in 1926.[38] In 1929, the AOA's official publication was the *Organizer*. The first issue of the *Journal of the American Optometric Association* was published in 1930, as volume 2, number 1 in bibliographic continuity with the *Organizer*.

The force behind the beginning of that publication was Minnesota optometrist Ernest H. Kiekenapp.[38,39,40] Kiekenapp became secretary of the AOA in 1922, a position he held for 35 years. He had wanted to start a journal after becoming secretary of the AOA, but due to opposition to the publication of a journal, he had started with the *Messenger*, and the *Organizer*, until he had the support to start a journal.[40] Kiekenapp was editor of the *Messenger* and the *Organizer*, and then served as editor of the *Journal* from its beginning in 1930 until his retirement in 1957. In the early years of the journal, Kiekenapp solicited papers from optometry school faculty members and leading optometrists. He estimated that he wrote over 300 editorials for the AOA publications.[41] Occasionally, he wrote under the pen name of Douglas Lincoln Young because if readers "saw nothing but the name Kiekenapp, they might be scared away."[41]

Kiekenapp graduated in 1912 from the Stone School of Optometry.[41] He practiced optometry until he served with the U.S. Army overseas during World War I. After the war he attended DeMars School of Optometry for a year and then reentered private practice in 1920. In a tribute article after his death, many optometrists were quoted as saying that he was extremely important in the activities and functions of the AOA during his years as secretary.[40] He also was a member of the Minnesota state optometry board and wrote their handbook and directory, and he was a secretary of the International Association of Boards of Examiners in Optometry.[42] He received two honorary degrees from the Northern Illinois College of Optometry and was given the AOA Distinguished Service Award at his retirement.[41,42]

Editors of the AOA's journal after Kiekenapp were Irving Bennett (1957-1964), Charles Margach (1964-1965), M ilton J. Eger (1965-1985), Jimmy D. Bartlett (1985-1990), John W. Potter (1990-1995), John G. Classé (1995-1997), Anthony A. Cavallerano (1997-1999), and Paul B. Freeman (1999-2012).[38,43]

In its first year, the *Journal* published articles based on educational presentations at the annual AOA meeting. Educational articles remained an important component of *Journal* content throughout its history.[38] Topical issues were common starting in the 1950s, with issues devoted to subjects such as contact lenses, pediatric optometry, ocular pharmacology, sports vision, diabetes, and low vision. Starting in 1958, there was an annual contact lens theme issue for over 25 years. In 1978, a journal review board was formed, and subsequently, papers submitted for publication were refereed. In 2000, the title of the journal was changed from *Journal of the American Optometric Association* to simply *Optometry*. In 2003, the AOA boasted that its journal was "the most widely circulated scholarly journal in the world."[44] However, only nine years later, the journal was discontinued. AOA president Dori Carlson cited "the realities of publishing costs and financial priorities" as a major reason for its discontinuance.[45] The last print issue was published in January 2012 (volume 83, number 1). A few more issues were published online with the last online issue being the June 2012 issue (volume 83, number 6).

One indication of the significance of the journals of the AAO and the AOA may be the results of a citation analysis done on the second edition of *Borish's Clinical Refraction*. The most cited optometry journal by a wide margin was *Optometry and Vision Science*, and the second most frequently cited optometry journal was *Optometry*.[46]

In a 2015 editorial in the British optometry journal *Ophthalmic and*

Physiological Optics, Elliott and Handley[47] traced some of the history of optometry journals and noted their importance for education, research, and support of clinical practice. They stated that despite the loss to the profession of the AOA journal's discontinuance, several foreign journals may help to keep the future of optometry journals bright. They mentioned, as examples, the *Canadian Journal of Optometry*, relatively new journals such as the *Journal of Optometry* (2008) from Spain and the *Scandinavian Journal of Optometry and Visual Science* (2008), and the renamed *African Vision and Eye Health* (2015).

SOME SPECIALIZED PERIODICALS

The periodicals examined so far have been general optometry periodicals, and all had started publication by 1930 or much earlier. Later in the twentieth century, some specialized optometric periodicals began, including some American optometric periodicals in contact lenses, vision therapy, optometric education, practice management, and optometry history.

CONTACT LENS JOURNALS

The first contact lens journal was *Contacto*, published from 1957 to about 1999, by the National Eye Research Foundation (originally the Eye Research Foundation).[48] Leonard Bronstein, a well-known contact lens practitioner who served as the first editor of *Contacto*, noted in its inaugural issue that: "the contact lens field is growing to such proportions that it needs an organ of communication."[49] *Contacto* published articles on cornea, contact lenses, orthokeratology, and related topics. It had two temporary title changes, to *Contacto Mini-abstracts* in 1984-1985, and *Global Contacto* in 1991-1992.

Many contact lens manufacturing companies started publishing newsletters and regular informational mailings in the late 1950s and early 1960s. For example, *Precision-Cosmet Digest* was published from 1960 to about 1977.[49]

International Contact Lens Clinic, with more emphasis on research papers, started publication in 1974. The year 1974 is notable in contact lenses because soft contact lenses were beginning to be popular. The first issue of *International Contact Lens Clinic* featured several articles on soft contact lenses, and one of the articles was titled "What should we call gel lenses?"[50] The article noted that they had been called "soft lenses, flexible lenses, hydrophilic lenses, hydroscopic lenses, as well as many generic and trade names." The founding editor of *International Contact Lens Clinic* was Robert B. Mandell, who received his OD from Los Angeles College of Optometry in 1956 and his PhD from Indiana University in 1962. A highly regarded contact lens researcher and educator, Mandell published the first edition of his widely used textbook, *Contact Lens Practice*, in 1965.

In 1985, *International Contact Lens Clinic* merged with *Optometric Monthly* to form *International Eyecare*, which was discontinued at the end of 1986. *International Contact Lens Clinic* resumed publication in 1987 and continued through 2000, when it was absorbed by *Contact Lens and Anterior Eye*, journal of the British Contact Lens Association.

Perhaps the most widely read contact lens periodicals have been *Contact Lens Forum* and *Contact Lens Spectrum*. *Contact Lens Forum* was started in 1976 with Neal J. Bailey as the editor. Bailey received his optometry and PhD degrees from The Ohio State University. He served on the optometry faculty at Indiana University from 1954 to 1958, when he returned to Columbus, Ohio, to start a private practice. He also taught at Ohio State and was a leading authority and writer on contact lenses.[51] *Contact Lens Forum* offered commentaries, reviews, case reports, and news items of interest to contact lens practitioners.

Contact Lens Spectrum published its first issue in January, 1986. Neal

Bailey left *Contact Lens Forum* to become founding editor of *Contact Lens Spectrum*. Of interest to optometric historians, in July 1987, *Contact Lens Spectrum* published a 64-page special issue on the past, present, and future of contact lenses, commemorating the 100th anniversary of contact lenses. In 1991, *Contact Lens Forum* was incorporated into *Contact Lens Spectrum*. Joseph T. Barr, who was editor of *Contact Lens Spectrum* from 1987 to 2007, saw it as providing "the most comprehensive information on contact lenses in a monthly journal."[52]

VISION THERAPY JOURNALS

The College of Optometrists in Vision Development (COVD) has published a journal since its formation about 50 years ago. COVD was formed in 1971 by the merger of three organizations: the National Society for Vision and Perception Training (NSVPT), the National Optometric Society for Developmental Vision Care, and the Southwest Developmental Vision Society. The NSVPT started publishing a journal with the title *Journal of Optometric Vision Therapy* in 1970, and COVD took it over in 1971 with the merger.[53] The name of the journal was changed to *Journal of Optometric Vision Development* in 1975 and then to *Optometry and Vision Development* in 2005, before ceasing after volume 43 in 2012.

The first editor of the journal was Robert M. Wold, who also served COVD in leadership roles for many years. Wold held OD and MS degrees from Pacific University and practiced in California.[54] Following him as editor were Martin Kane (1972-1986), James Bosse (1987-1991), Sidney Groffman (1992-2003), and Dominick Maino (2004-2012). The journal published editorials, research articles, literature reviews, book reviews, and COVD news. Leonard Press[55] noted that its annual reviews of the literature, which it published from 1976 to 2007, were "a highlight of the Journal."

The Optometric Extension Program (OEP), founded in 1928, for many years sent serialized writings in loose-leaf form to its members. These writings, frequently referred to informally as the "OEP papers," were often collected and published in softcover monographs. In the late 1980s, OEP decided to cease publication of the OEP papers and commence publication of a journal.[56] One of the motivations was to improve the standing of OEP in the academic community.[57]

In 1990, OEP launched the bimonthly *Journal of Behavioral Optometry*. The founding editor was Irwin B. Suchoff (1932-2018). Suchoff received a BS from New York University, and after serving in the U.S. Army as a pharmacist technician, he entered optometry school and earned his OD in 1960 from the Massachusetts College of Optometry.[57,58] Suchoff had a long career practicing vision therapy in private practice and serving as a staff member of the Optometric Center of New York and as a faculty member at the State University of New York (SUNY). In the 1980s at SUNY, Suchoff founded the first vision rehabilitation service for head trauma at an optometry school.[59] Suchoff also played a significant role in optometric residencies.[60] He was named Distinguished Service Professor at SUNY and was recipient of the COVD Skeffington Award for contributions to the optometric literature and the COVD Getman Award for work in developmental vision.

Suchoff served as editor of *Journal of Behavioral Optometry* from 1990 to 2007. W. C. Maples was editor from 2008 to 2011 and Marc B. Taub from 2011 to 2012 when it ceased publication after volume 23.

In 2013, OEP, COVD, and the Australasian College of Behavioural Optometrists embarked on a joint venture, the bimonthly peer-reviewed journal, *Optometry and Visual Performance*. It publishes research and clinical articles, case reports, literature reviews, and editorials. Marc Taub and Dominick Maino were initially co-editors, and later in its first year, Taub became sole editor-in-chief.

In 2014, COVD pulled out of the group effort publishing *Optometry and Visual Performance*, after deciding to publish its own journal. In 2015, it started the quarterly online peer-reviewed journal, *Vision Development and Rehabilitation*, which publishes research and clinical papers, case reports, book reviews, and editorials. Leonard J. Press has served as editor since its beginning.

OPTOMETRIC EDUCATION

The first issue of the *Journal of Optometric Education* appeared in Winter 1975, established by the Association of Schools and Colleges of Optometry. The inaugural issue listed a five-person editorial board, with Norman E. Wallis, president of the Pennsylvania College of Optometry, serving as its chairman. Wallis[61] explained that it was time for such a journal because there was a greater need than ever before for discussions of new teaching methodologies, curriculum, and effective administrative structures by faculty, students, and administrators as well as a united picture of optometric education for those outside the profession.

Later in 1975, Chester Pheiffer, then dean of the University of Houston College of Optometry, became chairman of the editorial board, followed by John F. Amos from 1978 to 1985. Subsequent editors have been John W. Potter (1985-1987), David A. Heath (1987-1991), Felix M. Barker (1992-1999), Roger Wilson (1999-2002), Lester E. Janoff (2002-2005), Elizabeth Hoppe (2005-2010), and Aurora Denial (2010-).

The title of the journal changed to *Optometric Education* beginning with volume 17, number 1 (Fall, 1991). The last print issue of *Optometric Education* appeared in Fall 2007, and starting with volume 33, number 2 (Spring 2008), it became available online only.

PRACTICE MANAGEMENT

The first practice management magazine for optometrists appears to have been *Optometric Practice Management*, edited by optometrist John Dickey and, published in October, 1964, but it lasted only one issue.[62] Soon thereafter, Optometric Management magazine started publication in January 1965, published by the company that produced *Dental Management*.

In 1970, Irving Bennett headed a group that purchased *Optometric Management* and turned it into a highly successful publication, which continues to operate.[63] Bennett was publisher and editor from 1970 to 1981. Under his leadership, the magazine included not only timely practice management information for optometrists but also a monthly column for paraoptometric personnel. Jack Runninger was editor from 1981 to 1989, and from 1994 to 2015, he wrote a regular column filled with wit and wisdom called "Lessons Learned."[64,65] From 1998, chief optometric editors have included Arthur B. Epstein, Neil Gailmard, Walter West, and Scot Morris.

OPTOMETRY HISTORY

The Optometric Historical Society was founded in 1969, and the first issue of its quarterly publication appeared in January 1970.[66,67,68,69] The publication had the title *Newsletter of the Optometric Historical Society*, from 1970 to 1991 (volumes 1-22), and then *Hindsight: Newsletter of the Optometric Historical Society*, from 1992 to 2006 (volumes 23-37). Starting in 2007, it was changed to a journal format and the title became *Hindsight: Journal of Optometry History*. Cumulative indexes were published for volumes 1-10, 11-20, 21-30, and 31-40. The first editor was Henry Hofstetter, who continued in that capacity for many years, with John R. Levene occasionally filling in for him in its early years and later Douglas K. Penisten serving as co-editor for several years. David Goss has served as editor since 1995.

In 1989, Hofstetter stated that the Optometric Historical Society's publication was "intended to be a documentary record of every possible detail of optometrically related history, a record to bring together the scattered and piecemeal bits of information that defy gathering otherwise."[70] With the shift to a journal format in 2007, *Hindsight* made a transition to publication of more formal articles than the previous newsletter.

In 1996, Hofstetter quoted an editorial in the February 1994 issue of *Smithsonian* magazine: "It is depressingly clear that we Americans are largely ignorant of our history," and he alleged that "like the *Smithsonian*, *Hindsight*'s role is to try to dispel our depressing ignorance of optometric history."[71] The 196 issues of the *Newsletter of the Optometric Historical Society*, and *Hindsight*, from 1970 through 2018, total more than 3,300 pages, representing a formidable compendium on optometry history.[69]

In 2013, back issues of the *Newsletter* and *Hindsight* were digitized and made available on IUScholarWorks, the digital repository service provided by the Indiana University Libraries. A few years later, *Hindsight: Journal of Optometry History* became one of the IUScholarWorks online journals, with current issues published on their website and print copies produced for Optometric Historical Society members who requested the print copies. The Optometric Historical Society was formed as an independent organization in 1970, but in 2015, the OHS became a program under Optometry Cares, the American Optometric Association Foundation.

Another periodical with content relating to optometry history is *Ophthalmic Antiques*, the publication of the Ophthalmic Antiques International Collectors Club. That organization is centered in the United Kingdom but has an international membership. The first issue was dated September 1982, and through the end of 2020, a total of 153 issues have been produced. Indexes have been published for issues 1-62, 1-85, 86-93, and 94-101.

STATE, REGIONAL, AND OTHER PERIODICALS

Numerous periodicals have been published by state optometric associations, regional optometric groups, optical companies, optometry school alumni organizations, and other entities. Some lasted for only a few issues or had changes in title, while others continued for decades. Notable regional journals, and their years of publication, include the *New England Journal of Optometry* (1949-1995), and the *Southern Journal of Optometry* (1959-1999).[49,72]

SOME SIGNIFICANT FOREIGN OPTOMETRY PERIODICALS

A few months after Frederick Boger started his first optometry periodical in New York in 1891, *The Optician* was started in London, England, to represent optical, scientific, and photographic instrument industries.[48] In 1896, the British Optical Association started publication of *The Dioptric and Ophthalmometric Review*. That periodical was the forerunner of the *British Journal of Physiological Optics*, which in turn was the forerunner of the present-day *Ophthalmic and Physiological Optics*.[48] In 1919, *Commonwealth Optometrist* was published in Australia. It became the *Australasian Journal of Optometry* in 1930, the *Australian Journal of Optometry* in 1959, and then *Clinical and Experimental Optometry* in 1986. The *Canadian Journal of Optometry* started in 1939.

Appendix 3: Notes

1. Hofstetter HW. *Optometry: Professional, Economic, and Legal Aspects*. St. Louis, MO: Mosby, 1948:399-400.
2. Hofstetter HW. Serial publications in the field of visual science. On file, Archives and Museum of Optometry, American Optometric Association.

3   Carlson P. Early ophthalmic English language journals and years of publication (a preliminary list). On file, Archives and Museum of Optometry, American Optometric Association.
4   International Library, Archives, and Museum of Optometry. History of early journals. On file, Archives and Museum of Optometry, American Optometric Association.
5   Ryer EL. From a sixty-year contributor. *Optical J Rev Optom.* 1966;103:111.
6   WorldCat online library catalog. www-worldcat-org.proxyiub.uits.iu.edu/title/keystone-a-monthly-journal-devoted-to-the-interests-of-the-watch-jewelry-and-optical-trades/oclc/2448120&referer=brief_results
7   Johnston JM. The really first optical journal, the "Eye-Echo." *Optical J.* 1909;25:115-117.
8   Hofstetter HW. Earliest exclusive optometric periodical? *Newsletter Optom Hist Soc.* 1978;9:18-19.
9   Hofstetter HW. The Johnston Eye-Echo. *Newsletter Optom Hist Soc.* 1978;9:19.
10 Johnston JM. *Eye Studies: A Series of Lessons on Vision and Visual Tests.* Chicago, IL: J. M. Johnston, 1892.
11 Hofstetter HW. Genealogy of the *Review of Optometry. Newsletter Optom Hist Soc.* 1978;9:20-21.
12 Hofstetter HW. A century ago. *Newsletter Optom Hist Soc.* 1979;22:31.
13 Boger F. Twenty years in optical journaldom. *Optical J.* 1909;25:40-42.
14 Herrin S. Herald of a revolution. *Rev Optom.* 1991;128(1):36-38.
15 The Optician. *Optical J Rev Optom.* 1966;103(2):62-63.
16 Price B. M. E. Cox, Sr., 96, retired publisher. http://articles.pilly.com/1997-03-13/news.
17 Maurice E. Cox retires from "Journal," *Optical J Rev Optom.* 1968;105(24):47.
18 OHS meeting. *Newsletter Optom Hist Soc.* 1985;16:1.
19 Anonymous. Lionel Topaz 1875-1942. *J Am Optom Assoc.* 1942;14:13.
20 Hofstetter HW. The Lionel Topaz Memorial Library. *Newsletter Optom Hist Soc.* 1984;15:36.
21 Newcomb RD. *Our History in Focus: The First 100 Years of The Ohio State University College of Optometry.* Columbus, OH: The Ohio State University, 2014:178-179.
22 Wheelock AP. Lionel Topaz. *Am J Optom Arch Am Acad Optom.* 1942;19:353.
23 To the memory of Lionel Topaz. *Optom Weekly* 1942;33:693, 734-737.
24 Gregg JR. *The Story of Optometry.* New York, NY: Ronald Press, 1965:185-186.
25 Kiekenapp EH. Obituary: Arthur E. Hoare. *J Am Optom Assoc.* 1971;42:1289.
26 Hofstetter HW. Arthur Hoare and oral history. *Newsletter Optom Hist Soc.* 1972;3:5-6.
27 Gregg JR. *Origin and Development of the Southern California College of Optometry, 1904-1984.* Fullerton, CA: Southern California College of Optometry, 1984:436,460,515.

28 Kendall R, Thal L. Optometry's screaming eagles. *California Optometrist* 2003;30(3):13-15; reprinted in *Hindsight* 2003;34:29-38.
29 Gregg JR. *History of the American Academy of Optometry 1922-1986.* Washington, DC: American Academy of Optometry, 1987:156-163.
30 Flom MC. How did our Academy journal start and become preeminent? *Optom Vis Sci.* 2005;82:1011-1013.
31 Leeds JP. Review of the Transactions of the American Academy of Optometry, 1922 to 1939. *Am J Optom Physiol Opt.* 1982;59:735-737.
32 Hirsch MJ, Weiner G. History of the *American Journal of Optometry. Am J Optom Arch Am Acad Optom.* 1968;45:43-57.
33 Peters HB. Dr. Carel C. Koch, November 23, 1896 – November 3, 1973. *Am J Optom Arch Am Acad Optom.* 1973;50:850-852.
34 American Optometric Association. *Directory of the American Optometric Association.* St. Louis, MO: Author, 1972:189.
35 Lyle WM. A time of change. *Optom Vis Sci.* 1996;135-137.
36 Newcomb RD, Eger M. *History of the American Academy of Optometry 1987-2010.* Washington, DC: American Academy of Optometry, 2012:45.
37 Borish IM. Tribute: William M. Lyle, editor. *Optometry and Vision Science,* 1978-1996. *Optom Vis Sci.* 1997;74:70.
38 Christensen JL. History of the *Journal of the American Optometric Association. J Am Optom Assoc.* 1985;56:852-858.
39 A journal interview: the incomparable Ernest Kiekenapp. *J Am Optom Assoc.* 1971;42:166-174.
40 Eger MJ. The passing of a legend. *J Am Optom Assoc.* 1973;44:680-684.
41 Oral history. Interviewee: Ernest H. Kiekenapp; Interviewer: Maria Dablemont. April 25, 1967. www.aoa.org/Documents/ArchivesMuseum/Oral_History/Kiekenapp_Ernest_H1967.pdf
42 American Optometric Association. *Directory of the American Optometric Association.* St. Louis, MO: Author, 1972:183.
43 Cavallerano AA. Editor's perspective: Where are they now (...or objects in the mirror are closer than they appear). *J Am Optom Assoc.* 1997;68:549-550.
44 American Optometric Association. *2003 Member Desk Reference: The Complete Guide to Your AOA.* St. Louis, MO: Author, 2003:42.
45 Carlson D. A message to readers. *J Am Optom Assoc.* 2012;83(1):np.
46 Goss DA. Literature and information in vision care and vision science. *Optom.* 2008;79:670-686.
47 Elliott DB, Handley N. A historical review of optometry research and its publication: Are optometry journals finally catching up? *Ophthal Physiol. Opt* 2015;35:245-251.
48 *IUCAT, Indiana University online library catalog.*
49 Bronstein L. The Eye Research Foundation: Its formation. *Contacto* 1957;1:10.

50 Mandell RB. What should we call gel lenses? *Internat Contact Lens Clin.* 1974;1:25-26.
51 Newcomb RD. *Our History in Focus: The First 100 Years of The Ohio State University College of Optometry.* Columbus, OH: The Ohio State University, 2014:109-110.
52 Barr JT. Happy 10th birthday, *Contact Lens Spectrum. Contact Lens Spectrum* January, 1996. www.clspectrum.com/issues/1996/january-1996.
53 Wold RM. COVD: The first twenty-five years. *J Optom Vis Dev.* 1995;26:177-189.
54 In memoriam: Robert M. Wold. *J Optom Vis Dev.* 2001;32:47-48.
55 Press L. COVD: Recapitulating 40 years of excellence. *Optom Vis Dev.* 2010;41:137-142.
56 Williams RA. Irwin Suchoff. *J Behav Optom.* 2008;19:4-5.
57 American Optometric Association. *Directory of the American Optometric Association.* St. Louis, MO: Author, 1972:343.
58 Haffner AN. Irwin Suchoff, OD, DOS. *J Behav Optom.* 2008;19:3.
59 Press LJ. In memoriam: Dr. Irwin Suchoff. *Vis Dev Rehab.* 2018;4:4-5.
60 Suchoff I. The first year-long optometric residency education program. *Hindsight* 2010;41:122-125.
61 Wallis NE. Why a journal. *J Optom Ed.* 1975;1:5.
62 Hofstetter HW. Almost simultaneous. *Hindsight* 1998;29:2.
63 Bennett I. The story behind *Optometric Management* magazine. *Hindsight* 2007;38:17-22.
64 From the Editor's desk: *Optometric Management*'s editors created the leading practice management publication. *Optom Management* 2015;50(Sept. 1):24-26,28.
65 Runninger J. 50th anniversary: Lessons learned – lessons to live by. *Optom Management.* 2015;50(Sept. 1):32.
66 Bennett I. The year that OHS began: Optometry in 1969. *Hindsight* 2019;50:13-16.
67 Myers RI. The origins of the Optometric Historical Society: A first-person account of OHS founders and contemporary events. *Hindsight* 2019;50:19-21.
68 Goss DA. 20/20 *Hindsight*: A history of the Optometric Historical Society chronicled in its newsletter and journal. *Hindsight* 2019;50:4-12.
69 Goss DA. OHS co-founder Henry W Hofstetter (1914-2002). *Hindsight* 2019;50:29-34.
70 Hofstetter HW. By way of explanation. *Newsletter Optom Hist Soc.* 1989;20:29-30.
71 Hofstetter HW. The OHS mission. *Hindsight* 1996;27:17-18.
72 Hébert K. Rare ophthalmic periodicals: The historiography of the profession at risk. *Hindsight* 2018;49:57-61.

Appendix 4
Notes on the History of Optometry Books

Optometry books are also a good source of information, not only on optometric practice but on its history. The first book which can be identified as encompassing the field of optometry at its time is the book by Daza de Valdes, published in Spain in 1623 and discussed in Chapter 1. There were several books in the late eighteenth century and into the nineteenth century, especially by English authors, on spectacles and vision that seem to have been written for the general public but which also could be used by those aspiring to provide optometric services. A prominent example is *An Essay on Vision* by George Adams Jr. (first edition, 1789), which presented information on the structure of the eye and the basic nature of vision and vision conditions with emphasis on the proper use and choice of spectacles for the "long-sighted" and the "short-sighted."[1] Other examples are *The Economy of the Eyes* by William Kitchener (1824-25), *A Treatise on the Nature of Vision, Formation of the Eye, and the Causes of Imperfect Vision* by Alexander Alexander (1833), and *How to Use our Eyes and How to Preserve Them by the Use of Spectacles* by John Browning (1883).[2] An example of a similar book by an American author is *The Human Eye, Its Use and Abuse* by Walter Alden (1866).

EARLY GENERAL OPTOMETRY AND REFRACTION BOOKS

What we might consider the first textbook written for optometrists by an American optometrist is *Handbook for Opticians* by William Bohne,[3] first published in 1888, with subsequent editions in 1892 and 1895. The title reflects the fact that the term *optometrist* was not yet in common usage. Similar American books appeared at about the same time, but they were designed, in part, to advertise their optical companies and were not as comprehensive as Bohne's book. The most notable of these was *How to Fit Glasses*, published in 1888 by the James Queen Company.[4] Bohne's third edition (1895) included theoretical background to go with the practical information on ophthalmic optics, refractive errors, and accommodation, along with consideration of a variety of other topics, including ocular anatomy, the ophthalmoscope, cataracts, emergency care for eye injuries, light sources, tears, and optical/optometric history.

Among the most important books in optometry in the early twentieth century were the instructional manuals by George A. Rogers and Robert M. Lockwood, who both had been educators before turning to optometry as a career. Both later spent some time on the faculty of the Northern Illinois College of Ophthalmology and Otology.[5] Rogers published two of the earliest books on retinoscopy (also known earlier as skiascopy, skiametry, or the shadow test), *Skiascopy: A Treatise on the Shadow Test in Its Practical Application to the Work of Refraction* (1899) and *The Shadow Test in Ocular Diagnosis* (1905). Rogers later wrote two books on optics, *Handbook of Fundamental Optics* (1915) and *Lenses and Mirrors* (1918), and a book on *The Muscles of the Eye* (1922). Lockwood's books, which were mostly published in a small 17 cm format and typically sold for 25 to 50 cents, were praised for being "so simply and clearly written that they have proven a delight to thousands of readers."[6] Among his books were *The Principles of Optometry* (1903), *The Trial Case and How to Use It* (1904), *Subjective Tests for Difficult Cases* (1904), *Frames and Lenses* (1905), *Skiascopy without the Use of Drugs* (1906), and *Transpositions: A Practical Treatise for Optometrists and Opticians* (1907).

In addition to the works by Rogers and Lockwood, other early books on retinoscopy included *A System of Ocular Skiametry* (1903) and *Dynamic Skiametry in Theory and Practice* (1911) by Andrew Jay Cross and *Dynamic Skiametry and Methods of Testing the Accommodation and Convergence of the Eyes* (1920) by Charles Sheard. Cross is credited with doing the most to popularize dynamic retinoscopy, and it was in Sheard's *Dynamic Skiametry* book that Sheard coined the term "lag of accommodation."[7]

Other important books in the first decades of the twentieth century were those by Lionel Laurance and Christian Henry Brown. Laurance was born in England and taught optometry in Canada and England.[8] His best books were *General and Practical Optics* (first edition, 1908) and especially *Visual Optics and Sight Testing* (first edition, 1912). *Visual Optics and Sight Testing* covered ocular anatomy, ocular optics, sensory aspects of vision, visual acuity, subjective testing, nature and management of refractive errors, phorias, strabismus, presbyopia, color vision, ophthalmic optics, keratometry, retinoscopy, ophthalmoscopy, retinal imagery, and spectacle frames. It was widely used throughout the world. Christian Henry Brown, an oculist, was co-founder of the Philadelphia Optical College in 1889 and its president until his death in 1933.[9] Brown's best-known book for optometrists was *The Optician's Manual*, a comprehensive textbook of practical optometry at the time. It was first issued in one volume in 1897, with later editions in two volumes starting in 1902. The 1921 edition had minimal changes in text from the previous edition, except that the title was changed to *The Optometrist's Manual*, and the term *optometrist* replaced the term *optician* throughout the text, reflecting the change in preferred terminology.

GEOMETRICAL AND VISUAL OPTICS

An optics book that should be mentioned is *Ophthalmic Lenses, Dioptric Formulae for Combined Cylindrical Lenses, The Prism Dioptry and Other Optical Papers* by Charles Prentice (first edition, 1900). It is a collection of his original papers and optical writings. Included are papers in which he described his concept of what we now call the *prism diopter* and how to calculate the prismatic effect of decentering lenses, now known as *Prentice's Rule*. He also described a tangent screen test for dissociated phorias, essentially the test that is now often referred to as the *modified Thorington test*. An important early twentieth century optics textbook was *Mirrors, Prisms, and Lenses* by James P. C. Southall (first edition, 1918). Southall was a physics professor at Columbia University and was director of the optometry school there for more than 25 years.[10]

Optics books by English authors that were widely used in optometry were *Optics* by W. H. A. Fincham (first edition, 1934); *Visual Optics* by H. H. Emsley (first edition, 1936); and *Clinical Visual Optics* by Arthur G. Bennett and Ronald B. Rabbetts (first edition, 1984), each of which continued through several editions. Other optics books written for optometrists include *Geometrical Optics* by Glenn Fry (1969); *Optics in Vision* by Henri Obstfeld (first edition, 1978); *Geometrical, Physical, and Visual Optics* by Michael P. Keating (first edition, 1988); *Optics of the Human Eye* by David A. Atchison and George Smith (2000); *Geometrical and Visual Optics* by Steven H. Schwartz (first edition, 2002); and *Introduction to the Optics of the Eye* by David A. Goss and Roger W. West (2002).

PHYSIOLOGICAL OPTICS/VISION SCIENCE

Following the lead of Hermann von Helmholtz's famous *Treatise on Physiological Optics*, the term *physiological optics* was considered synonymous with *vision science* for much of the twentieth century. Comprehensive physiological optics/vision science books included *Physiological Optics* by Charles Sheard (1918), *Physiological Optics* by W. D. Zoethout (first edition, 1927), and *Introduction to Physiological Optics* by Southall (1937). Among more recent vision science books by optometrists are *Visual Perception: A Clinical Orientation* by Steven H. Schwartz (1994) and *The Psychophysical Measurement of Visual Function*, edited by Thomas T. Norton, David A. Corliss, and James E. Bailey (2002).

EXAMINATION ROUTINE

In 1917, Charles Sheard published *Dynamic Ocular Tests*, in which he outlined his systematic optometric examination routine of 18 tests. The evolution of the Optometric Extension Program (OEP) 21-point examination, similar to Sheard's 18-test exam and discussed previously in Chapter 5, can be traced through A. M. Skeffington's *Procedure in Ocular Examination* (1928) and *Differential Diagnosis in Ocular Examination* (1931); and Sol K. Lesser's *Fundamentals of Procedures and Analysis in Optometric Examination* (first edition, 1933). Blur points were added to fusional vergence range tests, as advocated by Louis Jaques and George Crow in their 1934 book, *Applied Refraction with Special Reference to the Blur-out Point Technique*. Although the complete OEP 21-point examination routine and its analysis was published in many editions of a little soft-cover pocket-sized book, *Introduction to Modern Analytical Optometry* by S. K. Lesser (first edition, 1935), perhaps the first comprehensive text on it was the 1965 third edition of *Visual Analysis* by Leo Manas (first edition, 1958).

OPTOMETRY DICTIONARIES

Optometry dictionaries have served important roles as educational and reference tools. *Pocket Optical Dictionary* by James John Lewis was a small book that could fit into a shirt pocket. The year the first edition was published is uncertain, but the second edition appeared in 1907, and it continued to a ninth edition in 1946. A larger dictionary was *Oculo-Refractive Cyclopedia and Dictionary* by Thomas Atkinson (first edition, 1921). Atkinson was a doctor of medicine who served on the Northern Illinois College of Optometry faculty and wrote several other books for optometrists.[11] The first edition of *Dictionary of Visual Science* was published in 1960, with Max Schapero, David Cline, and Henry Hofstetter as editors, and its fifth edition appeared in 2000 with Henry Hofstetter, John R. Griffin, Morris Berman, and Ronald Everson as editors. Another dictionary is *Dictionary of Optometry* by Michel Millodot (first edition, 1986).

STATE OF THE OPTOMETRIC PROFESSION

In 1921, Eugene Wiseman published *Building Optometry*, in which he emphasized the importance of practicing professionally and having a good knowledge base. He discussed how to establish a professional practice, construction of the examination room, fees, optometric organizations, and the impact of optometric care.[12] E. E. Arrington published *History of Optometry* in 1929, examining not only optometry history but also then-current aspects of optometry, such as practice laws, state board examinations, optometric education, optometric procedures, organizations, and motorists' vision.

Optometry: Professional, Economic, and Legal Aspects was published by Henry Hofstetter in 1948. It contained information and data on a wide range of topics encompassing historical background, licensure, legal status, education, types and scope of practice, distribution and earnings of optometrists, and other matters relating to the practice of optometry.

In 1965, James R. Gregg published *The Story of Optometry*, an account of the history and current status of optometry. A contemporary review assessed it as "intended for the lay reader" but said that "optometrists should enjoy reading and owning this book."[13] A similar book, published in 1968, but with more emphasis on the functioning of an optometric practice and apparently more geared for an optometric audience was *The Optometric Profession* by Monroe J. Hirsch and Ralph E. Wick.[14]

VISION THERAPY

The book that we can identify as the first book on optometric vision therapy is *The Modern Treatment of Ocular Imbalances* by R.M. Peckham (1926).[15] Peckham's second edition was published in 1928, with the word *Ocular* in the title changed to *Binocular*. In the 1930s, T. J. Arneson published *The New Optometry: A New Technique for the Diagnosis and Treatment of Muscular Imbalances* (1932), and Louis Jaques published *Fundamental Refraction and Orthoptics* (1936). The 1950s saw the publication of *Corrective and Preventive Optometry* by Louis Jaques (1950); *Clinical Orthoptic Procedure* by William Smith (1950); and *Basic Orthoptics and Reconditioning* by George Crow and H. L. Fuog (1952).

More recent books on vison therapy procedures include *Binocular Anomalies* by John R. Griffin (first edition, 1976), *Vision Therapy in a Primary Care Practice* by Jerome Rosner and Joy Rosner (1988), *Applied Concepts in Vision Therapy* edited by Leonard J. Press (1997), and *Vision Rehabilitation: Multidisciplinary Care of the Patient Following Brain Injury* edited by Penelope S. Suter and Lisa H. Harvey (2011).

CONTACT LENSES

The first textbooks on contact lenses appear to have been *Contact Lens Technique* by L. L. Beacher (1941), *The Practice of Fitting Contact Lenses* by William Feinbloom (1942), and *Contact Lenses* by Theo. E. Obrig (1942), all of which dealt with scleral lenses. The advent of corneal lenses led to the appearance of many new books, including *Contact Lens Practice* by Newton K. Wesley and George N. Jessen (1953); *Corneal Contact Lenses* by William R. Baldwin and Charles R. Shick (1962); *Contact Lens Theory and Practice* by Theodore Grosvenor (1963); *Contact Lens Practice and Patient Management* by Irving P. Filderman and Paul E. White (1969); *Biomicroscopy for Contact Lens Practice* by Joe B. Goldberg (1970); *Contemporary Contact Lens Practice* by Theodore Grosvenor (1972); and *Rigid Gas-Permeable Contact Lenses* by Edward S. Bennett and Robert M. Grohe (1986). The online catalog for the Indiana University Libraries lists over 150 books published on the subject of contact lenses between 1980 and 2018.

Probably the most notable contact lens book is *Contact Lens Practice* by Robert B. Mandell, with a 471-page first edition published in 1965, and with each subsequent edition adding the latest developments, expanding to the 1,025-page fourth edition, published in 1988. A review of the fourth edition rated it "the definitive contact lens textbook" and said that it "represents a good balance between the scientific foundations of contact lens wear and clinical practice."[16]

PRACTICE MANAGEMENT

In 1941, E. LeRoy Ryer and Elmer E. Hotaling published *Optometric Procedure*. The book's purpose, as stated in the preface, was to set forth "the principles which it is believed should underlie the establishment and conduct of optometric practice." They stressed ethical professional practice, strong knowledge, a good professional library, an orderly complete examination, and paying as much attention to nearpoint function as to distance visual acuity. They discussed office floor plan, furnishings, and equipment, and gave examples of forms for appointment cards, billing, recall notices, and other communications.

How to Succeed in Optometry was published in 1948 by Ralph Barstow, who had a long career as an optometry practice management advisor after a background in business.[17] Barstow wrote about the nature of professional practice and how to achieve it, detailing how to start a practice; analyze a community; lay out and equip an office; determine and present fees; set up appointment, billing, and bookkeeping systems; establish a patient base; and other elements of practice management.

In 1963, *Optometric Practice Management* was published by California optometrist George P. Elmstrom. It contained information and data on distribution of optometrists and the U.S. population, locating and purchasing a practice, selecting and managing assistants, relations with patients and other professionals, optometric economics, collecting fees, and other aspects of administering a practice. It also had more than 50 photographs of the exteriors and interiors of several optometry practices. Subsequent practice management books have included *Rx for Success: Optometric Management* by Bob L. Baldwin, Bobby Christensen, and Jack W. Melton (1983); *The Koetting Touch: Optimum Management for the Progressive Practice* by R. A. Koetting (1985); *Management for the Eyecare Practitioner* by Irving Bennett (1993); and *Business Aspects of Optometry* by John G. Classé, Craig Hisaka, Donald H. Lakin, Ronald S. Rounds, and Lawrence S. Thal (first edition, 1997).

DEVELOPMENTAL VISION AND THE RELATION OF VISION AND LEARNING

A significant factor in the increased interest among optometrists, in the mid-twentieth century in this area of visual function was the publication of Darell Boyd Harmon's book, *Notes on a Dynamic Theory of Vision* in 1954. Harmon, who held a PhD in Experimental Education and did studies of the school performance of elementary school students, advocated proper viewing distance, posture, and lighting during reading, and optimal vision care to help children perform well in school.

Also important in this area was the work of optometrist Gerald Getman, whose book, *How to Develop Your Child's Intelligence*, was first produced in mimeograph form in the 1950s. An eighth edition was published in 1974 in soft cover. It was written for parents and discussed the importance of vision in learning, described developmental processes in childhood, and presented exercises for the development of basic movement skills, eye movements, vision-language relationships, and visualization. *Preschool Vision* by Richard J. Apell and Ray W. Lowry, Jr. (1959) was another influential book.

Books written in the 1990s in this area for optometrists include *Developmental and Perceptual Assessment of Learning-Disabled Children* by Sidney Groffman and Harold Solan (1994); *Optometric Management of Learning-Related Vision Problems* by Mitchell M. Scheiman and Michael W. Rouse (first edition, 1994); and *Optometric Management of Reading Dysfunction* by John R. Griffin, Garth N. Christenson, Michael D. Wesson, and Graham B. Erickson (1997).

ENVIRONMENTAL VISION AND PUBLIC HEALTH

In 1956, Henry Hofstetter published *Industrial Vision*, which offered information on industrial eye hazards and protection, vision testing for industrial settings, the relation of vision to industrial efficiency, and compensation for loss of vision in industry. *Guide to Occupational and Other Visual Needs* by Clark Holmes, Harry Jolliffe, James Gregg, Ian S. Cameron, and Robert Blyth (1958) analyzed visual requirements of many occupations. *Vision Screening for Elementary Schools: The Orinda Study* by Henrik L. Blum, Jerome W. Bettman, and Henry B. Peters (1959) helped to establish standards for vision screening. *Vision and Highway Safety* by Merrill J. Allen (1970) provided a comprehensive analysis of motorists' vision.

Several books have been written by optometrists on sports vision. Among them are *Vision and Sports: An Introduction* by James R. Gregg (1987); *Sports Vision* (volume 3, number 1 in the *Optometry Clinics* series), edited by John G. Classé (1993); and *Sports Vision: Vision Care for the Enhancement of Sports Performance* by Graham Erickson (2007).

A landmark in optometry's involvement in public health was the publication in 1980 of *Public Health and Community Optometry*, edited by Robert D. Newcomb and Jerry L. Jolley. A second edition, edited by Robert Newcomb and Edwin C. Marshall, appeared in 1990. *Ophthalmic Research and Epidemiology* by Stanley W. Hatch (1998) outlined the design of clinical research and public health applications.

A comprehensive examination of the topic of environmental vision is *Environmental Vision: Interactions of the Eye, Vision, and the Environment*, edited by Donald G. Pitts and Robert N. Kleinstein (1993). A guide for vision care for computer use, *Diagnosing and Treating Computer-Related Vision Problems*, was published by James E. Sheedy and Peter G. Shaw-McMinn in 2003.

PEDIATRIC AND GERIATRIC OPTOMETRY

The first widely used books with broad ranging coverage of pediatric and geriatric optometry appear to be those edited by Monroe J. Hirsch and Ralph E. Wick, *Vision of the Aging Patient* (1960) and *Vision of Children* (1963). Both of them featured chapters by well-known contributing authors on developmental/anatomical changes, psychological aspects, visual acuity, refractive changes, binocular vision, ocular disease, low vision, fitting and adjusting of spectacles, contact lenses, suggested further readings, and other age-appropriate matters.

Alfred A. Rosenbloom and Meredith Morgan contributed chapters for both of Hirsch and Wick's books, and some 25 years later, they recognized the need for updated and expanded books. With the help of more than 25 contributing authors on each of the books, they edited *Vision and Aging: General and Clinical Perspectives* (first edition, 1986) and *Principles and Practice of Pediatric Optometry* (1990). Other pediatric textbooks include *Pediatric Optometry* by Jerome Rosner (first edition, 1982) and *Clinical Pediatric Optometry* by Leonard J. Press and Bruce D. Moore (1993).

OPHTHALMIC OPTICS AND DISPENSING

In 1966, Margaret Dowaliby published *Fundamentals of Cosmetic Dispensing*. It discussed spectacle frame design and factors of importance in choosing shape, color, and size of spectacle frames. Dowaliby also wrote *Practical Aspects of Ophthalmic Optics* (first edition, 1972), which compiled information on the basic optics of spectacle lenses and on ophthalmic lens types and features, such as multifocal lens designs, plastic lenses, lens coatings, absorptive lenses, safety lenses, and other matters.

In 1979, *System for Ophthalmic Dispensing* by Clifford W. Brooks and Irvin M. Borish came out in its first edition. It contained the essentials of clinical ophthalmic optics and comprehensive coverage of frame selection and dispensing, including a remarkably extensive series of photographs of frame alignment, adjustment, and repair. A third edition of this popular textbook came out in 2007.

Clinical Optics by Troy E. Fannin and Theodore Grosvenor (first edition, 1987) contained more detail on spectacle lens optics than the Dowaliby book and the Brooks and Borish book. *Clinical Optics* looked at lens materials and physical characteristics, power measurement, prisms and decentration, correction of refractive error, aberrations, lens design, absorptive lenses and coatings, multifocal lenses, spectacle frames, anisometropia and aniseikonia, lenses for high refractive errors and for low vision, and optics of contact lenses.

LOW VISION

Among the textbooks written by optometrists for this important specialty area of optometry practice are *Low Vision Care* by Edwin B. Mehr and Allan N. Freid (1975), *The Art and Practice of Low Vision* by Paul B. Freeman and Randall T. Jose (first edition, 1991), *Primary Low Vision Care* by Rodney W. Nowakowski (1994), and *Essentials of Low Vision Practice* by Richard L. Brilliant (1999).

MORE GENERAL OPTOMETRY AND REFRACTION BOOKS

Earlier in this appendix, there was discussion of some general optometry and refraction books up through the 1920s. Later came the classic books by Irvin M. Borish. His first book, *Outline of Optometry* (1938), had 15 chapters on lenses and prisms, refractive errors, phorometry, retinoscopy, dynamic retinoscopy, and ophthalmometry, with additional chapters on ophthalmoscopy, external examination, perimetry, prescription bifocals, tinted lenses, and strabismus. The first edition of his *Clinical Refraction* was published in 1949, and a second edition appeared in 1954. For the third edition (1970), Borish enlisted the help of 19 collaborators, and it expanded to 1,381 pages. Each of the three editions was organized into five sections: I. Refractive Status of the Eye (including accommodation, presbyopia, and eye movements), II. Preliminary Examination, III. Refraction (including phorometry and dynamic retinoscopy), IV. Analysis and Prescription (including ophthalmic optics), and V. Monocularity and Strabismus. Twenty-eight years after the publication of the third edition of *Clinical Refraction*, the first edition of a new and completely rewritten book, *Borish's Clinical Refraction*, appeared under the editorship of William J. Benjamin. Borish was a consultant and one of the 46 authors for the new book. A second edition of *Borish's Clinical Refraction* came out in 2006.

Another classic general optometry textbook is *Primary Care Optometry* by Theodore Grosvenor (first edition, 1982). Material from his 1975 to 1981 column in *Optometric Weekly* and *Optometric Monthly* was used as the basis for chapters.[18,19] Grosvenor saw the concept of primary care optometry as representing the entry point into the vision care system, and he noted that optometry has always traditionally served that role. Grosvenor regularly produced new editions of *Primary Care Optometry*, culminating in the publication of the fifth edition in 2007, 25 years after the first edition came out. All five editions were organized in three parts: the first part providing background information on anomalies of refraction and binocular vision, and epidemiology of ametropia; the second part detailing optometric examination procedures; and the third part examining the diagnosis and management of anomalies of refraction and binocular vision.

When considering detailed vision analysis books, *The Principles and Practice of Refraction* by English optometrist George H. Giles should also be mentioned. The first edition was published in 1960 and the second in 1965. A review of the second edition said that "although the instruments illustrated by Giles, being of British manufacture, will often seem strange to American optometrists, this book will be a valued addition to our bookshelves."[22]

Diagnosis and Management in Vision Care, edited by John F. Amos (1987), is an informative, well-organized book containing chapters on 20 different vision conditions, with chapters divided into definition, classification, epidemiology, etiology, signs and symptoms, examination and diagnosis, course and prognosis, clinical management, and clinical summary. *Refractive Anomalies: Research and Clinical Applications*, edited by Theodore Grosvenor and Merton C. Flom (1991), summarized research on epidemiology, etiology, clinical course, and clinical management of refractive conditions. *Refractive Management of Ametropia*, edited by Kenneth E. Brookman (1996), featured information on diagnosis and management of refractive conditions. *Clinical Pearls in Refractive Care* by D. Leonard Werner and Leonard J. Press (2002) discusses aspects of conventional optometric wisdom and lessons learned from practice experience.

A number of monographs have been published on myopia, including treatises on possible etiologies and conference proceedings.[20] Among the books on myopia by optometrists are *Accommodation, Nearwork and Myopia* by Editha Ong and Kenneth J. Ciuffreda (1997); *Myopia and Nearwork*, edited by Mark Rosenfield and Bernard Gilmartin (1998); and *Clinical Management of Myopia* by Theodore Grosvenor and David Goss (1999).

Clinical Procedures in Optometry, edited by J. Boyd Eskridge, John F. Amos, and Jimmy D. Bartlett (1991), is an outstanding book, explaining the clinical use, available instrumentation, clinical procedure, and clinical implications of a wide range of refractive, ocular disease, pediatric, binocular vision, and low vision testing procedures in 84 chapters. Evidence of its wide usage comes from a citation analysis, which found it to be the most frequently cited book in the 2006 second edition of *Borish's Clinical Refraction*.[21]

Other texts on general optometry testing procedures include *Optometry*, edited by Keith Edwards and Richard Llewellyn (1988); *Clinical Procedures for Ocular Examination* by Nancy B. Carlson, Daniel Kurtz, David A. Heath, and Catherine Hines (first edition, 1990); and *The Ocular Examination: Measurements and Findings*, edited by Karla Zadnik (1997).

BINOCULAR VISION AND OCULAR MOTILITY

Some books with significant amounts of binocular vision content have been discussed earlier in this chapter in the General Optometry and Refraction sections and in the Examination Routine section. Other important binocular vision and ocular motility books by optometrists have been published since the 1970s.

Books summarizing research and clinical applications include *Vergence Eye Movements: Basic and Clinical Aspects*, edited by Clifton M. Schor and Kenneth J. Ciuffreda (1983); *Binocular Vision: Foundations and Applications* by Rogers W. Reading (1983); *Eye Movement Basics for the Clinician* by Kenneth J. Ciuffreda and Barry Tannen (1995); and *Foundations of Binocular Vision: A Clinical Perspective* by Scott B. Steinman, Barbara A. Steinman, and Ralph P. Garzia (2000).

Two outstanding books on diagnosis and management of binocular vision disorders are *Clinical Management of Binocular Vision: Heterophoric, Accommodative, and Eye Movement Disorders* by Mitchell Scheiman and Bruce Wick (first edition, 1994) and *Anomalies of Binocular Vision: Diagnosis and Management* by Robert P. Rutstein and Kent M. Daum (1998). The Rutstein and Daum book includes material on strabismus, while the Scheiman and Wick book does not. Scheiman and Wick explain vision therapy procedures in much more detail than the Rutstein and Daum book. A book by a British author on clinical testing and treatment is *Binocular Vision Anomalies* by David Pickwell (first edition, 1984).

My own entry in this area is *Ocular Accommodation, Convergence, and Fixation Disparity* (first edition, 1986), which I published after being tasked with teaching a course on the "graphical analysis" system of clinical accommodation and convergence case analysis, and realizing that there was no textbook available on the topic. The book covers the procedures for graphical display of clinical accommodation and convergence data and its attendant theoretical and patient management considerations, along with fixation disparity, normative analysis, and accommodative disorders.

One of my favorite books is *Optometric Management of Nearpoint Vision Disorders* by Martin H. Birnbaum (1993), and my assessment was echoed by a reviewer who declared it to be "a very thoughtful, comprehensive and generally successful text which analyzes the various theories and clinical approaches for optometric management of vision problems related to near visual task demands."[23] Birnbaum's firm advocacy for careful and complete evaluation of accommodation and convergence function can be seen in his statement in the book:

> Patients who present with impaired accommodative and binocular findings, but without asthenopia, are generally asymptomatic either because they have developed myopia or because they avoid reading. When asthenopia is absent, many practitioners assume that existing visual problems are insignificant and do not require treatment. Recognition that patients with functional vision disorder may be asymptomatic because they avoid or adapt leads the clinician to consider treatment in such cases, to eliminate the need for continued avoidance or further development of adaptive vision disorders.[24]

Some of the books discussed previously in this chapter have significant coverage of strabismus and amblyopia, such as *Binocular Anomalies* by Griffin and *Applied Concepts in Vision Therapy*, edited by Leonard J. Press.

Additional books on strabismus and amblyopia by optometrists include *Amblyopia* by Max Schapero (1971); *Amblyopia: Basic and Clinical Aspects* by Kenneth J. Ciuffreda, Dennis M. Levi, and Arkady Selenow (1991); and *Clinical Management of Strabismus* by Elizabeth E. Caloroso and Michael W. Rouse (1993).

OCULAR DISEASE AND PHARMACOLOGY

For many years, optometrists learned ocular disease mostly from books written by ophthalmologists for ophthalmologists. Some of the first ocular disease books written for optometrists were *Diseases of the Eye and How Recognized*, by C.W. Talbot (1910), and *Optometrist's Handbook of Eye Diseases*, by Joseph Pascal and Harold G. Noyes (1954). Talbot was an eye, ear, nose, and throat surgeon who was president of the Washington School of Optometry. Pascal was trained as both an optometrist and an ophthalmologist, and wrote other books, including *Modern Retinoscopy* (1930), and *Studies in Visual Optics* (1952).[11] Noyes was an ophthalmologist.

A Treatise on Blood Pressure in Ocular Work (1916), and *Ocular Symptomatology* (1924), were works by optometrist Eugene Wiseman, who was ahead of his time in addressing some matters relating to recognition of ocular and systemic disease. The first book on visual fields by an optometrist appears to have been *Visual Fields* (1936), by Theodore Brombach.[25] The first books on glaucoma by optometrists may have been *Synopsis of Glaucoma for Optometrists* (1959), by Arthur Shlaifer; and *Tonometry and Glaucoma Detection* (1969), by Jesse Rosenthal and D. Leonard Werner.

As optometrists became more involved in the diagnosis and management of ocular disease, the 1980s and 1990s saw the publication of the first editions of some significant books by optometrists on ocular disease and pharmacology. These include *Genetics for the Primary Eye Care Practitioner*, by Helene V. Fatt and John R. Griffin (1983); *Ocular*

Disease: Detection, Diagnosis, and Treatment, edited by Jack E. Terry (1984); *Ocular Assessment*, edited by Barry J. Barresi (1984); *Clinical Ocular Pharmacology*, edited by Jimmy D. Bartlett and Siret D. Jaanus (1984); *Primary Care of the Anterior Segment*, by Louis J. Catania (1988); *Primary Care of the Posterior Segment*, by Larry J. Alexander (1989); *Atlas of Primary Eyecare Procedures*, by Murray Fingeret, Linda Casser, and H. Ted Woodcome (1990); *Optometric Guide to Surgical Co-Management*, by Debra J. Bezan, Kathy Halverson, Kathleen Schaffer, and Pam Thomas (1992); and *Differential Diagnosis in Primary Eye Care*, by Debra J. Bezan, Frank P. LaRussa, John H. Nishimoto, David P. Sendrowski, Carl H. Spear, David K. Talley, and Tammy P. Than (1999).

MISCELLANEOUS

Some other books of note by optometrists are *Legalized Optometry and Memoirs of the Founder*, by Charles F. Prentice (1926); *My Fifty Years in Optometry*, by Albert Fitch (1955-59); *Optometric Instrumentation*, by David B. Henson (first edition, 1983); and *Computer Applications in Optometry*, by Joseph H. Maino, Dominick M. Maino, and David W. Davidson (1989). Various publishers have produced series of books. From 1959 to 1970, the American Academy of Optometry published a series of monographs with titles on glaucoma (by Shlaifer, mentioned earlier), contact lens fitting, optometric jurisprudence, legal aspects of contact lens practice, refractive state of the eye, and health science terminology. Chilton published its Principles of Optometry series in the 1960s. That series included *The Optometric Profession*, by Hirsch and Wick, and *Geometrical Optics*, by Glenn Fry.

Lippincott published its *Problems in Optometry* series of books with Richard London as series editor, beginning in 1989, with a book on *Ocular Emergencies*, and ending with the book *Ocular Vertical and Cyclovertical*

Deviations, in 1992. *Mosby's Optometric Problem-Solving Series* was a series of books published from 1995 to 1997, also with Richard London as series editor. Included in that series were books on special populations, low vision, prescription of prism, contact lenses, neurological disease, and geriatric optometry.

As we examine optometry books, we can identify publishers that seemed to have made a specialty of producing optometry books. Among them were Frederick Boger and Keystone in the early twentieth century, Professional Press extending from the 1920s to the 1980s, Chilton in the mid twentieth century, and Butterworth-Heinemann, which absorbed Professional Press, in the later twentieth century.

The longest continuing still-active publisher of optometry books appears to be the Optometric Extension Program (OEP), which has produced books since the 1930s, on a variety of topics centered on visual performance, binocular vision, vision-related learning problems, visual perception, vision development, and vision therapy. A list of some of the notable and most used of the numerous books published by OEP could include: *Practical Applied Optometry*, by A.M. Skeffington (1951-58, re-issued 1991); *Introduction to Clinical Optometry*, by A.M. Skeffington (first edition, 1964); *Optometric Case Analysis*, by Leonard C. Emery (first edition, 1968); *Strabismus and Amblyopia*, by Donald J. Getz (first edition, 1974); *The Full Scope of Retinoscopy*, by C laude A. Valenti (first edition, 1983); *Developmental Optometry*, by Gerald Getman (first edition, 1987); *Stress and Vision*, by Elliott B. Forrest (1988); *Computers and Vision Therapy*, by Leonard J. Press (1992); *NSUCO Oculomotor Test*, by W.C. Maples (1995); *Developing the Dynamic Vision Therapy Practice*, edited by Willard B. Bleything (1998); *Visual and Vestibular Consequences of Acquired Brain Injury*, edited by Irwin J. Suchoff, Kenneth J. Ciuffreda, and Neera Kapoor (2001); *Lens Power in Action*, by Robert A. Kraskin and edited by Paul A. Harris and Gregory Kitchener (2003); *Parallels Between Auditory and Visual Processing*, by Leonard J. Press (2012); and *Neuro-Visual Processing Rehabilitation*, by William V. Padula, Raquel Munitz, and W. Michael Magrun (2012).

There are undoubtedly many significant optometry books that have been inadvertently overlooked. For those seeking more information on the history of optometry books than the brief survey in this appendix, there are additional references that can be consulted.[26,27,28,29,30,31,32,33]

Appendix 4: Notes

1. Goss DA. George Adams Junior and his 1789 book *An Essay on Vision*. Hindsight 2009;40:63-68.
2. Goss DA. Nineteenth-century English optician John Browning and his book *How to Use Our Eyes*. Hindsight 2009;40:132-135.
3. Goss DA. William Bohne (1827-1906), Author of *Handbook for Opticians*, first textbook by an American optometrist. Hindsight 2011;42:14-16.
4. Aitken MJ. The incunabula of American optometry. Hindsight 2012;43:19-24.
5. Goss DA. Robert M. Lockwood and George A. Rogers, early twentieth-century optometry authors. Optom Vis Sci. 2010;87:190-194.
6. Tributes to the late Robert M. Lockwood as writer, editor, scholar, and educator: His great work for optometry. Optical J Rev Optom. 1920;45:666.
7. Sheard C. *Dynamic Skiametry and Methods of Testing the Accommodation and Convergence of the Eyes*. Chicago, IL: Cleveland Press, 1920:18.
8. Goss DA. Biographical notes on Lionel Laurance. Hindsight 2012;43:107-109.
9. Goss DA. Christian Henry Brown (1857-1933) and the Philadelphia Optical College. Hindsight 2010;41:114-121.
10. Goss DA. Biographical notes on James P. C. Southall. Hindsight 2013;44:9-12.
11. Goss DA. Some doctors of medicine who published optometry books and played significant roles in early twentieth-century optometric education. Hindsight 2011;42:20-28.
12. Goss DA. Eugene Wiseman (1885-1967), optometric practitioner, organizer, innovator, and writer. Hindsight 2010;41:71-78.
13. Hirsch MJ. Book review: *The Story of Optometry*. Am J Optom Arch Am Acad Optom 1965;42:152.
14. Goss DA. Biographical notes on Monroe Hirsch and Ralph Wick: Optometric leaders and co-authors of three significant books. Hindsight 2014;45:25-28.
15. Goss DA. Ray Morse Peckham (1876-1944) and his optometric writings. Hindsight 2010;41:9-14.
16. Efron N. Book review: *Contact Lens Practice*. Clin Exp Optom 1989;72:67.

17 Goss DA. Ralph Barstow (1884-1968), optometric practice management advisor and author of *How to Succeed in Optometry*. *Hindsight* 2011;42:94-96.
18 Goss DA. Biographical sketch: Darell Boyd Harmon (1898-1975). *Hindsight* 2018;49:81-83.
19 Grosvenor T. Clinical optometry textbooks. *Hindsight* 2007;38:40-46.
20 Goss DA. A historical survey of books on myopia. *Hindsight* 2014;45:85-95.
21 Goss DA. Literature and information in vision care and vision science. *Optom* 2008;79:670-686.
22 Hirsch MJ. Book review: The Principles and Practice of Refraction and its Allied Subjects. *Am J Optom Arch Am Acad Optom* 1965;42:202.
23 Leslie S. Book review: Optometric Management of Nearpoint Vision Disorders. *Clin Exp Optom* 1994;77:238-239.
24 Birnbaum MH. *Optometric Management of Nearpoint Vision Disorders*. Boston: Butterworth-Heinemann, 1993:56.
25 Goss DA. A history of the Distinguished Service Foundation of Optometry. *Hindsight* 2015;46:2-9.
26 Ketchum MB. Book studies for the optometrist. *Optical J Rev Optom* 1912;29:191-192.
27 Wiseman EG. *Building Optometry*. Philadelphia: Keystone, 1921:58-62.
28 Sutcliffe JH. *British Optical Association Library and Museum Catalogue*. London: The Council of the British Optical Association, 1932:1-296.
29 Cluxton HM. Some worthwhile optometric, optical, and ophthalmological books. *Am J Optom Arch Am Acad Optom* 1961;38:173-179.
30 Goss DA, Penisten DK. Most important 20th century optometry books. *Hindsight* 2004;35:36-40.
31 Goss DA. Rare book library catalogs with significant eye and vision content. *Hindsight* 2008;39:91-94.
32 Ayres J, Handley N. College of Optometrists Rare and Historical Books Collection. 2015. www.college-optometrists.org/uploads/assets/a95f0167-10d3-eb3e-0836ae6c5bfc60c3/Bibliography-of-the-historical-book-collection.pdf.
33 Aitken MJ. How an optometric collector became an optometric archivist. *Hindsight* 2019;50:79-80.

About the Author

David A. Goss holds a BA from Illinois Wesleyan University, BS and OD degrees from Pacific University, and PhD (physiological optics) and MLS degrees from Indiana University. Between optometry school and his PhD studies, he practiced optometry in the office of Drs. Allen Lande and Donovan Crouch in Storm Lake, Iowa. He was on the faculty of the College of Optometry at Northeastern State University in Tahlequah, Oklahoma from 1980 to 1992 and on the faculty of the Indiana University School of Optometry from 1992 to 2016. He was elected Fellow of the American Academy of Optometry (FAAO) in 1978 and Academic Fellow of the College of Optometrists in Vision Development (FCOVD-A) in 2001.

His teaching responsibilities included courses in binocular vision testing procedures and analysis, ocular motility, ocular optics, refractive development, refraction procedures, vision therapy, and vision development. At Northeastern State University, he was chief of the Myopia Clinic. At Indiana University, he was a consultant in the Binocular Vision/Pediatrics Clinic. Most of his research papers have been in the areas of myopia and other refractive errors, accommodation and binocular vision testing procedures, and optometry history. Throughout his career he involved optometry students in research, advising on 99 student research projects; many of these were subsequently published.

His published books include *Ocular Accommodation, Convergence, and Fixation Disparity*, 1986, 1995, 2009; *Eye and Vision Conditions in the*

American Indian, 1990 (with Linda L. Edmondson as co-editor); *Clinical Management of Myopia*, 1999 (with Theodore Grosvenor); and *Introduction to the Optics of the Eye*, 2002 (with Roger W. West). He has served as the editor of *Hindsight: Journal of Optometry History* since 1995 and was editor of the *Indiana Journal of Optometry* from 1998 to 2014. Service on journal review boards includes boards for the *Journal of the American Optometric Association*, *Optometry and Vision Development*, the *Journal of Behavioral Optometry*, and *Optometry and Visual Performance*.

He contributed chapters to several multi-author books, such as *Diagnosis and Management in Vision Care* (1987), *Refractive Anomalies* (1991), *Clinical Procedures in Optometry* (1991), *Refractive Management of Ametropia* (1996), *Myopia and Nearwork* (1998), and *Borish's Clinical Refraction* (1998, 2006). He was a member of the National Academy of Sciences Committee on Vision Working Group that produced the monograph *Myopia: Prevalence and Progression* (1989), and he was the principal author of the American Optometric Association Clinical Practice Guideline on *Care of the Patient with Myopia* (1997, 2001, 2006). He received the Faculty of the Year award for Research and Scholarly Activity from Northeastern State University in 1991, Teaching Excellence Recognition Awards from Indiana University in 1998 and 2010, and the Skeffington Award for optometric writing from the College of Optometrists in Vision Development in 2010.

Index

Abel, Oliver 209, 210
Abel, Stewart 238
Accelerated O.D. degree program 229–230
Accreditation Council on Optometric Education 215
Adams, Anthony 305
Adams, George, Jr. 319
Adams, George, Sr. 158
Adema, Joyce 120
Advertising in optometry 56, 71, 78, 80–82
Aegineta, Paulus 85
Afanador, Arthur 237
Ailman, John 36
Airlie House Conference 101
Airy, George Biddell 19
Albert, Richard I. 102
Alden, Walter 319
Alexander, Alexander 319
Alexander, E.B. 87, 149
Alexander, Larry J. 337
Allen, Merrill J. 214, 329
Alpern, Mathew 90
American Academy of Optometry 71–73, 77, 81, 87, 94, 100, 118, 121, 129, 132, 154, 200, 230, 232, 250, 253, 302, 303, 337
American Association of Opticians 39, 53–54, 55, 57, 59, 297
American Journal of Optometry 73, 132, 252, 253, 302–305
American Medical Association 82–83, 97, 124
American Optical Association 52, 54, 65, 77, 195
American Optical Project-O-Chart 154
American Optometric Association 39, 52, 53–54, 59, 60, 67, 70, 79, 81, 82, 98, 99, 101, 117, 118, 121, 123, 124, 127, 129, 130, 132, 177, 209, 214–215, 217, 226, 230, 232, 237, 250, 254, 272, 288, 297, 302, 306
American Optometric Foundation 75–77, 232
American Public Health Association 103, 129
American Optometric Student Association 118, 232
Amos, David M. 127
Amos, John F. 261, 312, 333
Apell, Richard J. 89, 328
Archives and Museum of Optometry 58, 75, 87, 254, 265
Armaignac, Henri 153
Armed Forces Optometric Society 120
Arneson, T.J. 87, 325
Arrington, E.E. 45, 324
Association of Regulatory Boards in Optometry 216
Association of Schools and Colleges of Optometry 127, 216–217, 232, 233, 273, 312
Astigmatism 18–21, 28, 42, 53, 84, 148, 154, 158, 161–162, 163, 164, 167, 168–169, 191, 193, 197
Atchison, David A. 322

Atkinson, Thomas 324
Autokeratometer 161, 178; see also Keratometer
Autorefractor 161, 170, 178

Bacon, Roger 5
Bailey, Ian 95
Bailey, James E. 323
Bailey, Neal J. 92, 309
Baldwin, Bob L. 327
Baldwin, William R. 100, 229, 326
Barker, Felix M. 312
Barr, F.P. 208
Barr, Joseph T. 310
Barresi, Barry J. 337
Barron, George A. 209, 210
Barstow, Ralph 259, 327
Bartisch, George 24, 85
Bartlett, Jimmy D. 261, 307, 333, 337
Bass, Cyrus 82–83, 98
Bausch, George R. 41
Bausch, John Jacob 14, 29
Bausch & Lomb 14, 29, 93, 153, 154, 155, 156, 161, 164, 170
Bayshore, Charles 92
Beacher, L.L. 326
Bellin, Lowell 104
Benjamin, William J. 259, 332
Bennett, Arthur G. 322
Bennett, Edward S. 326
Bennett, Irving 120, 136, 307, 313, 327
Bennett, Jack W. 227, 234
Berman, Morris 324
Bernell Corporation 90
Bestor, Harry Martin 203, 209, 210
Bettman, Jerome W. 329
Bezan, Debra J. 337
Bier, Norman 92
Bifocal, Franklin 15–17
Bifocals 87, 161, 332
  cemented 17
  fused 17
  invention of 15–17
Birnbaum, Martin H. 335
Bissell, W.W. 41
Bleything, Willard B. 338

Blood pressure, measurement by optometrists 177, 336
Bloom, Jacob C. 52
Blum, Henrik L. 329
Blyth, Robert 329
Boeder, Paul 75
Boger, Frederick 39, 41, 53, 249, 250, 297, 298, 315, 338
Bohne, William 14, 53, 255, 256, 297, 320
Book, by F.C. Donders 27–29, 86, 151
Book, first optometry 8–11
Borish, Irvin M. 92, 100, 104, 215, 257, 259, 260, 261, 330, 331–332
Borsch, John, Jr. 17
Borsch, John, Sr. 14, 17
Bosse, James 310
Bowen, Arthur H. 201
Bowman, William 163
Brilliant, Richard L. 331
Brock, Frederick 89
Brombach, Theodore A. 74, 336
Brookman, Kenneth E. 333
Brooks, Clifford W. 330
Brooks, Stephens H. 201, 202
Brown, Christian Henry 194, 195, 196, 199, 255, 321
Brown, C.S. 71
Brown, D.V. 194
Brown, H. Frank 209, 210
Browning, John 319
Buchanan, John 58
Bucklin, C.A. 295
Buffon, George Louis Leclerc 85
Bullimore, Mark 305
Burnett, Swan 38
Butterworth-Heinemann 338
Buzzelli, Andrew 238

Caloroso, Elizabeth E. 336
Cameron, Ian S. 329
Carlson, Dori 307
Carlson, Nancy B. 334
Carter, John H. 72, 229
Carter, Robert L. 227
Cary, William 18, 167
Casella, Benjamin 135

Casser, Linda 337
Casto, John 103
Catania, Louis J. 337
Cavallerano, Anthony A. 307
Chambers, David 159
Chambers, E.A. 159
Chilton Book Company 298, 299, 337, 338
Christensen, Bobby 327
Christensen, Jerry L. 228
Christenson, Garth W. 328
Ciuffreda, Kenneth J. 333, 334, 336, 338
Clark, B.B. 201
Clason, Milo B. 153
Clason Visual Acuity Meter 153, 154, 155, 156
Classé, John G. 307, 327, 329
Cline, David 324
College of Optometrists in Vision Development 120, 232, 310, 311
Columbia University 26, 210
  closure of optometry school 218–219, 221, 273
  optometry school 39, 94, 157, 201, 204–207, 211, 212, 257, 266, 272, 322
Comanagement 131, 162
Commercial practice of optometry 77–82
Committee on Public Health and Optometric Care 129
Conference on Optometric Practice (1966) 99
Contact lenses 84, 91–93, 94, 96, 97, 102, 116, 123, 132, 134, 158, 162, 176, 222, 232, 236, 254, 259, 307, 308–310, 326, 330, 331, 337
  corneal 91, 92
  scleral 91, 92
  Soflens 93
Contact Lens Forum (periodical) 309–310
Contact Lens Spectrum (periodical) 253, 309–310
Contacto (periodical) 308
Continuing education 101, 121, 177, 226, 235
Copeland, Jack C. 164
Corliss, David A. 323
Corneal topography 93, 162, 177

Coronet (magazine) 80
Correspondence courses 147–148, 174, 187, 191–194, 195–199, 207, 210, 250, 297
Costabile, John 103
Council on Optometric Education 100, 117, 127, 210, 214–215, 223, 301
Cox, Maurice E. 298
Cross, Andrew J. 30, 39, 40, 41, 45, 54, 55, 66, 71, 164, 165, 201, 202, 203, 205, 206, 255, 321
Crow, George 88, 323, 325
Cuignet, Ferdinand 163
Curriculum 177, 190, 202
  basic biological sciences 229, 233, 236
  length of optometric 134, 200, 201, 202, 207, 208, 210, 211, 214, 215, 217, 221–222
  ocular disease 134, 222, 226, 229, 235–236
  optometry school 129, 205, 208, 214, 221–222, 226, 228–229, 230, 233
  pathology 190, 201, 228, 236
  pharmacology 134, 222, 226, 228, 235–236
Cyert, Lynn 229

Dablemont, Maria 75, 119
da Brescia, Piero Ubertini 23
Dallos, Josef 91
da Pisa, Giordano 4
Daum, Kent M. 334
Davidson, David W. 337
da Vinci, Leonardo 91
Daza de Valdes, Benito 8, 166, 319
de Carle, John 92
de Chauliac, Guy 24
DeCook, Larry 233
Defense Officer Personnel Management Act of 1980 125
degli Armati, Salvino 5
Degree, Doctor of Optometry (O.D.) 65–70, 195, 207, 212, 217, 222
DeKeyser, A.P. 71, 209, 210
della Spina, Allesandro 5
DeMars, Louis L. 200, 209, 210

DeMars School of Optics 200, 209, 267, 272, 303
Denial, Aurora 312
Department of Health, Education, and Welfare 121
Descartes, René 91
DeVere, P.N. 124
De Zeng, Henry L., Jr. 164, 169–170, 173
Diagnostic pharmaceutical agents 84, 96–104
  first law for optometric use 102
Dickey, John 313
Dickinson, Frank 92
Diopter 10, 15, 36, 151–152, 168, 175, 199, 322
Dissociated phoria 147, 149, 150, 151, 171–176
Distinguished Service Foundation of Optometry 73–75
Doane, Howard C. 73, 209, 210
Doctor title 65–69
Dollond, Peter 158
Donders, Frans Cornelis 27–29, 42, 84, 86, 151, 152, 153, 163, 168, 174
Dowaliby, Margaret 330

Eames, Harold W. 206
Eberhardt, John C. 55, 57–59, 208, 267
Edwards, Keith 334
Eger, Milton J. 100, 307
Ellerbrock, Vincent 95
Ellis, John H. 57
Elmstrom, George P. 72, 327
Emery, Leonard C. 338
Emsley, H.H. 322
Environmental vision 84, 95–96, 129, 132, 329
Epstein, Arthur B. 313
Erickson, Graham B. 328, 329
Eskridge, J. Boyd 261, 333
Ethics, code of 55–56
Eure, Spurgeon B. 100
Everson, Ronald 221, 324
Ewalt, H. Ward, Jr. 100, 215, 226
Examination, optometric 77, 87, 147–151, 257, 323, 332
  late 20th century changes in 176–178
Examination, 21-point 77, 150–151, 176, 257, 323
Ezell Fellowships 75–77
Ezell, William C. 75, 76

Fannin, Troy E. 331
Fatt, Helene V. 336
Faye, Eleanor 95
Federal Trade Commission 81–82
Feinbloom, William 92, 94, 157, 326
Ferris, David W. 102
Ferris State University 227, 274
Fick, Adolph Eugen 91
Fielding, E.E. 71
Filderman, Irving P. 326
Fincham, W.H.A. 322
Fingeret, Murray 337
Finkelstein, Isidore 218
Fisher, Harold M. 100
Fitch, Albert 50, 51, 68, 99, 100, 212, 216, 337
Folsom, Laurence P. 73
Forrest, Elliott B. 338
Flax, Nathan 90
Flom, Merton C. 90, 304, 333
Fonda, Gerald 95
Franklin, Benjamin 12, 15–16, 158
Frantz, Don 155–157
Franzel, G.A. 228
Freeman, Paul B. 95, 307, 331
Freid, Allan N. 95, 331
Fronmüller, Georg 167
Fry, Glenn 90, 219, 220, 322, 337
Fulk, George 229
Fuog, H.L. 88, 325
Fusional vergence ranges 87, 90, 149, 150, 151, 174–176, 258, 323

Gailmard, Neil 313
Garzia, Ralph P. 90, 228, 334
Genensky, Sam 95
Gerhardt, William 14
Gesell, Arnold 88
Gesell Institute 88
Getman, Gerald N. 89, 328, 338

Getz, Donald J. 338
Ghazi-Birry, H.S. 238
Gilbert, Margaret S. 72
Giles, George H. 332
Gilmartin, Bernard 333
Girard-Teulon, Marc Antoine 169
Goldberg, Joe B. 92, 326
Goode, Henry 162
Goodlaw, Edward 92
Goodrich, Chauncey Enoch 20
Goodrich, Gregory 95
Goss, David A. 228, 313, 322, 333, 335
Grainger, Joseph W. 47
Grandfather clause 46–47, 77, 80
Greenstein, Tole 88
Gregg, James R. 325, 329
Griffin, John R. 90, 260, 324, 325, 328, 336
Groffman, Sidney 90, 310, 328
Grohe, Robert M. 326
Grolman, Bernard 157
Grosvenor, Theodore 162, 261, 326, 331, 332, 333

Haffner, Alden Norman 100, 103, 129, 134, 219, 226, 227
Haines, Howard 219
Hallock, William 205
Halverson, Kathy 337
Hamilton, Frederick 75
Harmon, Darell Boyd 259, 328
Harris, Paul A. 338
Harvey, Lisa H. 325
Hatch, Stanley W. 329
Haussmann, Otto 194
Havighurst Report 226–227
Havighurst, Robert J. 226
Hawkins, John Isaac 17–18, 19
Haynes, Harold 166, 213
Hazen, Edward 22, 23, 173
Hazlett, Richard 100
Heard, Thomas M. 28–29
Heart of America Congress 121
Heath, David A. 312, 334
Heath, Gordon G. 100
Hegeman, Sally 104

Henderson, F.L. 203
Henson, David B. 337
Hering, Ewald 72
Herschel, John F.W. 19, 91, 175
Hindsight (periodical) 74, 313–314
Hines, Catherine 334
Hirsch, Monroe 1, 72, 259, 304, 325, 330
Hisaka, Craig 327
Hitchcock, Hiram M. 46, 47
Hoare, Arthur E. 73, 300–301
Hoffman, Ellis 118
Hofstetter, Henry 90, 119, 214, 217, 219, 220, 237, 258, 313, 324, 329
Holmes, Clark 329
Hoppe, Elizabeth 238, 312
Hopping, Richard L. 233
Horology 61, 271
Hotaling, Elmer E. 87, 201, 202, 254, 258, 326
Houghton, George Stevens 73
House, Harry O. 228
Howard, Alison 305
Howard, P.H. 209, 210
Howlette, John L. 118
Hunter, Earle 235
Huston, William 55
Hutchinson, A.J. 190
Hutchinson, Ernest 209, 210, 217

Illinois College of Optometry 190, 221, 269, 273, 274, 275
Indiana University 70, 195, 213–214, 219, 220, 221, 224, 228, 235, 274, 314
Inskeep, Carey 159
Inskeep, Charles 159
Inter American University of Puerto Rico 237, 274
International Association of Boards of Examiners in Optometry 209, 215–216, 232
International Board of Boards 209, 210, 215, 277
International Contact Lens Clinic (periodical) 309

Jaanus, Siret D. 261, 337

Jackson cross cylinder 21, 28, 169
Jackson, Edward 21, 28, 164, 169
Jacobs, Robert J. 95
James Queen Company *see* Queen Company
Janney, David John 103
Janoff, Lester 312
Jaques, Louis 323, 325
Jarvis, John W. 13
Javal, Emile 84–85, 152, 159, 161
Jefferson, Thomas 12, 16
Jessen, George N. 92, 326
Jeweler optician 61
Jewelers' Circular Weekly (periodical) 53, 295–296
Jolley, Jerry L. 329
Jolliffe, Harry 329
Johnson, Chester 73
Johnston's Eye Echo (periodical) 249, 296–297
Johnston, J. Milton 249, 256, 296
Jose, Randall T. 95, 331
Journal of the American Optometric Association 79, 122, 136, 251, 253, 306–307
Journal of Behavioral Optometry 311
Journal of Optometric Education 253
Journal of Optometric Vision Development 310

Kalt, E. 91
Kane, Martin 310
Kapoor, Neera 338
Keating, Michael P. 227, 322
Keller, Jeffrey T. 127
Kenney, M.E. 41
Keratometer 158–162; *see also* Autokeratometer, Ophthalmometers
  Bausch & Lomb 161
  Javal-Schiotz 159, 160
Ketchum, Marshall B. 202–203, 276
Keystone (periodical) 296
Keystone Publishing Company 338
Kiekenapp, Ernest H. 73, 200, 306–307
Kindy, W.H. 78
King, Vincent 227
Kitchener, Gregory 338

Kitchener, William 319
Klein, August Andreas 190, 276
Klein School of Optics 187, 189, 190, 267, 272, 276
Klein, Theodore 209, 210
Kleinstein, Robert N. 329
Knapp, Herman 43
Koch, Carel C. 71, 200, 303
Koetting, Felix 129
Koetting, R.A. 327
Kohn, Harold 72
Korb, Donald 92
Kraskin, Robert A. 88, 338
Kratometer 173
Küchler, Heinrich 152
Kurtz, Daniel 334
Kurtz, Jack I. 303

LaGuardia Airport meeting 100–101
Lakin, Donald H. 327
Landolt, Edmond 57, 163, 174
LaRussa, Frank P. 337
Laurance, Lionel 257, 321
Lembke, Charles 21, 53–54
Lemoine, Albert N. 127
Lesser, Sol K. 88, 149, 323
Levene, John R. 313
Levi, Dennis M. 336
Lewis, James John 324
Licensure law, first optometry 46–47
Licensure laws, passage of optometry 47–52, 200
Llewellyn, Richard 334
Lockwood, Robert M. 164, 201, 202, 255, 257, 320
Lomb, Henry 14, 29
London, Richard 337
Long, William 228
Longstreth, Charles A. 53
Lovie-Kitchin, Jan 95
Low vision care 84, 93–95, 132, 232, 307, 330, 331
Lowry, Ray W., Jr. 328
Luckiesh, Matthew 73
Lyle, William M. 304–305

MacCracken, William P. 124
MacDonald, Lawrence 88
Mackeown, J.J. 40, 41
Mackintosh, Charles H. 77
Maddox, Ernest Edmund 86, 172, 173
Maddox, Mary 86
Maddox rod test 172
Magrun, W. Michael 339
Maino, Dominick M. 310, 311, 337
Maino, Joseph H. 337
Manas, Leo 259, 323
Mandell, Robert B. 92, 259, 309, 326
Maples, W.C. 311, 338
Margach, Charles 95, 213, 307
Marshall, Edwin C. 329
Mason, E.R. 41
Massachusetts College of Pharmacy and Health Sciences 238, 275
Maurolyco, Francesco 151
Mayer, Tobias 152
Mazow, Bernard 72
McAllister, Francis W. 13
McAllister, James Cook 13, 52
McAllister, John, Jr. 12, 13, 20, 21, 24, 52
McAllister, John, Sr. 12, 16
McAllister, Thomas H. 13
McAllister, William M. 13
McAllister, William Young 13, 25, 52
McBurnie, Thomas 73
McDonnell, C.N. 208
McFatrich, G.W. 71, 190, 209
McFatrich, James 190, 275
McGill, Frederick A. 298
Medicare, optometric parity in 130
Mehr, Edwin B. 95, 331
Melton, Jack W. 327
Méndez, Cristóbal 24
Meyer, J.H. William 190
Midwestern University 238, 275
Military Reorganization Act of 1947 124
Millodot, Michel 221, 324
Minchin, Howard D. 209, 210
Mittendorf, William F. 36
Modified Thorington test 172–173
Monoyer, Ferdinand 152, 152
Moore, Bruce D. 330

Morck, August 17
Morgan, Meredith 90, 330
Morris, Scot 313
Morrison, Robert 92
Mote, Herbert 219
Mulford, V.S. 298
Mullen, John 92
Muller, Friedrich 91
Munitz, Raquel 339
Myers, Raymond I. 118

Nagel, Albrecht 151, 152
National Association of Veterans Administration Optometrists 120
National Board of Examiners in Optometry 216, 232
National Eye Institute 133
National Optometric Association 118, 232
Needles, William B. 71, 164, 187, 209, 210, 275
Neill, John C. 92
Neuro-Optometric Rehabilitation Association 120
Newcomb, Robert D. 120, 329
New England College of Optometry 69, 70, 190, 229–230, 274, 276
New York Institute of Optometry 201, 204
Nishimoto, John H. 337
North Central States Optometric Council 121
Northeastern State University 128, 228, 229, 236, 274
Northern Illinois College of Optometry 69, 90, 211, 212, 272, 275
Norton, Thomas T. 323
Nott, Ivan 166
Nova Southeastern University 237, 275
Nowakowski, Rodney W. 95, 331
Noyes, Harold G. 336
Noyes, Henry D. 36
Nurock, E. C. 122

Obrig, Theo 92, 326
Obstfeld, Henri 322
Oculists 25, 42, 43, 44, 47

The Ohio State University 59, 70, 90, 207–208, 209, 211, 212, 219, 220, 222, 224, 273, 274, 300
Olin, Henry 190, 275
Ong, Editha 333
Ophthalmetron 170
Ophthalmic and Physiological Optics (journal) 252, 315
Ophthalmic Antiques (periodical) 314
Ophthalmologists 25–26, 82, 131
  attitudes toward spectacles 26–27
  spectacle prescribing by 25–26
Ophthalmometer, Chambers-Inskeep 159–161
Ophthalmometers 171, 198; *see also* Keratometer
Ophthalmoscope 160, 163, 169, 198
Optical Journal 52, 53, 195, 250, 297–298
Optical Journal and Review of Optometry 249, 251, 298
Optical Society of the State of New York 39, 41, 53, 70
The Optician (periodical) 249, 315
Optician 29
  description of 22
  refracting 29–30, 39–45
  types of 29–30
Optometer 57, 148, 170
Optometric education 226–227, 232–234, 254
  financing 234
  first conference to establish standards 209–212
Optometric Education (journal) 312
Optometric Extension Program 77, 87–89, 118, 121, 149–151, 176, 232, 311, 338
Optometric Historical Society 119, 136, 301, 313–314
Optometric Management (periodical) 136, 253, 313
Optometric research 70–77, 132–134, 233
Optometric scope of practice 96–105; *see also* Scope of practice expansion
Optometric technicians 122–123
Optometric Weekly (periodical) 89, 195, 250, 299–300

Optometric World (periodical) 300–301
Optometrists
  in Department of Veterans Affairs 126–127
  in the Indian Health Service 128
  net income 115–117
  numbers of 113–115, 223, 279–280
Optometry *see also* Scope of practice expansion
  adoption of term 56–60
  and Medicare 130, 136
  books 254–261
  degrees 65, 69–70, 122, 195, 207, 217
  in the Department of Veterans Affairs 126–127
  in the Indian Health Service 128
  military 80, 124–126
  periodicals 249–254, 295–315
  professional status of 39–49
Optometry and Vision Development (journal) 310
Optometry and Vision Science (journal) 73, 132, 134, 252, 253, 302–305
Optometry and Visual Performance (journal) 311
Optometry College Admission Test 225
Optometry residency programs 117–118
Optometry school applicants 225, 230–231
  women 230, 288–290
Optometry school enrollments 218, 223–224, 284
Optometry schools *see also* Curriculum
  accreditation of 215, 217, 284
  degrees held by faculty 219, 224–225, 226
  early 187–200
  list of extinct 265–270
  need for additional 223–224, 226, 234–235
  number of 225, 234, 237, 265
  number of graduates 223, 224, 272–273, 279–284
  present day 273–275
  1920s ratings of 210–212
Optometry students

indebtedness 239
minority 118, 238–239, 290–291
pre-optometry grade point averages 225, 287–288
pre-optometry studies of 97, 134, 200, 284–286
women 115, 288–290
Orthoptics 85–86

Pacific University 69, 74, 176, 213, 219, 221, 222, 225, 236, 274, 276–277
Padelford, Clinton R. 73
Padula, William 120, 339
Paré, Ambrose 85
Parkins, George A. 75
Parsons, J.R. 190, 271
Pascal, Joseph I. 209, 210, 336
Peale, Charles Willson 17
Peck, Carol 228
Peckham, R.M. 87, 258, 325
Peli, Eli 95
Penisten, Douglas K. 313
Pennsylvania College of Optometry 68, 69, 70, 94, 99, 103, 211, 212, 222, 269, 273, 274, 277
Pennsylvania Optical Society 52
Perimetry 95, 177, 332
Peters, Henry B. 126, 329
Petry, Ernest 71, 209, 210
Pheiffer, Chester H. 214, 228, 312
Philadelphia Optical College 65, 189, 194–200, 273, 321
Phoria, von Graefe 172, 193
Phoropter 169, 173
  Bausch & Lomb Greens' 170
  De Zeng 170
Physiological optics, M.S. and Ph.D. degrees in 219–221
Pickwell, David 334
Pierce, Samuel 158
Pike, Benjamin, Jr. 14
Pike, Benjamin, Sr. 14
Pike, Daniel 14
Pine, Harry, Jr. 13, 79
Pine, Harry, Sr. 13
Pitts, Donald G. 329

Plácido, Antonio 162
Polarization, use in testing 157
Policoff, William W. 94–95
Potter, John W. 307, 312
Porterfield, William 18, 57, 170
Powell, C. Clayton 118, 119
Prentice, Charles F. 14–15, 30, 36–45, 54, 57, 66, 94, 173, 175, 188, 205, 206, 256, 297, 322, 337
Prentice's Rule 15, 322
Prentice, James 14, 21, 30
Press, Leonard J. 325, 330, 333, 335, 338, 339
Press, T. Channon 40, 41
Prisms, Risley 173, 175
Professional Press 191, 299, 304, 338
Profession, characteristics of 35–36
Projectors
  for vision examination 153–154, 155–156
  remote controlled 157
  vectographic slide for 157

Queen Company 20, 168, 320
Queen, James 13, 21, 25, 52

Rabbetts, Ronald B. 322
Radde, Carl A. 72
Ramsden, Jesse 158–159, 167
Ramsey, Walter S. 103
Readers Digest 78–80
Reading, Rogers W. 334
Refraction, optometric expertise in 48, 102
Retinoscope 164, 165
Retinoscopy 147, 150, 163–166, 193, 198, 320, 321
  dynamic 39, 150, 165, 166, 176
Review of Optometry (journal) 249, 251, 253, 297–299
Richardson, Edmund 279
Richardson, William 12
Richman, Jack 90
Ring, M.M. 276
Risley, S.D. 175
Rittenhouse, David 12

Robinson, John 103
Rochester School of Optometry 201–204, 209, 211, 270, 273
Rogers, E.E. 75
Rogers, George A. 164, 255, 298, 320
Roosa, D. B. St. John 38, 41
Rosen, Edward 4
Rosenbloom, Alfred A. 95, 226, 330
Rosenfield, Mark 333
Rosenthal, Bruce P. 95
Rosenthal, Jesse 336
Rosner, Jerome 90, 325, 330
Rosner, Joy 325
Rounds, Ronald S. 327
Rouse, Michael W. 328, 336
Ruddy, T.J. 276
Runninger, Jack 313
Rutstein, Robert P. 334
Ryer, E. LeRoy 70, 87, 88, 201, 202, 254, 257, 258, 326

Sanders, Sunny 238
Santiago, Hector C. 238
Scarlett, Edward 151
Schaffer, Kathleen 337
Schapero, Max 324, 336
Scheiman, Mitchell M. 328, 334
Schiotz, Hjalmar August 159
Schor, Clifton M. 334
Schrock, Ralph 88
Schwartz, Steven H. 322, 323
Scope of practice expansion 84–105, 135–136, 228, 233
  arguments against 100, 102, 104
  efforts for 99–104
  ophthalmological opposition 98
  reasons for 97–99, 100, 101–102
Second floor office 56
Seger, Charles 100, 226
Seid, Reuben 275
Selenow, Arkady 336
Sendrowski, David P. 337
Shastid, Thomas Hall 26
Shaw-McMinn, Peter G. 329
Sheard, Charles 71, 73, 87, 148, 149, 175, 207, 210, 214, 257, 300, 301, 321, 323

Sheedy, James E. 329
Sheridan, John W. 125
Shick, Charles 92, 326
Shlaifer, Arthur 72, 336
Silver, Edwin H. 73
Silverman, Morton W. 102
Sissons, Jeremiah 158
Skeffington, A. M. 87, 89, 149, 323, 338
Skiascopy *see* Retinoscopy
Skiametry *see* Retinoscopy
Skuza, Burton H. 129
Sloan, Clark 208
Sloan, Louise 95
Smith, George 322
Smith, Lincoln 50
Smith, William 325
Snell, Clifton A. 47
Snellen, Herman 153
Solan, Harold 90, 328
Sommer, Balthasar, widow of 12
Söhnges, Wilhelm 92
Southall, James P.C. 73, 257, 322
South Bend College of Optics 147, 174, 189, 191–194, 250, 270
Southern California College of Optometry 127, 270, 274, 276
Southern College of Optometry 69, 131, 212, 222, 273, 274
Southern Council of Optometrists 121
Spear, Carl 337
Spectacle peddler 60–61
Spectacles 4–8, 12–18, 166–167
  early 6–8
  in China 6
  in colonial America 12–15
  invention of 4–6
State University of New York 219, 221, 227, 231, 274
Steinfeld, Morris 71
Steinman, Barbara A. 334
Steinman, Scott B. 334
Stelmack, Thomas J. 127
Stevens, George 43
Stewart, Charles R. 76, 214
Stifler, W.W. 205
Stoddard, Kenneth 217, 220

Index   353

Stokes, George Gabriel 21, 169
Stokes lens 21
Streff, John 89
Subjective refraction 147, 148, 149, 150, 166–171, 193
Suchoff, Irwin B. 311, 338
Suckow, Melissa 238
Summit on Optometric Education 232–234
Sutcliffe, John 161
Sutcliffe, Robert 161
Suter, Penelope S. 325
Sweningson, Alexander 47

Talbot, C.W. 336
Talley, David K. 337
Tannen, Barry 334
Taub, Marc B. 311
Terry, Jack E. 337
Test charts 152–153
Thal, Lawrence S. 327
Than, Tammy P. 337
Therapeutic pharmaceutical agents 84, 96–105, 125, 128, 129, 177
  first law for optometric use 103, 135
Thomas, Pam 337
Thomson, H.A. 147, 191
Thorington, James 164, 173
Tonometer 157
Topaz, Lionel 250, 299–300
Treganza, Amorita 120
Treleaven, Clifford 217
Trial lens set 167, 171
Trifocals, invention of 17, 19
Tuohy, Kevin 92
Twa, Michael 305

Uglum, John R. 74
Uniformed Services Health Professions Revitalization Act of 1972 125–126
University of Alabama at Birmingham 219, 221, 225, 274
University of California at Berkeley 70, 90, 211, 212, 219, 220, 222, 224, 229, 273, 274
University of Houston 69, 76, 214, 219, 221, 222, 225, 274
University of Missouri at St. Louis 228, 274
University of Pikeville 238, 275
University of the Incarnate Word 238, 275
Upham, Frank A. 47

Valenti, Claude A. 338
van Nus, Frederick 120
Van Veen, Hank 228
Verschoor, J.W. 57
Videokeratoscopes 162, 177
Vision Development and Rehabilitation (journal) 312
Vision Educational Foundation 131
Vision therapy 84–91, 132, 232, 254, 258, 325
Visual acuity 152
Vodnoy, Bernard E. 90
Volunteer Optometric Services to Humanity 120
von Arlt, Ferdinand Ritter 25
von Graefe, Albrecht 172
von Helmholtz, Hermann 159, 219, 322
von Jaeger, Eduard 152
von Rohr, Moritz 94
Voorhees, Lorraine 235

Wahl, James F. 74, 213
Wallis, Norman E. 100, 229, 312
Walls, Lesley L. 104, 228, 238
Ware, James 25, 168
Weiner, Grace 305
Weiss, Ephraim 60
Wells, David W. 86
Wells, George Washington 29
Wells, John Soelberg 152
Wells, William Charles 168
Welzmiller, Louis R. 205
Werner, D. Leonard 333, 336
Wesley-Jessen Photo-Electronic Keratoscope 162
Wesley, Newton K. 92, 213, 326
Wesson, Michael D. 328
West, Roger W. 229, 322

West, Walter 313
Western University of Health Sciences 238, 275
Whatley, George 16
Wheelock, Arthur P. 154
Whewell, William 20
White, Paul E. 326
Wichterle, Otto 92
Wick, Bruce 334
Wick, Ralph 1, 122, 259, 325, 330
Wickham, M. Gary 228
Wild, Bradford W. 82
Williams, Henry Willard 26
Williams, T. David 305
Williams, W. Reed 194
Wilson, Roger 312
Wiseman, Eugene 71, 72, 254, 258, 324, 336
Wolcott, Claude 210
Wold, Robert M. 310
Woll, Frederic A. 73, 201, 202, 205, 210
Women in optometry 115, 288–290
Woo, George 95
Wood, Casey 26
Woodcombe, H. Ted 337
Worrell, Burton E. 118
Worth, Claude A. 85–86

Young, Thomas 18, 91, 152, 170

Zadnik, Karla 334
Zahn, Johann 167
Zentmayer, Joseph 14, 20, 29, 256
Zoethout, W.D. 323

www.ingramcontent.com/pod-product-compliance
Lightning Source LLC
Chambersburg PA
CBHW030316100526
44592CB00010B/449